Quick Reference to
CLINICAL TOXICOLOGY

Quick Reference to CLINICAL TOXICOLOGY

Edited by

IRWIN B. HANENSON, M.D.

Professor of Medicine and Pathology,
Departments of Medicine and Pathology;
Director, Clinical Toxicology;
Associate Director, Division of Laboratory
Medicine, University of Cincinnati College of
Medicine, Cincinnati, Ohio

With 23 Contributors

J. B. Lippincott Company
Philadelphia • Toronto

1   3   5   6   4   2

Library of Congress Cataloging in Publication Data
Main entry under title:

Quick reference to clinical toxicology.

   Includes index.
   1. Poisoning. 2. Toxicology. I. Hanenson, Irwin B.
[DNLM: 1. Toxicology. QV600.3 Q62] RA1211.Q53
615.9   79-26400
ISBN 0-397-50418-7

The authors and publisher have exerted every effort to ensure that drug selection and dosage set forth in this text are in accord with current recommendations and practice at the time of publication. However, in view of ongoing research, changes in government regulations, and the constant flow of information relating to drug therapy and drug reactions, the reader is urged to check the package insert for each drug for any change in indications and dosage and for added warnings and precautions. This is particularly important when the recommended agent is a new or infrequently employed drug.

CONTRIBUTORS

W. Fraser Bremner, M.B., Ch.B., Ph.D.
Associate Professor of Medicine
Department of Medicine
University of Cincinnati College of Medicine
231 Bethesda Avenue
Cincinnati, Ohio

Diana Burton, B.S. Pharm.
Menoral Medical Center
4949 Rock Hill Road
Kansas City, Missouri

Alastair Connell, M.D.
Dean and Professor of Medicine
University of Nebraska College of Medicine
42nd Street and Dewey Avenue
Omaha, Nebraska

Edward C. Conradi, M.D.
Associate Professor of Medicine and Pharmacology
Department of Pharmacology
Medical University of South Carolina
171 Ashley Avenue
Charleston, South Carolina

T. Douglas Cowart, Pharm.D.
Assistant Professor of Pharmacology and Clinical
   Pharmacology
Department of Pharmacology
Medical University of South Carolina
171 Ashley Avenue
Charleston, South Carolina

Thomas Elo, M.D.*
Emergency Medical Services
University of Washington
Seattle, Washington

**Edward A. Emmett, M.B., B.S., M.S.,
F.R.A.C.P.**
Professor of Environmental Health Sciences
Director, Division of Occupational Medicine
Johns Hopkins University School of Hygiene and
   Public Health
Department of Environmental Health Sciences
615 North Wolfe Street
Baltimore, Maryland

David Fedders, M.D.
Assistant Clinical Professor of Psychiatry
University of Cincinnati College of Medicine
231 Bethesda Avenue
Cincinnati, Ohio

Peter Frame, M.D.
Assistant Professor of Medicine and Pathology
Departments of Medicine and Pathology
University of Cincinnati College of Medicine
231 Bethesda Avenue
Cincinnati, Ohio

Paul Hammond, D.V.M., Ph.D.
Professor of Environmental Health
Department of Environmental Health
University of Cincinnati College of Medicine
231 Bethesda Avenue
Cincinnati, Ohio

Irwin B. Hanenson, M.D.
Professor of Medicine and Pathology
Departments of Medicine and Pathology
Director, Clinical Toxicology
Associate Director, Division of Laboratory Medicine
University of Cincinnati College of Medicine
231 Bethesda Avenue
Cincinnati, Ohio

Michael Hassan, B.S.
Supervisor, Toxicology Laboratory
Division of Laboratory Medicine
Department of Pathology
University of Cincinnati College of Medicine
231 Bethesda Avenue
Cincinnati, Ohio

Richard Kozera, M.D.
Associate Professor of Medicine
Chief, Medical Services
Veterans Administration Hospital
3200 Vine Street
Cincinnati, Ohio

Richard Levy, M.D.
Associate Professor of Emergency Medicine
Division of Emergency Medicine
University of Cincinnati College of Medicine
231 Bethesda Avenue
Cincinnati, Ohio

Charles L. Mendenhall, M.D., Ph.D
Associate Professor of Medicine
Chief, Digestive Disease
Veterans Administration Hospital
3200 Vine Street
Cincinnati, Ohio

*Deceased.

Donald P. Morgan, M.D., Ph.D.
Associate Professor of Preventative Medicine and
  Environmental Health
Department of Preventative Medicine and
  Environmental Health
University of Iowa School of Medicine
Iowa City, Iowa

E. Don Nelson, Pharm.D.
Assistant Professor of Pharmacology/Cell
  Biophysics
Assistant Professor of Experimental Medicine
Drug and Poison Information Center
University of Cincinnati College of Medicine
231 Bethesda Avenue
Cincinnati, Ohio

Edward J. Otten, M.D.
Resident, Division of Emergency Medicine
University of Cincinnati College of Medicine
231 Bethesda Avenue
Cincinnati, Ohio

Amadeo J. Pesce, Ph.D.
Professor of Pathology and Experimental Medicine
Departments of Pathology and Medicine
University of Cincinnati College of Medicine
231 Bethesda Avenue
Cincinnati, Ohio

William J. Rietscha, Pharm.D.
Resident, Department of Pharmacy
University of Cincinnati Hospital
234 Goodman Street
Cincinnati, Ohio

Leonard T. Sigell, Ph.D.
Associate Professor of Pharmacology/Cell
  Biophysics
Associate Professor of Experimental Medicine
Director, Drug and Poison Information Center
University of Cincinnati College of Medicine
231 Bethesda Avenue
Cincinnati, Ohio

Jeffrey B. Spears, Pharm.D.
Assistant Administrator for Clinical
  Pharmacy Services
Department of Pharmacy
Jackson Memorial Hospital
1611 N.W. 12th Avenue
Miami, Florida

Robert E. Weesner, M.D.
Assistant Professor of Medicine
Division of Digestive Disease
Veterans Administration Hospital
3200 Vine Street
Cincinnati, Ohio

Robert Yokel, Ph.D.
Assistant Professor of Pharmacology
College of Pharmacy
University of Kentucky Medical Center
Lexington, Kentucky

PREFACE

Although chemical intoxication has been a significant medical problem throughout history, clinical toxicology has failed to achieve the recognition and interest of other clinical specialities. Explanations for this are many and varied. Physicians have an ambivalent attitude toward the suicide attempt, particularly with drugs, since both the act and the means are in conflict with fundamental professional tenets. Also, despite extensive basic toxicological research, clinical investigation in this area has been limited by the difficulty in designing experiments which satisfy ethical considerations. Finally, but certainly not of least importance, is the lack of agreement in defining clinical toxicology. It should include not only intentional and accidental overdoses, but all harmful effects of drugs and nontherapeutic agents, including adverse drug reactions and drug interactions.

This book is intended as a concise reference which will provide physicians with a readily accessible source of information for the identification and management of toxic effects of drugs and other harmful agents. Chapter 1 contains general information for the management of intoxication. This is followed by chapters on drugs and nontherapeutic agents which group together compounds on the basis of their pharmacological and chemical similarities. The concluding three chapters deal with adverse drug interactions (Chap. 23), locating toxicologic information (Chap. 24), and analytical toxicology (Chap. 25).

No attempt has been made to provide a comprehensive bibliography. There are selected references which serve to document the text. Chapter 24, Locating Toxicologic Information, provides additional resources available for more intensive review of a subject.

In conclusion, it should be emphasized that a major goal of this book is to apply rational principles to the diagnosis and management of toxicological problems. Its value will be in direct relationship to the degree to which this objective is achieved.

I.B.H.

ACKNOWLEDGEMENTS

For the success of a book, an editor depends on the quality of his contributors and publisher. I have indeed been fortunate in both respects.

It is a pleasure for me to express sincere appreciation to my colleagues who have so generously contributed their time and expertise to make this volume possible.

An equal debt of gratitude is owed to Mr. Stuart Freeman, of the J. B. Lippincott Company, and to Mr. Louis Reines for their continuing support and motivation. I would also like to thank Ms. Lisa Biello for her gracious help with the manuscript.

During the preparation of this book, we lost one of its most enthusiastic and dedicated authors, Dr. Thomas Elo. I am gratified that he had already completed his chapter before his untimely death, but very much saddened that he was denied the satisfaction of seeing it in print.

Finally, I would like to dedicate this book to my wife, Judith, and daughter, Nina, for their confidence and encouragement from inception to completion.

CONTENTS

Quick Reference to
CLINICAL TOXICOLOGY

1. GENERAL PRINCIPLES IN THE MANAGEMENT OF ACUTE POISONING

Irwin B. Hanenson, M.D.

The treatment of acute intoxication by therapeutic or nontherapeutic agents may be divided into three phases. They include first aid, which for the most part consists of therapeutic measures that can be instituted before professional support is available, supportive life-sustaining treatment, which entirely or in part includes basic therapeutic adjuncts generally applicable to all forms of poisoning, and finally, specific measures which are applicable to reverse the harmful effects of the specific toxic agent. It should be emphasized that these three components are not exclusive of each other but often overlap and must be combined for optimum management of the patient.

I. FIRST AID

This phase refers to the emergency treatment recommended by a trained professional, usually a physician, to assist a lay person in the initial management of any form of intoxication before the subject can reach a medical facility.

A. HISTORY

Advice regarding therapeutic management requires information concerning the toxin (e.g., name or description, time of intoxication, age of subject). It is helpful, if the agent is available, to request that a sample be brought with the patient to assist with identification by physical properties and analysis.

B. INGESTED TOXINS

Nonprofessionals, unless specially trained, should not treat comatose or convulsing subjects.

1. Administer an emetic to remove agent from the stomach before significant absorption can occur (syrup of ipecac: children 15 ml., adults 30 ml.), followed by a glass of water.

2. Do not administer if patient has ingested corrosives (acids or alkalies) or petroleum products.

C. INHALED TOXINS

1. Immediately remove subject to a toxin-free environment.

2. Artificial respiration (mouth-to-mouth preferable with patient's head extended and mouth open) at a rate of 15–20 per minute.

D. SKIN CONTAMINATION

1. Remove clothing and wash skin thoroughly with large amount of water. In addition, cleanse with soap when available.

2. Use no chemical antidotes.

E. EYE CONTAMINATION

Separate eyelids and rinse eyes with water.

F. ANIMAL BITE

1. Immobilize patient. Take particular care to limit movement of the area of the bite.

2. Transport patient carefully and rapidly to a medical facility for specific treatment (e.g., antivenin).

II. SUPPORTIVE TREATMENT

This portion of the program includes the basic elements for life support following the patient's arrival at a medical facility. Certain procedures may have already been completed or may be in progress at the time of arrival.

A. CLINICAL EVALUATION

1. History

a. Identification of poison. Information obtained from relative or other person accompanying the patient, physician, pharmacist, available sample of poison or poison container.

b. Time of ingestion or contact with poison.

c. Psychiatric and social history including information containing previous suicide attempts, agents used, etc.

It should be noted that the reliability of the history is uncertain. For example, in multiple drug ingestions the accuracy of identification of the ingested material may be as low as 33%. Even a sample of the alleged poison or the container may provide false or only partially correct information.

2. Clinical Assessment of the Patient

a. Observe for diagnostic features associated with ingestion of certain poisons. For example, in tricyclic antidepressant overdose, look for loss of consciousness, dilated pupils, bladder distention, absent bowel sounds, cardiac arrhythmias, and pyramidal tract involvement. The knowledge of drug toxicity or toxic reactions associated with various nontherapeutic agents can assist in identifying the toxin and aid in the initiation of therapy prior to the availability of laboratory identification. To help in providing this information, every emergency medical facility should have an available source of information, e.g., text books, relevant articles. Additional information may be obtained by calling poison information centers (see Chap. 24).

b. Record vital signs—blood pressure, heart rate, respirations, and temperature.

c. Ascertain the level of consciousness:

Grade 1: drowsy but responds to verbal commands.

Grade 2: unconscious but responds to mild painful stimulus.
Grade 3: unconscious and responds only to maximum painful stimulus.
Grade 4: unconscious without response to painful stimulus.

---

d. The standard painful stimulus is rubbing the patient's sternum firmly with knuckles of a clenched fist.

B. EMERGENCY THERAPY

Priorities in the management of acute poisoning are determined by the intoxicating agent, its mode of entry into the body, and the clinical condition of the patient. In most instances, a number of therapeutic adjuncts are employed concurrently rather than in a sequential fashion. Stimulating agents (analeptics) are contraindicated. They are of no benefit and have been responsible for deaths. Not infrequently, seizures accompany their use.

1. Removal of Toxin

a. Ingested Poisons

(1) Emesis is only employed in fully conscious patients with an intact gag reflex.

(a) Give syrup of ipecac (adults, 30 ml.; children, 15 ml. orally).

(b) Give Apomorphine (0.06 mg./kg. I.V. or S.C.). Terminate with naloxone (Narcan) 0.4 mg./I.V.

(c) Administer one to two glasses of water with the emetic. Employ emesis within 4–6 hours of drug ingestion except for salicylates which may still be recovered up to 10 hours after ingestion.

(2) Gastric lavage is employed if the patient is unconscious or lacks a gag reflex. Endotracheal intubation should be performed before lavage is attempted to prevent aspiration. Following intubation, place the patient in the left lateral position with head dependent. Introduce, through either the nose or mouth, a #30–

36 French Ewald tube into the stomach. Rinse the stomach repeatedly with 100–200 ml. aliquots of warm water until the recovered fluid is clear. In case of lipid soluble agents, e.g., glutethimide, lavage fluid should consist of equal quantities of water and olive oil. At the end of lavage 30–60 ml. of olive oil should be left in the stomach.

(3) Activated charcoal should be administered as a slurry after lavage or emesis. Since the charcoal absorbs ipecac, it should not be given prior to or with the emetic. The amount administered is determined by the quantity of toxic agent ingested (15–60 gm.; 30 gm. if amount unknown).

Agents adsorbed include:

Salicylic acid	Quinine
Barbiturates	Quinidine
Phenytoin	Chloroquine
Propoxyphene	Glutethimide
Morphine	Methyl Salicylate
Opium	Chlorpheniramine
Strychnine	Iodine
Atropine	Tricyclic Antidepres-
Mercuric chloride	sants
Phenol	Ipecac
Sulfonamides	Cocaine
Dextroamphetamine	Camphor
Primaquine	Organophosphates
Colchicine	(malathion, parathi-
Nicotine	on)
Alcohol	Metals (antimony,
Probenecid	arsenic, selenium,
Quinacrine	silver)
Phenothiazine	Penicillin
Meprobamate	Digitalis

(4) After lavage or emesis administer 30 gm. sodium sulfate in 250 ml. water as a cathartic.

(5) Special considerations and reservations in use of gastric lavage and emesis include:

(a) With corrosives such as strong acids or bases, lavage or emesis may lead to perforation.

(b) Convulsions may be induced by emesis and increased in frequency and severity by lavage.

(c) Ingestion of paraffin, kerosene, or other petroleum distillates, because of their low surface tension and high vapor pressure, can lead to severe pneumonitis on aspiration of even a few milliliters into the respiratory passages.

b. Skin Decontamination

Toxic agents which penetrate or damage the skin must be removed as quickly as possible. These include alkalies, acids, pesticides, hydrocarbons, and cyanide. Thoroughly wash all skin areas with tincture of green soap, if available, since it is effective in removing substances soluble in alcohol and will hydrolyze organophosphates. Plain soap is less effective but useful in the absence of green soap. It is particularly important that such relatively unaccessible areas as the umbilicus, undernails, ears, and groin be thoroughly cleansed. However, the effort should not be so vigorous as to produce skin abrasion.

During the process of surface cleansing, the person performing the decontamination should be careful to avoid skin contact with the toxic agent. Proper clothing should be worn, and all materials with which the patient comes in contact should be identified and cleansed or discarded immediately.

c. Respiratory Depression

It is essential to maintain a clear airway to support respiration and prevent aspiration.

(1) Clean mouth and fauces of any debris.

(2) Turn patient on left side with head dependent to avoid inhalation of vomitus or secretions.

(3) With absent gag reflex or depressed level of consciousness, insert a cuffed en-

dotracheal tube and provide respiratory assistance with mechanical ventilation if necessary. Oxygen administration should be guided by measurement of arterial blood gases.

d. Aspiration

Aspiration generally occurs following emesis or regurgitation of the toxic material and rarely during ingestion. There may be no physical signs after aspiration, and chest x-ray may be negative for several hours. Conservative treatment is recommended. Steroids have not been documented to be of benefit. Antibiotics should be withheld until there is clinical evidence of infection. Identification of the organism is helpful in selecting the appropriate drug.

e. Shock

Shock following acute intoxication is not the result of loss of volume, but rather a decrease in effective circulating volume. There is a disproportion between vascular capacity and fluid volume. This is the result of a combination of dilatation of the vascular bed and reduction in venous return of the blood to the heart with consequent decrease in cardiac output and blood pressure.

For practical purposes, shock exists when the systolic blood pressure is below 80 mm. Hg. This is generally associated with a urine output less than 25 ml. per hour. Treatment of shock should include general supportive therapy for associated complications such as coma, respiratory depression, pain, and acidosis (sodium bicarbonate). Specific therapy is directed toward the relative hypovolemia, which requires the intravenous administration of sufficient fluid volume to reestablish an adequate level of blood pressure.

(1) Place the patient in a supine position with elevation of lower extremities.

(2) Start an intravenous infusion of normal saline or 5% glucose in half normal saline through an 18-gauge venous catheter. At the same time, a catheter

should be inserted for the measurement of central venous pressure. Guides for fluid administration are arterial blood pressure, central venous pressure, and urine output. To assure accurate measurement of urine output, an in-dwelling Foley urethral catheter should be inserted. Fluid administration may require 500 ml. to 1 liter per hour for blood pressures below 80 mm. Hg and 100–200 ml. per hour when blood pressures are 80 mm. Hg or above.

Should this program fail to produce a satisfactory increase in blood pressure without an abnormal elevation of central venous pressure, an intravascular volume expander, such as plasma or 5% normal human serum albumin, may be employed. Rapid infusion up to a volume of 2 liters within two hours may be administered. This infusion should be discontinued when arterial pressure reaches acceptable levels or central venous pressure is elevated.

(3) Inability to raise blood pressure or progressive deterioration of blood pressure in spite of the above regimen of fluid replacement may require the use of pressor agents. It should be emphasized that these drugs should be reserved for those situations in which blood pressure does not respond to volume expansion. The regimen suggested is either the intravenous infusion of norepinephrine, 8 mg., and phentolamine, 10 mg. in 500 ml. 5% glucose in water, or metaraminol, initially I.M. 5 mg. at 20-minute intervals. Administer these drugs in amounts that will maintain systolic blood pressure at 100 mm. Hg or above.

(4) For those patients who remain refractory, steroids may be added to the therapeutic regimen, although there is insufficient evidence to support their efficacy. Hydrocortisone, 100 mg. I.V. every four to six hours, is suggested.

(5) In some cases, since hypotension may be accompanied by arterial constriction, vasodilator drugs may be helpful. The patients most likely to benefit would be those who fail to improve after admin-

istration of intravenous fluid and manifest abnormal increments in central venous pressure. In such cases, the administration of phenoxybenzamine, 1 mg./kg. I.V., may produce a reduction in central venous pressure accompanied by an increase in blood pressure, cardiac output, and urine flow.

f. Convulsions

(1) General measures include support of respiration, restraint of patient to avoid personal body injury, quiet environment, and avoidance of any procedures such as emesis or gastric lavage that may further stimulate the patient.

(2) Specific treatment includes administration of anticonvulsants to stop the seizures.

    (a) Diazepam, 5–10 mg. I.V. Repeat if necessary.

    (b) Barbiturates

        i. Thiopental, 2.5% solution I.V. at slow rate; maximum dose, 0.5 ml./kg.

        ii. Pentobarbital, 2.5% solution I.V.; maximum rate, 1 ml. per minute.

        iii. Phenobarbital, 1 mg./kg. I.M.; dose not to exceed 5 mg./kg.

    (c) Succinylcholine, 10–50 mg. I.V. at a slow rate; respiratory assistance *must* be maintained during use of this drug.

g. Delirium

Delirium occurs particularly following intoxication with stimulant drugs. This condition is characterized by physical hyperactivity and hallucinations which make it extremely difficult to control the patient. Give chlorpromazine (Thorazine), 25–50 mg. I.M. Repeat every four to six hours if needed.

h. Methemoglobinemia

This is produced by a number of chemicals, e.g., nitrites, chlorates, amino and nitro-organic compounds and certain drugs, e.g., acetanilid, phenacetin.

(1) General treatment includes administration of oxygen and removal of toxin.

(2) Antidote

    (a) Methylene blue, 0.1 mg./kg. of 1% solution I.V. over a 10-minute period. This is administered if methemoglobin concentration is over 40% or patient is experiencing symptoms.

    (b) Ascorbic acid, 1 gm. I.V., if methylene blue not available.

    (c) Methemoglobin levels below 30% may not require therapy.

i. Body Temperature Regulation

(1) For hyperthermia, apply cool, wet towels and, if necessary, immerse the extremities in water at 72°F (25°C).

(2) For mild hypothermia (temperature above 95°F, 35°C) apply blankets and keep patient in a warm environment. For severe hypothermia (less than 95°F, 35°C), immerse body or extremities in hot water not exceeding 107.6°F (42°C) and apply blankets.

j. Laboratory Studies

(1) General

Laboratory studies including chemistry, hematology, electrocardiography, chest x-ray, and arterial blood gases are determined by the clinical condition of the patient. Laboratory information may be of direct and immediate benefit or may be helpful in providing a baseline for comparison with subsequent analytical procedures to follow the clinical course or determine the prognosis.

(2) Specific

Body fluid samples may be obtained for the identification of the toxic agent.

(a) Advantages

    i. To accurately identify the drug or nontherapeutic agent.

    ii. To predict the clinical course of the patient by identifying the toxic agent. For example, the tricyclic antidepressant drugs are known to be cardiotoxic, and if they are present, their identification alerts the physician to the potential risk of the development of cardiac abnormalities.

(b) Limitations

i. Screening procedures for drug identification are lengthy, often requiring several hours. Patients acutely ill must be treated before the results are available. In such instances, supportive therapy and any antidotes suggested by the history or clinical picture of the patient should be instituted.

ii. Quantitative measurements of the drug or chemical in serum or blood may not correlate with the clinical manifestations. This is due not only to individual variation but also to many other factors including age, interactions with other drugs or nontherapeutic agents, clinical status of patient prior to intoxication, prior exposure to the intoxicating agent.

(c) The body fluid samples to be collected for analysis are as follows:

i. Gastric: In patients who have ingested the toxic material; samples of the vomitus or lavage fluid useful for identification of the parent compound.

ii. Urine: Easily obtainable in large quantities; useful for identification of the toxin. Because of the variability in urine concentration and the presence of metabolites, quantitative estimates on urine are generally of little value.

iii. Blood or serum: Used for quantitation of the toxic agent. It may also be used for identification; contains both the parent compound and metabolites.

III. SPECIFIC THERAPEUTIC MEASURES

A. Antidotes and antagonists.

B. Specific agents to expedite removal from the body of heavy metals and organophosphates.

1. ANTAGONISTS AND ANTIDOTES

a. Opiates

Naloxone (Narcan), 0.4 mg. I.V. It can also be given I.M. or S.C. The dose may be repeated at 2–3 minute intervals if the desired improvement is not observed within 1–2 minutes. In contrast to other antagonists, naloxone is effective against pentazocine (Talwin). Although sufficient evidence of efficacy is not yet available, naloxone should also be used in propoxyphene (Darvon) overdoses. If naloxone is ineffective, other antagonists should be tried, although lack of effectiveness may be a clue to incorrect diagnosis. If naloxone is not available, use nalorphine hydrochloride (Nalline), 5–10 mg. I.V., or levallorphan tartrate (Lorfan), 0.3–1.2 mg. I.V. These are less desirable since they are partial agonists. Give these drugs every 15 minutes until clinical status of patient is satisfactory.

b. Cyanide

Kit available and should be in the emergency unit. Sodium nitrite, 10 ml. of 3% solution I.V. 2.5–5.0 ml. per minute. Follow with 50 ml. 25% sodium thiosulfate I.V. at 1.5–5.0 ml. per minute. Repeat if symptoms reappear.

c. Organophosphates (Weed Killer, Insecticides)

Treat within four hours. Atropine 2 mg. I.M. every 15–40 minutes until there is clinical evidence of atropinization, i.e., flushed face, dry mouth, widely dilated pupils, fast pulse, absent bowel sounds. Repeat dose as necessary to maintain signs of atropinization. When patient atropinized, give pralidoxine in aqueous solution 1 gm. I.V. Dose may be repeated twice within 24 hours and within an interval of 30 minutes if necessary. Rate of administration should not exceed 50 mg. per minute.

d. Anticholinergic Drugs (Tricyclic Antidepressants, Atropine, Scopolamine)

Physostigmine, 1–4 mg. I.V. should be administered depending on severity of intoxication. Repeat I.V. or I.M. as needed but no more frequently than every 20–30 minutes.

e. Nitrites and Nitrates

Give methylene blue, 0.2 ml./kg. I.V. over 5 minutes. Prepare as 1% solution in 5% dextrose or 0.9% sodium chloride.

f. Amphetamines

Give chlorpromazine, 0.5–1.0 mg./kg. I.M.

g. Phenothiazines

Give diphenhydramine (Benadryl), 2.5–5.0 mg./kg. P.O. for extrapyramidal symptoms.

h. Acetaminophen

Blood sample should be analyzed 4 hours or later following ingestion. Samples obtained prior to 4 hours are of little prognostic value. Patients with elevated serum levels should be treated within 12 hours of the time of ingestion.

(1) Methionine

(a) Oral: 5 gm. initially with additional 5 gm. every 4 hours until the patient has received a total dose of 20 gm.

(b) Intravenous: initial loading dose of 5 gm. over a 10-minute period followed by infusion of 5 gm. in the next 4 hours and 5 gm. in each of the subsequent 8-hour periods for a total of 20 gm.

(2) N-Acetylcysteine

Prepare a 5% solution with water or flavored drink. Administer an oral loading dose of 140 mg./kg. followed by a maintenance dose of 70 mg./kg. every 4 hours over a period of 68 hours (i.e., 17 maintenance doses). If patient vomits a loading or maintenance dose within 1 hour of dosing, repeat the dose.

i. Carbon Monoxide

Provide 100% oxygen by mask.

2. AGENTS TO REMOVE DRUG FROM BODY

a. Arsenic and Mercury

Administer dimercaprol (BAL) within 4 hours. Give 10% solution in oil at rate of 3–4 mg./kg. I.M. every 4 hours for 2 days and then every 12 hours for 10 days.

b. Lead, Mercury, Copper, Nickel, Zinc, Cadmium, Cobalt, Beryllium, and Manganese

Administer EDTA (Versene), 15–25 mg./kg. in 250–500 ml. 5% glucose and water I.V. over 1–2-hour period twice daily. If CSF pressure is elevated, give 50 mg./kg. daily I.M. of 20% solution in 0.5–1.5% procaine.

c. Iron

Administer deferoxamine (Desferal), 2 gm. in 10 ml. water I.M. STAT. In addition, begin an I.V. infusion at a rate of no more than 15 mg./kg. per hour. The maximum dose by this route is 80 mg./kg. per 12 hours. The intramuscular injection of deferoxamine may be repeated at 12-hour intervals according to clinical status and plasma iron levels. An iron level above 800 μg./100 ml. in an adult within 4 hours of ingestion indicates severe poisoning.

C. Forced diuresis (Table 1-1).

D. Peritoneal dialysis and hemodialysis.

1. Agents removed by dialysis include:

Alcohols	Fluorides
Chloral hydrates	Iodides
Ethylene glycol	Quinidine
Barbiturates	Quinine
(particularly	Strychnine
long-acting)	Anilines
Meprobamate	Antibiotics
Paraldehyde	Boric acid and its salts
Acetaminophen	Carbon tetrachloride
Salicylates	Chlorates
Phenacetin	Dichromates

Amphetamines	Ergotamine
Arsenicals	Isoniazid
Calcium	Nitrobenzenes
Lithium	Nitrofurantion
Magnesium	Phenytoin
Potassium	Sulfonamides
Bromides	Thiocyanates

2. Dialysis is of limited or no value in removing the following agents:

Tricyclic antidepressants	Hallucinogens
	Heroin
Antihistamines	Methaqualone
Atropine	Methyprylon
Chlordiazepoxide	Ethchlorvynol
Diazepam	Oxazepam
Digitalis	Phenothiazines
Glutethimide	Propoxyphene

E. Charcoal hemoperfusion: This is a procedure where blood from the patient

Table 1.1. **Agents Eliminated by Forced Diuresis***

Amphetamines (elimination increased by acid urine)[†]
Quinine (elimination increased by acid urine)[†]
Salicylates (elimination increased by alkaline urine)[‡]
Barbiturates (elimination increased by alkaline urine)[‡] (long-acting)
Alcohol
Ethylene glycol
Bromide
Lithium
Sulfonamides
Penicillin
Quinidine
Aniline
Isoniazid
Strychnine
Phencyclidine

*10% mannitol, 5–10 ml. per minute. Maintain urine flow at about 5 ml. per minute. Avoid volume overload. Intake should equal urine flow plus insensible loss.
[†]Maintain urinary pH < 6.5 beginning with solution of 500 ml. 5% G/W containing 1.5 gm. NH_4Cl.
[‡]Maintain urinary pH ≥ 7.5 beginning with solution of 500 ml. 1.25% $NaHCO_3$.

passes through a cannister containing activated charcoal and is then returned to the subject. Chemicals adsorbed by activated charcoal are effectively removed from the blood. However, caution must be exercised with this procedure because other normal constituents of the blood, such as platelets, glucose, and divalent cations, may also be removed. However, it is an effective adjunct when used in a hospital setting with careful monitoring.

F. Tricyclic antidepressant overdose: Following gastric lavage, remove the Ewald tube, insert a #17 nasogastric tube, and aspirate gastric contents by low Gomco suction for a maximum of 24 hours or until patient's condition is satisfactory.

BIBLIOGRAPHY

Arena, J. M.: Poisoning. 3rd. ed. Springfield, Ill. Charles C Thomas, 1974.

Baselt, R. C., et al: Therapeutic and toxic concentrations of more than 100 toxicologically significant drugs in blood, plasma, or serum: a. 1. tabulation. Clin. Chem., 21:44, 1975.

Crane, G. E.: Cardiac toxicity and psychotropic drugs. Dis. Nerv. Syst., 31:534, 1970.

Davies, B. S., and Prichard, B. N. C. (eds.): Biological Effects of Drugs in Relation to Their Plasma Concentration. New York, University Park Press, 1973.

Davis, J. M., et al.: Overdose of psychotropic drugs: a review Dis. Nerv. Syst., (Part I) 29:157, 1968; (Part II) 29:246, 1968.

Dimijian, G. G., and Radelat, F. A.: Evaluation and treatment of the suspected drug user in the emergency room. Arch. Intern. Med., 125:162, 1970.

Fowler, N. O., et al.: Electrocardiographic changes and cardiac arrhythmias in patients receiving psychotopic drugs. Am. J. Cardiol., 37:223, 1976.

Freeman, J. W., et al.: Management of patients unconscious from drug overdosage. Med. J. Aus., 2:1165, 1970

Gard, H., et al.: Qualitative and quantitative studies on the disposition of amitriptyline and other tricyclic antidepressant drugs in man as it relates to the management of the overdose patient. Clin. Toxicol., 6:571, 1973.

Gleason, M. N., et al.: Clinical Toxicology of Commercial Products. 3rd ed. Baltimore, Williams & Wilkins, 1969.

Knepshield, J. H., et al.: Dialysis of poisons and drugs. Trans. Am. Soc. Artif. Intern. Organs, 19:590, 1973.

Matthew, H.: Acute Barbiturate Poisoning. Amsterdam, Excerpta Medica, 1971.

Matthew, H.: Acute poisoning: some myths and misconceptions. Br. Med. J., *1:*519, 1971.

Peterson, R. G., and Rumack, B. H.: Treating acute acetaminophen poisoning with acetylcysteine. J.A.M.A. *237:*2406, 1977.

The Poisoned Patient: The Role of the Laboratory. Ciba Foundation Symposium 26. Amsterdam Associated Scientific Publishers, 1974.

Prescott, L. F., Sutherland, G. R., Park, J., et al.: Cysteamine, methionine, and penicillamine in the treatment of paracetamol poisoning. Lancet, *2:*109, 1976.

Shubin, H., and Weil, M. H.: Shock associated with barbiturate intoxication. J.A.M.A., *215:*263, 1971.

2. TRANQUILIZERS

David Fedders, M.D.

Phenothiazines are the most prevalent major tranquilizers used in self-poisonings, followed by the buterophenones and thioxanthenes. Of the minor tranquilizers, the benzodiazepine group alone or in combination accounts for the majority of all hospitalized drug overdoses.

The mortality from this type of self-poisoning is low and rarely associated with residual impairment. The degree of morbidity is variable, but the usual case, when appropriately managed with conservative and supportive treatment, fully recovers without complication.

The tranquilizers are often taken in combination with alcohol. Other frequent combinations include phenothiazine with an antiparkinson agent or a tricyclic antidepressant.

In this chapter phenothiazines and benzodiazepines serve as prototypes for the major and minor tranquilizers. Because the variability among drugs within these two prototypes is minimal in terms of clinical management, other tranquilizers will be discussed in terms of their relationship to these two groups to avoid repetition.

I. MAJOR TRANQUILIZERS

A. PHENOTHIAZINES

The toxic effects of phenothiazines primarily involve the three components of the nervous system: central (CNS), autonomic (ANS), and extrapyramidal (EPS).

The three subgroups of phenothiazines vary some in terms of their likelihood of demonstrating one or more of the major clinical features described in Table 2-1.

1. Clinical Features (Fig. 2-1)

a. Mild Intoxication

(1) CNS. Sedation, ataxia, slurred speech, disorientation. Paradoxical agitation or hyperactive behavior occurs particularly in children or senescent persons following ingestion of the piperazine (least-sedating) group. Seizure activity has also been noted on rare occasions during this period of excitability from lowering the seizure threshold.

(2) EPS. Usually there are no symptoms in the mild overdose except abnormal salivation. Signs include extrapyramidal involvement, e.g., decreased eye blinking. Generally there is no noticeable muscle stiffness. Dystonic reactions are rare at this level of involvement but are quite frightening to the patient when they do occur.

In general, EPS symptoms are most significant when the patient is conscious, and although they are more likely to occur with deeper levels of sedation, they are not as significant once the subjective component is removed by loss of consciousness.

(3) ANS.

Skin. Temperature and color change: warm, cold, flushed, or pallid with hyperhidrosis.

ENT. Nasal and sinus congestion, xerostomia.

Eye. Blurred vision, mydriasis, accommodation difficulties, and precipitation of glaucoma.

G.I. Paralytic ileus, constipation, and fecal impaction; cholestatic hepatosis.

G.U. Urinary retention, urinary hesitancy, aggravation of prostatism; tran-

Table 2-1. **Clinical Features of Phenothiazines**

Phenothiazine Subgroup	CNS	EPS	ANS
	SEDATION	PARKINSON'S	HYPOTENSION
Aliphatic group (chlorpromazine)	+4	+2	+4
Piperazine group (fluoperazine, fluphenazine, perphenazine)	+1	+4	+1
Piperidine group (thioridazine)	+2	+1	+2

sient erectile, ejaculatory, or orgasmic inhibition.

Cardiovascular. Orthostatic hypotension with associated vertigo, syncope, or head trauma; dysrhythmias with tachyarrhythmias more common than bradyarrhythmias; conduction disturbances, hypotension, and shock.

b. Moderate Intoxication

(1) CNS. The patient is comatose but responds to painful stimuli. The duration of this state will depend on the type of phenothiazine. It will be longest for the aliphatic group. The additional presence of alcohol or hypnotics is important in the evaluation.

(2) EPS. The patient exhibits muscle stiffness, e.g., cog-wheeling upon passive movement of the neck, biceps, or quadriceps, and excessive salivation or drooling. Dystonic reactions occur but are not threatening because the patient is asleep. There is oculogyric crisis and dyskinesias of the tongue. Laryngospasm is the only life-threatening manifestation.

(3) ANS. Toxic manifestations of the gastrointestinal and gastrourinary tracts become more severe, e.g., acute urinary retention, paralytic ileus, and fecal impaction. Dysrhythmias and hypotension are more common.

c. Severe Overdose

(1) CNS. In coma the patient is unarousable to both verbal and painful stimuli.

(2) EPS. Salivation, blepharospasm, and cog-wheel stiffness of the extremities; hyperactive DTRs; and Babinski sign may be present. Dystonic reactions may occur most commonly of the head and neck and involving cranial nerves. There is a greater possibility of laryngospasm. There may also be torticollis and opisthotonus, especially with mild temperature elevation.

(3) ANS. Shock and dysrhythmias are the most life-threatening complications. There may be precipitation of an acute glaucoma attack. Acute renal shutdown, acute urinary retention, and paralytic ileus may occur.

d. Extraneurological Toxicity

(1) ECG abnormalities include left axis deviation and negative T waves. Though thioridazine is thought to have a direct effect on the heart, causing T-wave inversion, the phenothiazines as a group probably exact their ECG effects by altering electrical conductivity through potassium regulatory mechanisms. With phenothiazine administration there is a decrease in both serum and urinary potassium indicating a relative intracellular shift. This mechanism may also be relevant to the mechanism of altered seizure threshold.

(2) Cholestatic hepatosis is another clinically significant toxic complication. The symptoms resemble those of extrahepatic obstructive jaundice, and the laboratory pattern consists of elevated alkaline phosphatase, transaminases, prothrombin

Major Tranquilizers

Trade Name (Generic Name)	Classification	Approximate Equivalent (mg. to 100 mg. chlorpromazine)	Usual Daily Dosage Range for Antipsychotic Effect (mg.)	EPS Effects	Sedation and Hypotension Effects
Haldol (haloperidol)	buterophenone	2	2-15		
Navane (thiothixene)	thioxanthine	2	10-60		
Prolixin (fluphenazine)	piperazine ∮	2	5-20		
Stelazine (trifluoperazine)	piperazine ∮	5	10-40		
Quide (piperacetazine)	piperadine ∮	10	40-160		
Trilafon (perphenazine)	piperazine ∮	10	12-64		
Compazine (prochlorperazine)	piperazine ∮	15	30-150		
Tindal (acetophenazine)	piperazine ∮	20	40-120		
Vesprin (triflupromazine)	aliphatic ∮	25	30-150		
Serentil (mesaridazine)	piperadine ∮	70	150-400		
Sparine (promazine)	aliphatic ∮	100	150-800		
Toractan (chlorprothixene)	thioxanthene	100	75-600		
Mellaril (thioridazine)	piperadine ∮	100	75-800		
Thorazine (chlorpromazine)	aliphatic ∮	100	100-2,000		

Fig. 2-1. Comparative effects of major tranquilizers on sedation-hypotension and the EPS for phenothiazines, buterophenones, and thioxanthenes. (∮ = phenothiazine.)

time, and BSP retention. The course is usually benign but is protracted over a 4–6-week period without residual cirrhosis or injury, except in patients with pre-existing liver disease.

2. Treatment

a. General Measures

The basic treatment of the phenothiazine toxic person is conservative and supportive, and follows the principles outlined in Chapter 1.

b. Specific Measures

Table 2-2 summarizes the treatment for neurological toxicity.

(1) Mild Overdose. Hospitalization is not necessarily indicated for this type of overdose. The patient can frequently be managed as an outpatient provided some family or support structure exists during

the interim. A psychiatric consultation may be helpful in assessing continued life risk. The CNS depression needs to be diagnosed as stable before release from medical observation. Observation for an hour or two should show no progression to the moderate or severe category.

The autonomic signs and symptoms are usually transient and mild and require no treatment. The patient and family should be advised about orthostatic hypotension emphasizing the importance of rising slowly and wearing support stockings.

The patient and family should also be informed about the possible appearance of dystonic reactions; however, if a dystonic reaction has not occurred before the point of clinical stabilization, it is doubtful that it will occur.

(2) Moderate Overdose. The depressed level of consciousness requires medical supervision and hospitalization for supportive therapy and monitoring. Shock and hypotension occur rarely at this level of involvement. Forced diuresis and dialysis are ineffective.

Dystonic reactions, particularly in muscles innervated by the cranial nerves, are likely and are usually reversed by 1.0 to 2.0 mg. benztropine (Cogentin) I.V. or I.M. If there is no response to benztropine, endotracheal intubation is indicated to maintain a patent airway. Oculogyric crisis and tongue dyskinesia may also occur.

Urethral catheterization is indicated for acute urinary retention.

(3) Severe Overdose. The patient is comatose and requires hospitalization. Airway and cardiopulmonary status require constant monitoring. Shock is usually managed adequately with I.V. fluids and monitoring of central venous pressure and urinary output to safeguard against fluid overload. Pressor agents should be avoided since they may produce a hypertensive crisis.

Fever poses a difficult differential diag-

Table 2-2. **Treatment for Neurological Toxicity**

Clinical Problem	Treatment
CNS	
Seizure; hyperactivity	Diazepam, up to 10 mg. I.V.; restraints when necessary
EPS	
Muscle rigidity; hypersalivation	Benztropine, 1 mg., I.V. or I.M.; supportive care
Dystonic reaction; akathisia	Benztropine, 1–2 mg., I.V. or I.M.; restraints
ANS	
Hypotension	I.V. fluids with central venous pressure monitoring
Nasal and sinus congestion	0.25% neosynephrine drops or spray
Blurred vision	No treatment, counseling
Glaucoma	Local cholinergics, ophthalmology consultation
Urinary retention	Catheterization
Constipation	Cathartics

nostic problem in the comatose patient. To rule out temperature elevation as an EPS symptom, 1 mg. benztropine may be given without serious risk, and the temperature monitored. Dystonic reactions occur in severe cases but are usually not life threatening and reverse with clearance of the toxic drug. For psychological reasons, benztropine treatment may be required as the patient approaches the hypnotic awakening state.

Urinary catheterization is indicated for both urinary retention and to monitor urinary output.

B. Nonphenothiazine Major Tranquilizers

1. Thioxanthenes and Buterophenones

The thioxanthenes and buterophenones are two significant groups of nonphenothiazines. Extrapyramidal effects are dystonic

Table 2-3. Benzodiazepines

Generic Name	Trade Name	Usual Dose Range (mg.)
Chlordiazepoxide	Librium	15–100
Diazepam	Valium	6–40
Oxazepam	Serax	30–120
Clorazepate dipotassium	Tranxene	12–60
Flurazepam HCl	Dalmane	15–30

reactions, which respond to benztropine or other centrally acting anticholinergics. Hypotensive complications are minimal. Because of the low sedating qualities, there may be transient hyperactivity prior to coma, and recovery may be complicated by akathisia.

II. MINOR TRANQUILIZERS

A. MEPROBAMATE

It is still not clear whether meprobamate (Miltown), which predates the benzodiazepines, should be classified as a major or minor tranquilizer. It is a derivative of mephenesin, a muscle relaxant, and was discovered to have tranquilizing effects without extrapyramidal and autonomic side effects. However, it appears to have an addictive potential similar to that for barbiturates, with a lethal-to-therapeutic dose ratio of about 1:8, again similar to barbiturates. It is further difficult to demonstrate from the literature that the clinical side effects are any fewer than with barbiturates or benzodiazepines. Treatment is supportive (Chap. 1). Dialysis may be helpful in life-threatening situations.

B. BENZODIAZEPINES

Variations on the 1.4-benzodiazepine nucleus constitute a group of minor tranquilizers that are the most widely used drugs in the practice of medicine. In 1972 more than 75 million prescriptions for benzodiazepine derivatives were filled in the United States, two-thirds of which were for diazepam (Valium). Five derivatives are available in the United States, and a sixth, nitrazepam (Mogadon), is popular elsewhere.

In view of the extremely high use of this group of drugs, complications and toxicity are exceedingly low. However, they top the list of therapeutic agents used for suicide attempts.

Table 2-3 contains the identifying information for the benzodiazepines.

1. Clinical Features

The toxic effects of benzodiazepines range from oversedation and ataxia to coma (Table 2-4). Toxic effects on other organ systems are rare. The autonomic nervous system is only mildly affected, and cardiopulmonary function is impaired only with very large doses. The exact dosage required to cause cardiopulmonary impairment has not been determined but is probably beyond 100 times the therapeutic dose. Approximately 15–20 times the therapeutic dose usually produces ataxia, drowsiness, dysarthria, sleep without coma, hypotension, hyporeflexia, or abnormal neurological reflexes.

Studies by the Boston Collaborative Drug Surveillance Program (1973) have demonstrated that coincidental cigarette smoking and age have a significant effect on the toxicity of benzodiazepine. The greater the number of cigarettes smoked per day, the less common were CNS effects. They were more common in advancing age whether the person smoked or not. Increased metabolism with cigarette smokers and decreased metabolism in older patients were thought to be the cause.

Benzodiazepines are frequently combined with alcohol in suicidal attempts. They act synergistically and significantly worsen the prognosis.

In summary, the toxic effects of benzodiazepines are almost exclusively de-

Table 2-4. **Classification of Clinical Severity of Benzodiazepine Toxicity**

Classification	CNS Involvement	Treatment
Mild	Ataxia, drowsiness, arousal to verbal stimuli	Outpatient and emergency room management; psychiatric consultation
Moderate	Arousal to painful but not verbal stimuli	Medical supervision; possible hospitalization
Severe	Unarousable to painful stimuli	Hospitalization; conservative and supportive management

pression of the CNS, as with the phenothiazines, but uncomplicated by ANS and EPS symptoms.

2. Treatment

In general, a conservative and supportive medical regimen is indicated with cardiovascular monitoring and neurological observation. Hospitalization is indicated for coma. Physical indicators of possibly unfavorable or complicated recovery are: older age, presence of alcohol, and dosage exceeding 20 times the therapeutic dose.

Hypotension rarely occurs and can successfully be managed with I.V. fluids.

BIBLIOGRAPHY

Barry, D., Meyskens, F. L. Jr., and Becker, C. E.: Phenothiazine poisoning: a review of 48 cases. Calif. Med., *118*:1, 1973.

Boston Collaborative Drug Surveillance Program; Boston University Medical Center: Clinical depression of the central nervous system due to diazepam and chlordiazepoxide in relation to cigarette smoking and age. N. Engl. J. Med., *288:* 277, 1973.

Greenblatt, B. J., et al.: Rapid recovery from massive diazepam overdose. J.A.M.A., *240:*1872, 1978.

Gupta, J. M., and Lovejoy, F. H., Jr.: Acute phenothiazine toxicity in childhood: a five year survey. Pediatrics, *39:*771, 1967.

Hollister, L. E.: Overdoses of psychotherapeutic drugs. Clin. Pharm. Ther., *7:*142, 1966.

3. HYPNOTICS

Jeffrey B. Spears, Pharm.D., and Irwin B. Hanenson, M.D.

Hypnotic drugs are most often prescribed for insomnia. When insomnia becomes severe or chronic, it may be a symptom of a serious psychological illness such as depression. Hypnotics are dangerous drugs in the hands of a depressed patient because of the risk of suicide.

A portion of the population abuses hypnotic drugs. Like the depressed insomniac, the abuser uses both barbiturate and nonbarbiturate hypnotics (see Table 3-1). However, problems usually arise from miscalculation of a "safe dose" rather than a suicide attempt.

I. ACUTE INTOXICATION— BARBITURATES

Although not the case anymore, formerly the agents most commonly responsible for deaths from poisonings were barbiturates. It was estimated in 1949 that 25% of the cases of acute poisonings admitted to general hospitals were due to barbiturates. More recently, the estimate is 20%.

The most commonly abused barbiturates are phenobarbital, pentobarbital, secobarbital, and amobarbital. The clinical problems differ depending on whether the intoxication is acute or chronic.

Acute barbiturate poisoning results from either intentional or accidental ingestion of excessive amounts of the drug. The former is usually a suicidal attempt or gesture and often includes other central nervous system depressant drugs, especially alcohol. These multiple drug ingestions can be particularly dangerous because of synergism.

Barbiturates are known to depress all excitable tissues. However, not all tissues are equally susceptible, with the central nervous system being the most sensitive. Attempts at localization of the site of action have failed. Nonetheless, eventually all excitable tissues will be affected, and death, when it occurs, is usually due to respiratory failure and circulatory collapse.

A. CLINICAL FEATURES

The signs and symptoms vary in onset and duration with the drug ingested. The differences usually parallel the traditional classification of short-, intermediate-, and long-acting barbiturates (see Table 3-2). Generally, larger amounts of long-acting barbiturates are needed to produce a depth of coma comparable to that of a short-acting barbiturate. Mortality is usually greater among those intoxicated with long-acting barbiturates because of the complications of prolonged coma.

1. Mild Intoxication

(1) The patient is usually in Grade 1 or 2 coma.

(2) The symptoms resemble those of acute alcohol intoxication, except that the face is *not* flushed, the conjunctiva are *not* suffused, and there is *no* odor of alcohol on the patient's breath (unless concomitantly ingested).

(3) The patient may think slowly and be somewhat disoriented.

(4) Lability of mood, impairment of judgment, slurred speech, drunken gait, and nystagmus may be present.

(5) Reflexes and vital signs are not usually affected.

2. Moderate Intoxication

(1) The level of consciousness is more severely depressed; patients are usually in Grade 3 coma.

(2) Respirations may be decreased but are usually still adequate.

(3) The blood pressure usually remains normal.

Table 3-1. **Hypnotic Drugs**

Generic Name	Trade Name	Street Name
Barbiturates		Barbs, idiot pills, candy, courage pills, seggy, peanuts, sleepers, downers
Amobarbital	Amytal (capsules)	Blue heaven, blue birds, blue devils
Amobarbital in combination with secobarbital	Tuinal	Rainbow, double trouble
Pentobarbital	Nembutal	Nemmies, canary, yellows, yellow jackets
Secobarbital	Seconal	F-40s, reds, red devils, red birds
Chloral hydrate	Noctec	Joy juice
Chloral hydrate in combination with alcohol		Mickey Finns
Ethchlorvynol	Placidyl	
Flurazepam	Dalmane	
Glutethimide	Doriden (tablets)	CD
Methaqualone	Sopor, Parest, Quaalude	Sopors, rorer 714s, ludes
Methaprylon	Noludar	

(4) Deep tendon reflexes may be depressed or even absent.

In moderately severe intoxication, respirations may be rapid, shallow, or of the Cheyne-Stokes variety. The patient may or may not be rousable. If awakened, the patient frequently drifts back into coma.

3. Severe Intoxication

(1) The patient is usually in Grade 4 coma.

(2) Initially the face is reddened, then ashy pale, or cyanotic.

(3) Respirations are shallow and slow or rapid or irregular, or both.

(4) Pulmonary edema may be present.

(5) Pupils may show hypoxic dilatation but usually remain reactive to light.

(6) Deep tendon reflexes are usually absent. In most cases, the corneal reflex is lost before the deep tendon reflexes, but there is no consistent pattern. Laryngeal and tracheal reflexes may also vanish, leading to accumulation of secretions that, if not treated, may precipitate respiratory failure.

(7) Body temperature may fall to hypothermic levels (30°C).

(8) Pulse is often thready and rapid.

(9) Blood pressure may decrease to shock levels, complicating the problem.

4. Complications

a. Skin Lesions

Some patients who have ingested enough barbiturates to produce moderate to severe intoxication develop sweat gland necrosis and bullous cutaneous lesions. The lesions do not seem to be the result of hypersensitivity reactions or hypothermia. They appear within 24 hours and are usually on the extremities. The etiology is uncertain but is believed to be a direct toxic effect of the drug.

1. Dusky, erythematous plaques
2. Tense vesicles, surmounting erythematous, indurated bases
3. Large, tense, clear bullae, surrounded by a narrow rim of erythema

It has been reported that these lesions occur in up to 6% of all patients intoxicated with barbiturates. It is interesting to note that no patient has been reported to develop bullae, unless that patient was at one time comatose from barbiturate in-

Table 3-2. **The Barbiturates**

Short-acting Barbiturates
Pentobarbital
Secobarbital

Intermediate-acting Barbiturates
Amobarbital
Butabarbital

Long-acting Barbiturates
Phenobarbital
Mephobarbital

toxication. The bulla fluid has been shown to contain barbiturate.

Bullae and the other skin lesions have been found with intoxication with other agents (carbon monoxide, methadone, tricyclic antidepressants, meprobamate, and chloral hydrate) and are no longer valid as a diagnostic criteria for barbiturate intoxication.

b. Coma

(1) Pulmonary Complications. Pulmonary edema secondary to overhydration or cardiac failure. Patients intoxicated with barbiturates may also aspirate vomitus and develop an aspiration pneumonia.

(2) Renal Complications. Acute tubular necrosis secondary to shock. A rare complication is that of myoglobinuria with renal damage as a result of ischemic muscular necrosis.

(3) Electroencephalogram. The EEG in the comatose patient shows typical signs of depression. In mild intoxication, the normal activity is replaced by fast activity most prominent in the frontal regions. The amplitudes are augmented and the frequency is reduced as the severity of poisoning increases. In severely poisoned patients, the tracing may be flat.

(4) Thrombophlebitis and Pulmonary Embolism. A rare complication in severe cases with prolonged treatment.

B. DIAGNOSIS

The diagnosis of barbiturate intoxication may be difficult and is very often a diagnosis of exclusion. History and physical examination are important. When a patient is in a coma, the usual differential diagnosis must be considered. However, there are few conditions that cause coma with flaccid paralysis, reactive pupils, hypothermia, and hypotension. Multiple drug ingestions present problems, however, and ultimately the diagnosis must rely on laboratory confirmation. There is a variable correlation between serum concentration of barbiturate and toxicity.

C. TREATMENT

The treatment of acute barbiturate poisoning depends on the severity of intoxication. There is no antidote. Therapy is supportive with maintenance of vital signs.

1. Supportive Therapy (Refer to Chap. 1)

a. Respiratory Support

(1) Clear mouth and fauces of any debris.

(2) Turn patient on left side, head dependent, to prevent aspiration of vomitus or secretions.

(3) If patient respirations are depressed as in coma, or gag reflex is absent, insert a cuffed endotracheal tube and if necessary, provide ventilatory assistance.

b. Circulatory Support

(1) Correct dehydration and volume deficit.

(2) Administer pressor agents if volume replacement is inadequate.

c. Hypothermia

(1) Mild (above 35°C, or 95°F). Apply blankets and keep in warm room.

(2) Severe (less than 35°C, or 95°F). Immerse body or extremities in hot water (42°C, or 107.6°F) and apply blankets.

2. *Other Measures*

a. Prevention of Absorption

(1) Emesis should be induced only in fully conscious patients with syrup of ipecac. Apomorphine may be used if syrup of ipecac does not work. Apomorphine emesis can be terminated with naloxone.

(2) Gastric lavage should be used in unconscious patients or those who lack a gag reflex; insert a cuffed endotracheal tube before attempting lavage. Gastric lavage after four to six hours from the time of ingestion is rarely of value.

(3) Activated charcoal should be administered as a slurry of 15–60 gm. after lavage or emesis.

(4) After emesis or lavage and charcoal administration, induce catharsis with a cathartic (e.g., sodium sulfate or magnesium citrate).

b. Elimination of the Drug From the Body

(1) Forced diuresis with osmotic agents (e.g., mannitol) has been shown to be effective for the removal of phenobarbital, but not for the other barbiturates.

(2) Alkalinization of the urine above pH 7.5 may increase the excretion of phenobarbital.

(3) Hemodialysis removes barbiturates from the body approximately four times faster than peritoneal dialysis. The addition of albumin to the dialysis fluid nearly doubles the amount of drug removal.

(4) The use of charcoal hemoperfusion is also effective in removing barbiturates from the blood.

II. ACUTE INTOXICATION— NONBARBITURATES

A. BROMIDE INTOXICATION

Bromism occurs from the ingestion of bromoureides, bromide salts, and contaminated water supplies.

1. *Clinical Features*

The therapeutic and toxic effects of the bromide ion result from displacement of chloride in body fluids. Bromide in the central nervous system produces a nonspecific, reversible depression. The biological half-life of the bromide ion is approximately 10–14 days. Continuous use may produce intoxication from accumulation of the drug. Ingestion of 16.5 mEq. daily (maximum recommended therapeutic dose) could result in toxicity within 8 days. Renal insufficiency leads to more rapid accumulation.

Acute bromide intoxication is rare. Toxic doses produce gastric irritation with nausea and vomiting to decrease drug available for intestinal absorption. Chronic intoxication, or bromism, is more likely to be seen. Symptoms include rash, confusion, irritability, tremor, anorexia, weight loss, ataxia, stupor, and coma.

2. *Diagnosis*

The diagnosis of bromism is based on history, symptomatology, and serum concentration. Toxicity is usually seen when serum levels are above 1,000 μg./ml. Lower concentrations may produce toxicity in certain persons. Although the potential exists, bromide intoxication is rare from bromoureides or hydrobromide salts of other drugs.

3. *Treatment*

The drug should be discontinued or the source of bromide avoided (e.g., contaminated water supplies). Withdrawal symptoms and signs have not been reported. Chloride intake should be increased to at least 6 gm. per day in divided doses. This reduces the half-life of bromide ions by as much as 75%. Renal excretion of bromide is increased by the use of diuretics. Hemodialysis is also effective in removal of bromide from the body.

B. Chloral Hydrate Intoxication

Chloral hydrate is the oldest member of the hypnotic drugs marketed today. Knock-out drops or "Mickey Finns," considered to be highly toxic, are a mixture of chloral hydrate and alcohol. Chloral betaine and triclofos sodium are chloral derivatives, and their toxic properties resemble those of chloral hydrate. Chloral hydrate is rapidly reduced to trichloroethanol in the body. It is believed that the central nervous system depression from chloral hydrate is due to trichloroethanol.

1. Clinical Features

Acute chloral hydrate intoxication resembles acute barbiturate intoxication. Chloral hydrate is irritating to the skin and mucous membranes. Nausea and vomiting and, rarely, gastric necrosis occur secondary to gastric irritation. Other clinical manifestations include bullous skin lesions, pinpoint pupils, and hepatic damage with icterus. Transient cardiac arrythmias have also been reported.

2. Diagnosis

The diagnosis of acute chloral hydrate poisoning is made from the history, clinical features, and laboratory confirmation of chloral hydrate metabolites.

3. Treatment

The treatment for acute chloral hydrate poisoning is the same as for acute barbiturate intoxication.

C. Paraldehyde Intoxication

Paraldehyde has been used in medicine for treatment of abstinence phenomena, convulsive disorders, and as a hypnotic since the 1880s. Despite its long use, little is known of its pharmacology, metabolic fate, or toxicology. It is a rapidly acting hypnotic, inducing sleep usually within 10–15 minutes after an oral dose. The unpleasant odor and taste of paraldehyde are probably responsible for the low rate of use.

1. Clinical Features

Acute poisoning with paraldehyde typically produces a confused, nauseated patient with the odor of paraldehyde on the breath. In addition there is rapid, labored breathing which is believed to be caused by the effects of paraldehyde itself or its breakdown products on the lung, or the acidosis that accompanies paraldehyde intoxication. Respiratory depression, cardiovascular irritability, azotemia, oliguria, albuminuria, and leukocytosis also have been reported.

2. Diagnosis

The diagnosis of paraldehyde intoxication is based on the history, clinical features, and the odor of paraldehyde on the breath. Laboratory confirmation may be helpful; blood levels of 500 μg./ml. have been reported to be fatal.

3. Treatment

The treatment of acute paraldehyde intoxication is the same as for acute barbiturate intoxication.

D. Glutethimide Intoxication

Glutethimide was introduced in 1954 as a hypnotic drug. Within a year, it became the sixth most prescribed hypnotic because it was promoted as non-addicting.

1. Clinical Features

The signs and symptoms of acute glutethimide poisoning resemble those of acute barbiturate poisoning. Respiratory depression is usually less marked than in barbiturate intoxication; however, cardiovascular depression is often more severe. Glutethimide possesses anticholinergic activity, causing xerostomia, paralytic ileus, atony of the bladder, and long-lasting mydriasis. Spasms, twitchings, and seizure activity also may occur.

Patients intoxicated with glutethimide may exhibit cyclic episodes of wakefulness and coma. This is attributed to the enterohepatic recycling of glutethimide. Plasma half-lives have been noted to be as long as 105 hours in acute intoxication, with an average of approximately 40 hours. In addition, an active metabolite (4-OH-glutethimide) has been reported to contribute to toxicity.

2. Diagnosis

The diagnosis of acute glutethimide intoxication is based on the history, clinical features, including anticholinergic effects, and laboratory confirmation.

3. Treatment

The treatment of acute glutethimide intoxication is the same as that for acute barbiturate poisoning.

E. ETHCHLORVYNOL INTOXICATION

Ethchlorvynol has been available for use as a hypnotic drug since 1955. It, too, has been widely used for the same reasons as glutethimide.

1. Clinical Features

Acute intoxication with ethchlorvynol resembles barbiturate poisoning and is characterized by prolonged deep coma, respiratory depression, hypotension, bradycardia, and hypothermia. Other clinical features associated with ethchlorvynol poisoning include peripheral neuropathy and pancytopenia. Pulmonary edema occurs rarely and is believed to be due to capillary damage.

2. Diagnosis

The diagnosis of ethchlorvynol intoxication is based on the history, signs and symptoms, and laboratory confirmation.

3. Treatment

The treatment of acute ethchlorvynol intoxication is the same as for acute barbiturate intoxication.

F. METHYPRYLON INTOXICATION

Methyprylon has also been marketed since 1955.

1. Clinical Features

The clinical features of acute methyprylon and barbiturate toxicity are similar. Hypotension and shock are usually more of a problem than respiratory depression.

2. Diagnosis

The diagnosis of acute methyprylon intoxication is based on the history, clinical features, and laboratory confirmation.

3. Treatment

The treatment of acute methyprylon intoxication is the same as for acute barbiturate poisoning.

G. METHAQUALONE INTOXICATION

In recent years, methaqualone has become a major drug of abuse. It was introduced to the United States in 1965 and promoted as a safe and nonaddicting sedative–hypnotic.

1. Clinical Features

Usual hypnotic doses often produce a sensual and somewhat euphoric state. The body may develop a tingling sensation and then become extremely relaxed. Inhibitions disappear. A feeling of intimacy develops, and some claim an aphrodisiac effect from methaqualone. This has led to the increased use and abuse of methaqualone.

The hypnotic action of methaqualone resembles that of barbiturates. The sensual manifestations, however, suggest a different mechanism. Mild toxic effects of methaqualone include headache, hangover, torpor, restlessness, anxiety, dry mouth, foul-smelling perspiration, blurred vision, and unsteady gait. Central nervous system depression parallels amount of drug ingested.

With moderate to severe intoxication, muscular hypertonicity, hyperreflexia, and myoclonia often develop. These signs may be prominent enough to be of diagnostic value. Unlike other hypnotics, cardiovascular and respiratory depression is usually not severe with methaqualone intoxication. Bleeding tendencies from thrombocytopenia and prolonged prothrombin times and excessive salivation may also occur.

2. Diagnosis

The diagnosis of acute methaqualone intoxication is based on the clinical features, history, and laboratory confirmation.

3. Treatment

The treatment of acute methaqualone intoxication is supportive as for the other hypnotics.

H. FLURAZEPAM INTOXICATION

Flurazepam, introduced for use as a hypnotic in 1970, has become the most widely prescribed hypnotic drug in the United States.

1. Clinical Features

Flurazepam belongs to the benzodiazepine class of antianxiety agents. Adverse reactions include hangover and motor and intellectual function impairment. Headache, dry mouth, bitter or metallic taste, and swelling of the tongue have also been reported.

Severe toxicity usually does not develop from flurazepam alone. However, when used in combination with other central nervous system depressants, a serious clinical problem may result due to synergism.

2. Diagnosis

The diagnosis of flurazepam intoxication is based on the history, clinical features, and laboratory confirmation.

3. Treatment

The treatment of acute flurazepam intoxication is supportive. If mixed drug in-

gestion has occurred, it may be helpful to hasten the excretion of the other drugs, if possible.

III. CHRONIC INTOXICATION

Most of the hypnotic drugs are both psychologically and physically addicting. Chronic intoxication with hypnotic drugs resembles chronic alcoholism with respect to addiction, tolerance, and especially the withdrawal syndrome.

A. CLINICAL FEATURES

They are similar to mild acute barbiturate poisoning. Mental acuity is diminished; dress and personal habits become untidy. Neurological signs are also present.

B. DIAGNOSIS

The diagnosis of chronic hypnotic intoxication is based on history, clinical features, and laboratory confirmation.

C. TREATMENT

Treatment of chronic intoxication (i.e., detoxification) is primarily concerned with the withdrawal syndrome and should be carried out in a hospital.

BIBLIOGRAPHY

Almeyda, J., and Levantine, A.: Cutaneous reactions to barbiturates, chloral hydrate and its derivatives. Br. J. Dermatol., *86:*313–316, 1972.

Greenblatt, D. J., Allen, M. D., Noel, B. J., and Shader, R. I.: Acute overdosage with benzodiazepine derivatives. Clin. Pharmacol. Ther. *21:*497–514, 1977.

Hansen, A. R., Kennedy, K. A., Ambre, J. J., and Fisher, L. J.: Glutethimide poisoning: a metabolite contributes to morbidity and mortality. N. Engl. J. Med., *292:*250–252, 1975.

Maher, J. F.: Determinants of serum half-life of gluthethimide in intoxicated patients. J. Pharmacol. Exp. Ther., *174:*450–455, 1970.

Mandy, S., and Ackerman, A. B.: Characteristic traumatic skin lesions in drug-induced coma. J.A.M.A., *213:*253–256, 1970.

Matthew, H., and Lawson, A. A. H.: Acute barbiturate poisoning: a review of two years experience. Q. J. Med., *35:*539–552, 1966.

Moeschlin, S.: Clinical features of acute barbiturate poisoning. *In* Matthew, H. (ed.): Acute Barbiturate Poisoning: pp. 117–128. Amsterdam, Exerpta Medica, 1971.

Pleasure, J. R., and Blackburn, M. G.: Neonatal bromide intoxication: prenatal ingestion of a large quantity of bromides with transplacental accumulation in the fetus. Pediatrics, *55:*503–506, 1975.

Reidt, W. U.: Fatal poisoning with methaprylon (Noludar): a nonbarbiturate sedative. N. Engl. J. Med., *255:*231–232, 1956.

Teehan, B. P., Maher, J. F., Carey, J. J. H., Flynn, P. D., and Schreiner, G. E.: Acute ethchlorvynol (Placidyl) intoxication. Ann. Intern. Med., *72:*875–882, 1970.

4. ANALGESICS AND ANTIPYRETICS

E. Don Nelson, Pharm.D.

I. NARCOTIC ANALGESICS

Narcotic overdose usually is the result of a pediatric accidental ingestion, an overdose of street drug, or a medication error. Narcotic analgesics are metabolized in the liver and eliminated in the bile and urine. In the body, heroin is rapidly hydrolyzed to morphine. Thus, the laboratory may only detect morphine after an injection of heroin, and problems may be caused by factors other than the heroin itself, e.g., quinine used to "cut" the heroin, microorganisms in the street drug, particulate matter, other drugs taken along with the heroin, such as barbiturates, diazepam, or alcohol. Patients may be "dumped" at the emergency unit by friends or others who do not want to "get involved." The overdosed patient should be carefully examined for trauma and other effects from street first aid measures such as salt or milk injection and broken ribs from blows to the chest to increase respirations. The terminal event in most narcotic overdose deaths is respiratory depression. However, many addicts collapse immediately after injecting street heroin. It is speculated that the terminal event in these cases has an allergic, idiosyncratic, or vasovagal etiology because of the nature and rapidity of onset of symptoms. A drug abuse history may be invaluable if it can be obtained.

A. Clinical Features

Symptoms include nausea and vomiting, dizziness, itching, and flush, especially with heroin or morphine (due to histamine release). Sleepiness, drowsiness, and respiratory distress are common.

Signs of narcotic overdose are varying degrees of coma, analgesia, sedation, lethargy, slow, shallow, or absent respirations (Fig. 4-1), convulsions, miosis with most narcotics, and rarely midriasis with meperidine. Pupil size is an unreliable index of the intensity of narcotic overdose. Another sign is being sedated but easily arousable (on the nod). Cyanosis, weak pulse, contraction of smooth muscles of the gastrointestinal tract (e.g., sphincter of Oddi), hyporeflexia, hyperpyrexia, hypotension, and pulmonary edema are also typical findings in narcotic overdose. Fresh needle marks on any part of the body with central nervous system (CNS) depression are suggestive of narcotic overdose. A response toward normal to I.V. naloxone (Narcan) is diagnostic.

B. Laboratory

Blood, urine and gastric contents are useful in identification of the specific narcotic involved. Quinine may be detected in body fluids since it is frequently used to "cut" street heroin.

C. Treatment

Establish and maintain a patent airway. Monitor arterial blood gases and maintain oxygen level consistent with good tissue perfusion. An intravenous line should be inserted and kept open to administer naloxone and fluids. Give naloxone (Narcan), 0.01 mg./kg. I.V. Repeat in 5 minutes if no response. Large doses (up to 40 mg.) may be necessary if a large narcotic overdose has been taken. Naloxone is a competitive antagonist with almost no agonist (narcoticlike) activity of its own. Since the narcotic (Table 4-1) will usually last longer (4–48 hours) than the antagonist (0.5–2 hours), repeated doses or an I.V. naloxone drip may be necessary. Do not release any seriously narcotic overdosed patient as soon as he wakes up following a dose of naloxone because the action of naloxone is short-lived. Remove swallowed drug via lavage or emesis if level of consciousness permits. It may be useful to leave charcoal in the stomach after lavage to absorb remaining ingested narcotic. Pulmonary edema usually resolves with the injection of naloxone. If it does not, further measures are indicated, including the administration of furosemide (Lasix) I.V. The administration of naloxone may precipitate narcotic withdrawal in a narcotic addict. This can be prevented by using a naloxone drip to titrate the level of intoxication.

II. NONNARCOTIC ANALGESICS

Salicylates are used more frequently in overdoses than any other group of minor analgesics. However, recently, changes in patterns of use have resulted in a higher percentage of overdoses with other minor analgesics, e.g., acetaminophen (Tylenol). The toxicity of the nonsteroidal anti-inflammatory drugs is similar but not identical to that of the salicylates (Table 4-2). The toxic manifestations of salicylate intoxication derive largely from two actions of the salicylates:

1. Uncoupling of oxidated phosphorylation with increased oxygen consumption, increased glucose consumption, increased production of lactate and pyruvate, production of ketone bodies, and other disturbances of carbohydrate metabolism
2. Direct stimulation of the respiratory center early in the intoxication, and depression of the center in late intoxication

The typical course of intoxication in patients up to 5 years of age is (0.5–4 hours) respiratory alkalosis followed by a metabolic acidosis in about 4 hours. This temporal relationship may or may not be present in a particular case. This clinical course is less frequent in adolescent and adult patients who may be alkalotic during their entire period of intoxication.

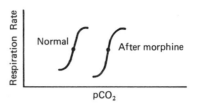

Fig. 4-1. Comparison of respiration rates before and after administration of morphine.

Acute minor analgesic intoxication is more life-threatening in pediatric than in older patients. The child up to age 5 is the one at greatest risk of suffering morbidity and mortality from minor analgesic intoxication, usually secondary to electrolyte and acid-base disturbances. Chronic poisoning is most likely to occur in the patient with a prolonged illness and nausea, vomiting, diarrhea, and fluid loss leading to dehydration. A high index of suspicion is required to make the diagnosis of chronic salicylism since the history of salicylate intake may be obscured by concern about the patient's primary illness(es). A serum salicylate level can be very helpful.

Table 4-1. **Drug Half-Lives at Therapeutic Doses**

Drug	Half-Life at Therapeutic Dose* (hours)
Morphine	2
Heroin	2
Meperidine (Demerol)	2–3
Codeine	2
Dihydrocodeinone (Hyrodan)	2–3
Oxycodone (Percodan)	2–3
Hydromorphone (Dilaudid)	2–3
Pentazocine (Talwin)	3
Propoxyphene (Darvon)	3
Butorphanol (Stadol)	2–4†
Methadone (Dolophine)	12+
LAAM (investigational)	24+

*Half-life in overdose is invariably longer, but exact times vary.
†Preliminary data suggests great variability.

Table 4-2. **Complications and Toxicity of Salicylate Therapy**

Plasma Salicylate Level		Toxicity
Intoxication	90 mg./100 ml.	Renal failure
	80 mg./100 ml.	Cardiovascular collapse
	70 mg./100 ml.	Anemia, hypoprothrombinemia fever, coma
	60 mg./100 ml.	Metabolic acidosis
	50 mg./100 ml.	Respiratory alkaosis, occasional tetany
	40 mg./100 ml.	Hyperventilation—first symptom of intoxication
Rheumatic Fever	30 mg./100 ml.	Irritability, psychosis
		Central nausea and vomiting, deafness, headaches, vertigo tinnitus (most frequent and reliable symptom of salicylism)
	20 mg./100 ml.	
Rheumatoid Arthritis		Peptic ulcer (reactivation not uncommon)
	10 mg./100 ml.	Gastrointestinal bleeding (frequent)
		Gastric intolerance (frequent)
Analgesic Range		Idiosyncrasy (rare, mostly in asthmatics)
	0	

A. SALICYLATE INTOXICATION

1. Clinical Features

Respiratory alkalosis (usually seen early in intoxication) produced by stimulation of the respiratory center. The body attempts to compensate for lost carbon dioxide by excreting bicarbonate in the urine. This period of intoxication is characterized by tachypnea, flushed face, nausea, vomiting, tinnitus, and occasionally central nervous system symptoms such as excitation and/or delirium.

A more serious and usually later phase of salicylate intoxication is metabolic acidosis. This is produced by the following combination of factors:

1. Previous renal elimination of bicarbonate during metabolic alkalosis
2. An anion gap produced by the presence of salicylate acid and other salicylate metabolites
3. Decreased renal excretion of sulfate, phosphate, and other acidic moieties
4. Production of acetoacetic and other ketone acids due to the metabolic derangement

Metabolic acidosis is frequently the terminal event in patients who die from salicylate intoxication.

Increased glucose utilization, in patients with inadequate hepatic glycogen stores, may lead to hypoglycemia. In large doses (see Table 4-2), salicylates interfere with the production of vitamin-K-dependent clotting factors by the liver, and, there may be hypoprothrombinemia and bleeding. Fluid imbalances and dehydration may lead to oliguria. A serum salicylate level can be diagnostic.

2. Treatment

Remove drug from the body (refer to Chap. 1). Since metabolic alkalosis is usually self-limiting, in most cases there is no need to treat the increase in respiratory rate. Metabolic acidosis should be treated with I.V. sodium bicarbonate. Glucose may be required to correct hypoglycemia. Serial electrolyte determinations are necessary to monitor and guide treatment of the fluid and electrolyte abnormalities. Administration of fluids should be carefully monitored in seriously poisoned patients with the placement of a CVP line.

Bleeding may be corrected by administration of whole blood, administration of vitamin K_1, or both.

Hyperthermia should be treated with physical means since drug interventions are not effective.

Blood levels of salicylate should be

Table 4-3. **Non-salicylate Minor Analgesics**

Drug	T ½ (hours)	Usual Therapeutic Dose per Day (gm.)
Fenoprofen	2 – 3	1.2 – 2.4
Ibuprofen	2 – 3	0.6 – 1.6
Naproxen	10 – 17	0.3 – 0.5
Tolmetin	1 – 3	0.6 – 1.8
Sulindac	6 – 8	0.1 – 0.2

*The active compound may be the sulfide metabolite, which has a T½ of about 16 hours at therapeutic doses.

followed during the clinical course. Therapy should be based on a combination of clinical manifestations and blood salicylate determinations.

Sodium salicylate and its metabolites can be removed from the body by osmotic, alkaline diuresis, peritoneal dialysis, or hemodialysis (refer to Chap. 1). Exchange transfusion may be necessary in pediatric patients who have taken life-threatening doses of salicylate.

III. ANTIINFLAMMATORY AGENTS

Relatively little is known about the acute toxicity of the other nonnarcotic, nonsalicylate, antiinflammatory analgesic compounds. These compounds include fenoprofen (Nalfon), ibuprofen (Motrin), naproxen (Naprosyn), tolmetin (Tolectin), and sulindac (Clinoral). The half-life at therapeutic doses of each of the agents is given in Table 4-3. For naproxen, the T½ at doses of 4 gm. per day does not seem to differ significantly from the T½ therapeutic doses.

A. CLINICAL FEATURES

These consist mainly of gastrointestinal irritation, skin rash, hematologic abnormalities (anemia, leukopenia), somnolence, dizziness, confusion, and insomnia.

B. TREATMENT

Remove drug from body (refer to Chap. 1). Relieve symptoms.

IV. ACETAMINOPHEN, PHENACETIN

The target organ of acetaminophen toxicity is the liver. Hepatotoxicity results from the transformation of acetaminophen into toxic metabolites that form covalent bonds with hepatic tissue. This process can be limited or prevented by the administration of methionine or N-acetylcystine, which act as a "chemical sink" for the toxic metabolites formed in the liver by the cytochrome P-450 mixed function oxidase system.

Phenacetin is usually encountered in a multiple drug intoxication. It most often occurs in combination with salicylates. Acute toxicity in these cases is related to the other drugs (e.g., salicylates).

A. CLINICAL FEATURES

Nausea and vomiting may follow the ingestion of large amounts of acetaminophen. Hepatic toxicity may not be evident until 12 – 24 hours after ingestion. It is dose dependent. Early clinical manifestations are not diagnostic or indicative of the severity of the intoxication. It is necessary, therefore, that blood levels of drug be known within 10 hours for appropriate treatment to be instituted. The efficacy of antidote administered more than 10 to 12 hours after ingestion of acetaminophen is questionable.

B. TREATMENT

Remove drug from body (refer to Chap. 1). Glutathione substitute drugs, such as methionine and N-acetylcysteine (Mucomyst), should be administered to patients who:

1. Have 4-hour postingestion blood levels above 300 µg/ml.
2. Have 4-hour postingestion blood levels of 150 µg/ml. to 300 µg/ml. and plasma acetaminophen half-lives of greater than 4 hours as determined by serial blood levels

Figure 4-2 relates hepatic toxicity to plas-

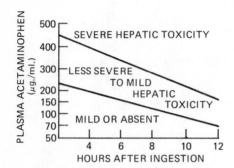

Fig. 4-2. Nomogram relating hepatic toxicity to plasma concentration of acetaminophen and time after drug ingestion.

ma acetaminophen level, and can be used as a guide to the treatment of acetaminophen toxicity with glutathione substitute agents according to severity.

Treatment should be instituted within 10 to 12 hours following ingestion of drug. The following regimen is recommended:

1. Methionine, 5 gm. P.O. every 4 hours repeated four times
2. N-acetylcystine (Mucomyst), 140 mg./kg. P.O. in an acidic soft drink, juice, or water as a loading dose; then 70 mg./kg. every 4 hours P.O. for 68 hours

V. PHENYLBUTAZONE, OXYPHENBUTAZONE

The toxicity of these agents is similar to that of aspirin, but in addition there may be bone marrow suppression and renal toxicity.

A. CLINICAL FEATURES

Symptoms include nausea, vomiting, rapid breathing, flushed facies, tinnitus, and hearing loss. There may be gastrointestinal erosion, epigastric pain, hematemesis, proteinuria, hematuria, anuria,

and, in fatal cases, acute nephritis. Other signs include hepatitis with increased enzymes and bilirubin, lethargy, coma, convulsions, edema secondary to sodium retention, agranulocytosis, and aplastic anemia.

B. TREATMENT

Remove drug from body (refer to Chap. 1). Osmotic alkaline diuresis. Serum electrolytes should be closely monitored, especially potassium. The half-life of phenylbutazone and oxyphenbutazone at therapeutic doses is 50 to 100 hours; the half-life is longer in overdose.

VI. CINCOPHEN

A lethal dose is 5–30 gm.

A. CLINICAL FEATURES

Nausea and vomiting, epigastric pain, loss of appetite, diarrhea. Heart failure late in intoxication, and toxic hepatitis.

B. TREATMENT

Emesis or lavage followed by activated charcoal.

BIBLIOGRAPHY

Bates, T.: Phenylbutazone. *Pediatrics, 17:*967, 1956.
Bender, J. K.: Salicylate intoxication. *Drug Intell. Clin. Pharmacol., 9*(7):350, 1975.
Brem, J. and Miller, T. B.: Salicylates in spinal fluid. *N. Engl. J. Med., 298:*744, March, 1978.
Done, A. K.: Salicylate intoxication: significance of measurements of salicylates in blood in cases of acute ingestion. *Pediatrics 26:*800, 1960.
Hill, J. B.: Salicylate intoxication. *N. Engl. J. Med., 288:*1110, 1973.
Peterson, R. G., and Rumack, B. H.: Treating acute acetaminophen poisoning with acetylcysteine. *J.A.M.A., 237:*2406, 1977.
Prescott, L. F., Sutherland, G. R., Park, J., et al.: Cysteamine, methionine, and penicillamine in the treatment of paracetamol poisoning. Lancet, 2:109, 1976.
Temple, A. R., et al.: Salicylate poisoning complicated by fluid retention. *Clin. Toxicol., 9:*61, 1976.

5. ANTIDEPRESSANTS

Richard Levy, M.D.

I. TRICYCLIC ANTIDEPRESSANTS

The tricyclic antidepressant (TCA) drugs have become the most widely used medications for the treatment of depression. Imipramine (Tofranil), desipramine (Norpramin), amitriptyline (Elavil), protriptyline (Vivactil), nortriptyline (Aventyl), and doxepin (Sinequan) are common examples of TCAs. Because of their wide availability and generous use of prescriptions for depressed patients, these drugs are frequently employed in suicide attempts.

The efficacy of TCAs in depression was established during the 1960s and 1970s. A biogenic amine theory of depression gained increasing acceptance, although definitive evidence is still lacking. According to this hypothesis, norepinephrine and serotonin are related to depression. Mammalian neurons are separated by a synaptic cleft into which these neurotransmitters are released. TCAs are presumed to block the reuptake of neurotransmitters at the presynaptic terminal. If depression is the result of norepinephrine and serotonin deficiency, the increased concentration of neurotransmitters available at the postsynaptic terminal might account for TCAs' therapeutic effect.

When taken as recommended, TCAs become effective in two to three weeks. Prior to that, the patient feels sleepy, anxious, and more unhappy. Since depression can be accentuated during this initial period, the drug must be given with extreme caution. Nonlethal amounts should be prescribed during this critical time.

TCAs are well absorbed from the gastrointestinal tract resulting in a rapid onset of action. Most of the parent compound and active metabolites of TCAs are quickly bound to plasma and tissue proteins. Only a small amount remains unbound in the plasma. Demethylation, hydroxylation, and oxidation of the central ring are the major pathways of metabolism. Enterohepatic recirculation and gastric secretion occur. Most of the metabolites are excreted in the urine within 72 hours. The ingestion of 10–20 mg./kg. of body weight is usually toxic, and 30–40 mg./kg. can be fatal.

A. CLINICAL FEATURES

1. Mild Intoxications

Systemic anticholinergic actions of TCAs may occur when taken in therapeutic amounts. Significant effects include blurred vision, dry mucous membranes, tachycardia, constipation, and urinary retention. Less common side effects are mania, convulsions, tremors, hypotension, cholestatic jaundice, bone marrow depression, peripheral neuropathy, and cardiac dysrhythmias.

2. Severe Intoxications

In addition to the central and peripheral anticholinergic signs already described, severe poisonings may cause hypertension, ataxia, dysarthria, myoclonus, hyperreflexia, extrapyramidal rigidity, coma, mydriasis, respiratory depression, and hyperpyrexia. Cardiac dysrhythmias are the most likely cause of death even in the treated overdose patient. Several pathophysiologic mechanisms are responsible for the atrial, nodal, and ventricular disturbances. Tachycardia is an anticholinergic effect. The enhanced adrenergic stimulation of the myocardium and direct toxic effects of TCAs on the myocardium contribute to the development of dysrhythmias. Acidotic patients have a greater fraction of unbound drug and are therefore at greater risk. Potentially fatal dysrhythmias such as ventricular fibrillation usually occur within 12 hours of ingestion, although they have been reported to occur days after other signs and symptoms have disappeared.

B. TREATMENT

Initial treatment of acute poisonings depends on whether the patient is alert or comatose. If the patient is alert, emesis should be induced with 30 ml. of syrup of ipecac. If the patient is comatose, adequate ventilation must be provided immediately and may require endotracheal intubation. Once a patent airway has been assured, the patient is connected to an electrocardiographic monitor. An intravenous catheter is inserted for fluid administration. Arterial blood gases should be measured. Blood and urine specimens are collected for serum electrolyte and toxicological analyses. Gastrointestinal evacuation of the drug is accomplished as promptly as possible through a large-bore (#30–36 French Ewald) gastric tube passed orally or nasally, and the stomach lavaged with 100–200 ml. aliquots of tap water until the aspirate is clear. The aspirate should be saved for toxicological analysis. To bind drug remaining in the stomach, administer a slurry of 30 gm. activated charcoal. To accelerate elimination of any remaining drug in the gastrointestinal tract, a cathartic such as 30 gm. sodium sulfate should be administered. The insertion of a small-bore nasogastric tube, passed with gentle continuous suction, will remove TCAs and their metabolites which are secreted back into the stomach.

Physostigmine, a reversible cholinesterase inhibitor that crosses the blood-brain barrier, is useful in some TCA poisonings. When peripheral and/or central anticholinergic signs are suggestive of a TCA poisoning but historical evidence is missing, a diagnostic trial of physostigmine is warranted. Physostigmine can also be helpful in those patients too drowsy to be given syrup of ipecac but too awake to lavage with an endotracheal tube in place. In these patients, physostigmine can temporarily improve the level of consciousness so that emesis can be induced. If physostigmine is to be given, it should be diluted 2 mg. in 10 ml. and administered intravenously over a minimum of two minutes. Physostigmine may produce bradycardia, seizures, and bronchoconstriction. Consequently, it should be used cautiously.

Supportive care is essential for the effective treatment of TCA poisonings. Few patients succumb when good intensive care is provided. Hypotension may occur and is treated with intravenous fluids. The use of vasopressors should be avoided because of the possibility of producing arrythmias secondary to drug-induced myocardial sensitivity. Treat seizure activity with diazepam (Valium) or a short-acting barbiturate. Dilantin should be avoided because it may compromise myocardial function. Cardiac dysrhythmias are difficult to treat after TCA ingestion since the response to drugs varies with the etiology. For example, physostigmine may be effective if the dysrhythmia is due to anticholinergic vagal blockade. If the dysrhythmia is due to the direct myocardial effect of the TCA, sodium bicarbonate, potassium, lidocaine, or propranolol may prove beneficial. Cardioversion and transvenous myocardial pacing should be employed if drug therapy does not appear to be effective.

Hospitalization is not necessary for every patient taking a TCA. Patients who are evacuated early and do not require intensive supportive care may be observed for a short time in the hospital emergency department. If after 10 hours of cardiac monitoring the patient does not exhibit any signs of myocardial intoxication, i.e., dysrhythmias or prolonged QRS complex, and remains alert, discharge may be considered. However, in intentional overdoses a psychiatric evaluation should be obtained before the patient is released from the emergency department.

II. MONAMINE OXIDASE INHIBITORS

Monamine oxidase inhibitors (MAOI) include such drugs as tranylcypromine (Parnate), isocarboxazid (Marplan), nialamide (Niamid), and phenelzine (Nardil). This group of drugs was introduced for treatment of depression in 1957. They are used infrequently at present because of their adverse effects and because of the availability of other, more effective drugs.

MAOI have been employed primarily to treat endogenous depression. Less often they have been used in the therapy of hypertension and angina pectoris. MAOI work by inactivation of MAO, resulting in an intracellular buildup of biogenic amines. Consequently, more amines are available at nerve endings, producing pharmacological effects.

A. CLINICAL FEATURES

Toxic effects may occur within hours and they may last for days. The most commonly seen adverse effects are anticholinergic and include blurred vision, dry mucous membranes, constipation, and urinary retention. Orthostatic hypotension as well as paradoxical hypertensive crises following ingestion of tyramine-containing foods can be seen. Other toxic effects following overdose are anxiety, confusion, hallucinations, hyperreflexia, convulsions, and hyperpyrexia.

B. TREATMENT

Treatment of acute intoxications should be aimed at maintaining normal vital signs. The conservative approach of early evacuation of ingested drug coupled with supportive therapy is usually successful. If hypertensive crisis occurs it is best treated with an alpha-adrenergic-blocking agent such as phentolamine.

BIBLIOGRAPHY

Bickel, M. H.: Poisoning by tricyclic antidepressant drugs. J. Clin. Pharmacol., *11*:145–176, 1975.

Biggs, J. T.: Clinical pharmacology and toxicology of antidepressants. Hosp. Prac. *13*:79–84, 1978.

Byck, R.: Drugs and the treatment of psychiatric disorders. *In* Goodman, L. S., and Gilman, A. (eds.): The Pharmacological Basis of Therapeutics, pp. 174–179. New York, Macmillan, 1975.

Gard, H., Knapp, D., Walle, T., Gaffney, T., and Hanenson, I.: Qualitative and quantitative studies on the disposition of amitriptyline and other tricyclic antidepressant drugs in man as it relates to the management of the overdosed patient. Clin. Toxicol., *6*:571–584, 1973.

Schildkraut, J. T.: The catecholamine hypothesis of affective disorders: a review of supporting evidence. Am. J. Psychiatry, *122*:509–522, 1965.

Walker, W. E., Levy, R. C., and Hanenson, I. B.: Physostigmine: its use and abuse. Journal of American College of Emergency Physicians, *5*:436–439, 1976.

6. STIMULANTS

Robert Yokel, Ph.D.

The compounds discussed in this chapter produce similar toxicities in that they are all stimulants of the central nervous system. Toxicity results in increased levels of mental and physical activity. Cocaine is discussed separately from the amphetamine-type compounds because of its rapid action and route of administration.

I. AMPHETAMINE AND RELATED DRUGS

This section includes many drugs that are qualitatively but not quantitatively similar in their actions and toxicity. The main difference is related to their central versus peripheral toxicity. The drugs are amphetamine and its optical isomers, methamphetamine, phenmetrazine, methylphenidate, diethylpropion, phentermine, clortermine, pemoline, mazindol, propylhexedrine, phenylpropanolomine, ephedrine, and pipradol. Because there have been more poisonings with amphetamines, more is known about amphetamine toxicity than the other compounds. Discussion will focus on amphetamine as the prototype.

Although toxicity has been seen with therapeutic doses, these drugs have a fairly broad margin of safety between therapeutic (10–15 mg. amphetamine per day in adults) and lethal doses (single doses of over 100 mg. amphetamine in adults). The major toxic signs are due to sympathomimetic effects on the cardiovascular and central nervous systems and a schizophreniclike paranoid psychosis. The most life-threatening signs are hypertension, hyperthermia, convulsions, and cardiovascular collapse.

Some basic principles are as follows:

1. The repeated use of amphetamines results in considerable tolerance to most of its effects.
2. Toxicity is 50 times more likely with intravenous than oral use.
3. These drugs are used nonmedically to remain alert, to enhance performance, as euphoriants, to prevent the lethargy and depression resulting from their withdrawal, to reverse the depression of barbiturates and alcohol, and to get "high."
4. The drugs are administered and abused by nearly all routes: intravenous, inhalation of powder or smoke, and intranasal.

A. ACUTE INTOXICATION

1. Clinical Features and Diagnosis

Due to tolerance, physical examination may be normal in drug abusers. Onset of action for routes other than intravenous is about 15 minutes, peak effects usually occurring in 30–60 minutes, with a duration of greater than 4 hours depending on the amount taken.

a. Mild Intoxication

(1) Cardiovascular System. Changes are commonly seen in intoxication and are the most life-threatening of the effects produced by these drugs. Both *d*- and *l*-amphetamine are equiactive and equitoxic on the cardiovascular system.

(a) Tachycardia is usually present. If over 150 it is most likely due to an amphetamine rather than another type of drug (e.g., anticholinergic). This may progress to reflex bradycardia.

(b) Palpitations may be experienced by the patient.

(c) Hypertension, systolic and diastolic, is usually present, particularly in early phases of intoxication. Headache may result.

(d) As a result of hypertension and hyperthermia, patient may be flushed.

(2) Central Nervous System. Toxic effects are commonly seen and more often produce management problems or threatening, irresponsible behavior rather than directly threaten the patient's life.

(a) Insomnia and increased activity are initially seen. This may progress to restlessness and tenseness.

(b) Children may demonstrate self-destructive behavior, blank staring, or purposeless movements. Adults may be agitated, demonstrating labile inappropriate affect (e.g., intense need for kindness and affection without the ability to demonstrate same), or suicidal-homicidal tendencies. Stereotyped obsessive-compulsive behavior (repetition of mechanical tasks) is seen particularly in chronic drug users.

(c) Hyperthermia may result from increased activity and as a direct effect of these drugs.

(d) Increased activity results in hyperreflexia, evidenced by hyperactive deep tendon reflexes.

(e) Reactive dilated pupils are usually seen. Blurred vision may be experienced. These drugs increase intraocular pressure, even at therapeutic doses.

(f) Decreased pain sensation may result from the analgesic effects of these drugs.

(g) Toxicity is increased by sensory input stimulation from light, sound, heat, and the presence of other people.

(h) A psychoticlike state characterized by euphoria and paranoia followed by dysphoria and depression may develop, particularly after chronic use (see section on chronic intoxication). It can be differentially diagnosed from true paranoid schizophrenia by physical evidence or history of drug abuse, and by dissipation of the psychosis 1–2 days after termination of drug intake. Blood levels do not correlate with the degree of psychotic behavior. Be aware of potential for violence by such a stimulated, agitated patient.

(i) *d-* Amphetamine is more active and tonic than the *l-* isomer (2–3 times) on the central nervous system.

(3) Muscular System. Muscular dyskinesias and stereotyped movements are seen at therapeutic and higher doses. These may manifest in lip smacking, facial grimacing, abnormal head, jaw, or neck movements, or choreoathetoid head, arm, or leg movements. Some of these movements (especially jaw grinding) are controllable with conscious effort.

(a) Goose bumps may be present.

(b) Muscle and joint pain have been reported following high-dose intravenous use.

(4) Respiratory System. Pulmonary stimulation may result in rapid shallow breathing.

(5) Gastrointestinal System. May manifest as nausea, vomiting, diarrhea, and abdominal cramps. Some intoxicated persons have complained of a metallic taste in the mouth. Gastric emptying time is delayed, and gastrointestinal motility is decreased.

(6) Genitourinary System. Urinary retention with pain and difficulty in micturition may result from contraction of the urinary bladder sphincter. Uterine tone may be increased.

(7) Hypersensitivity (urticaria, atopic and nonspecific dermatitis) is uncommon.

b. Moderate Intoxication

(1) Cardiovascular System. Signs and symptoms seen in mild intoxication may have progressed to:

(a) Pallor or cyanosis with chills

(b) Anginal chest pain

(c) Hypotension may develop after the peak hypertensive effects and lead to circulatory collapse.

(2) Central Nervous System

(a) A psychotic state, as mentioned above, may be present. Additionally, the patient may be confused and delirious, symptoms not usually seen in simple amphetamine-induced psychosis.

(b) The dilated pupils may now respond only sluggishly to light.

(c) The patient may be ataxic and demonstrate nystagmus.

(d) Tremors and clonic jerks in all extremities can occur and progress to convulsions.

(e) Profuse sweating

c. Severe (Life-Threatening) Intoxication

(1) Cardiovascular System

(a) Acute hypertensive crisis with cerebrovascular hemorrhage and death

(b) Ventricular fibrillation

(c) Chest (anginal) pains after large intravenous doses

(2) Central Nervous System

(a) Convulsions, leading to circulatory collapse, respiratory failure, coma, and death.

(b) Dilated nonreactive pupils.

(c) Temperatures above 43°C (109°F) which are usually lethal.

(3) Pulmonary System

(a) Aspiration of vomitus and asphyxia are common, serious complications.

(b) Embolic pneumonia, as well as pneumonia from intravenous drug use, may occur.

(4) Systemic Acidosis

2. Dose-Effect Relationships

a. Low therapeutic doses may produce severe idiosyncratic reactions.

b. Above 20 mg. is potentially lethal to a child.

c. Tolerant persons can survive a much larger single dose. In nontolerant persons, the lethal dose is probably less than 3 mg./kg. orally, and 1 mg./kg. intravenously.

3. Useful Laboratory Tests

a. Blood glucose. Hypoglycemia may develop in moderate intoxication.

b. Blood gases. Acidosis can occur in severe intoxication.

c. Urine analysis should demonstrate the presence of amphetamine as 40% is excreted unchanged at normal urine pH (60% in chronic amphetamine users). Amphetamine may be found in urine up to one week after drug discontinuation when large amounts are consumed. Routine hospital urine toxicological analysis for amphetamine will not detect presence of related drugs. Analysis of these drugs requires specific methods.

d. Blood amphetamine levels peak one to two hours after oral doses, and may range up to 0.1 μg./ml. with therapeutic doses. Toxicity is usually seen at higher levels in nontolerant persons.

4. Treatment

The use of antipsychotic drugs as antidotes is described below.

a. For a large dose oral ingestion within one hour in a conscious, nonconvulsing patient, induce vomiting or perform gastric lavage. This may retrieve tablet fragments due to the delaying effect of these drugs on gastric emptying time. (For emetics and procedures, see Chap. 1.)

b. Follow with a saline cathartic (e.g., sodium sulfate, 30 gm. in 250 ml. of water or juice for adults; 200 mg./kg. for children).

c. Blood pressure must be monitored and controlled. If elevated, give phentolamine, 5 mg. intramuscularly or intravenously. Be aware that the duration of phentolamine action is less than most of these drugs. If patient is in shock, treat as discussed in Chapter 1.

d. Temperature. Keep below 39°C (102°F) with ice baths, alcohol baths, or a hypothermic blanket. Chlorpromazine may decrease body temperature if patient is in a cool room, and it also inhibits shivering.

e. Convulsions should be controlled with intravenous diazepam, 5–20 mg. Repeat every 15–20 minutes as needed. Do not use barbiturates (see section on complications). Monitor respiratory status and blood pressure during such treatment.

f. Reduce sensory input by maintaining low, constant illumination, keeping manipulations of the patient to a minimum, and housing the patient in a cool, quiet environment. Reduce the patient's activity by restraints if necessary to protect patient and medical personnel, especially if the patient is in an agitated psychotic state. Otherwise avoid restraints. For children, use a padded crib or bed railings.

g. Osmotic diuresis (mannitol) with acidification of the urine increases amphetamine excretion. The usefulness of urinary acidification has not been assessed with stimulants other than amphetamines. They are weak bases with pKa's between 8.5 and 10.5 and are excreted more rapidly in acidic urine. The half-life of amphetamine at urine pH 7 is 20 hours, whereas the half-life is 12 hours at pH 6 and 5–6 hours at pH 5.

(1) Ammonium chloride, 1 gm. every 2 hours for 8 hours, then 1 gm. every 6 hours.

(2) Urine pH 5 is desirable but may not be obtainable if patient is hyperventilating enough to produce respiratory alkalosis.

h. Monitor electrolytes. Although profound disturbances are not usually seen, amphetamine does increase sodium loss. Electrolyte imbalance is more common in chronic drug abusers than in acute intoxication.

i. Sedation. Administer diazepam, 10–20 mg. orally or intravenously.

j. Dyskinesias (especially dystonic grimacing, ticlike movements of the mouth, tongue, and jaws). Administer diphenhydramine, 25 mg. orally or intramuscularly.

5. Antipsychotic Drugs as Antidotes

Consider dopamine-blocking antipsychotic agents as "antidotes" if amphetamine or similar stimulant is the only drug involved (see complications below concerning other drug involvement). The antipsychotics must be given before the end of the agitated phase of intoxication to be useful.

a. Dopamine-blocking antipsychotics

decrease the hypertension, hyperthermia, tachycardia, agitation and aggression, euphoria and psychosis, hypoglycemia, and perhaps the incidence of convulsions produced by the amphetamines. The antipsychotics may increase the depression that follows the stimulation phase of these drugs.

(1) Chlorpromazine, 0.5–1.0 mg./kg. intravenously or intramuscularly followed by 0.5 mg./kg. orally every 30 minutes until the patient responds.

(2) Haloperidol, 2.5–5 mg. intramuscularly. Repeat as needed. May be used instead of chlorpromazine.

(a) Haloperidol is less effective than chlorpromazine in reducing hypertension, but more effective on tachycardia.

(b) Haloperidol may be better than chlorpromazine in reducing the psychotic effects of the amphetamines.

(c) Haloperidol does not inhibit amphetamine metabolism as do high doses of chlorpromazine and thioridazine.

These drugs produce central nervous system effects within a few minutes, but sympathomimetic effects occur less rapidly (especially hypertension). Observe the patient because symptoms may recur hours after administration of the antipsychotic, and sedation of the antipsychotic may increase poststimulant sedation. Monitor for hypotension, decreased seizure threshold, and anticholinergic effects when antipsychotics are used.

6. Complications

a. Due to other drugs

(1) CNS depressants

(a) CNS depression is potentiated by the dopamine-blocking antipsychotic drugs.

(b) Amphetamine-barbiturate combinations are prescribed (and abused) to counteract some of each other's effects. In combined stimulant-barbiturate intoxication, the excitation phase usually precedes depression caused by the barbiturate. The hazard of barbiturate toxicity exists because of the large doses of barbiturate necessary to partially control amphetamine effects and the combined poststimulant and barbiturate depression. Barbiturates induce a drunken, emotionally labile state increasing stimulant behavioral toxicity (especially violence). Barbiturates have potentiated stimulant hypertension, and they do not reduce amphetamine psychosis. Use of neuroleptics in stimulant-depressant ingestions should be one-half of above suggested doses.

(2) Anticholinergics. The dopamine-blocking neuroleptics potentiate atropine-like intoxication.

(3) Tricyclic antidepressants may interfere with amphetamine metabolism to increase brain amphetamine levels.

(4) Chronic lithium therapy attenuates amphetamine euphoriant and CNS-stimulating effects.

(5) Dopamine-blocking antipsychotics may produce hypotension with amphetamine analogues such as STP, MDA, DMT.

(6) Monoamine oxidase inhibitors potentiate amphetamine pressor effects and toxicity.

(7) Marijuana has additive effects with amphetamine to increase heart rate and amphetamine stimulation.

(8) Less than 50% of drugs sold illicitly as amphetamine contain amphetamine as the only active drug; many also contain caffeine and ephedrine. These are sold as: uppers, speed, crystal, diet pills, pep pills, white crosses, and cross tops.

b. Hypertension may produce subdural and subarachnoid hemorrhage from aneurysms or arteriovenous malformations. Intracerebral bleeding, cerebrovascular thrombosis, and multiple microhemorrhages also occur.

c. Hyperthermia may produce coagulation defects and reversible renal failure.

d. Stroke syndromes have been reported as complications of acute intoxication.

e. Injection of impure substances using nonsterile techniques and equipment can lead to hepatitis (infectious, Type A; and serum, Type B), tetanus, endocarditis, cellulitis, and superficial abscesses at the site of injection. Intravenous injection of crushed tablets containing talc (e.g., methylphenidate) leads to talc deposition in the eyes, lungs, liver, and spleen (Richter, 1975; Jaffe and Koschmann, 1970).

f. Inadvertant intraarterial injection produces immediate severe burning pain and rapid blanching in the extremity distal to the injection. Thrombosis, vasospasm, and gangrene may result. Sympathetic ganglionic blockade, heparinization, continuous intermittent positive pressure limb compression (to 40–50 mm. Hg 30 of each 60 seconds) and surgical removal of thrombus and fasciotomy for tense extremity may be necessary.

7. Prognosis

a. Recovery is likely if the patient survives the first six hours.

b. Death is likely if temperatures exceed 43°C.

c. Aphasia or paralysis occur similar to that seen after cerebrovascular accident.

d. Hyperpyrexia and cardiovascular collapse usually precede death.

e. Death among regular amphetamine users is usually a complication of intravenous injection. There are less than 50 reports in the world literature of death directly attributed to amphetamines. Death from violent behavior, hepatitis, and trauma related to amphetamine is more frequent. Drug-related deaths are usually due to direct drug action in persons not regularly using stimulants in large amounts, or due to secondary complications resulting from the route of administrations in persons regularly using large amounts.

B. Chronic Intoxication

1. Clinical Features and Diagnosis

See above discussion of acute intoxication for discussion of many problems also present during chronic intoxication. Most of the toxicity of chronic intoxication is manifested by central nervous system signs and symptoms.

a. Central Nervous System

(1) Acute anxiety reaction

(2) Depression

(3) Social withdrawal and stereotyped or choreiform movements preceding psychosis.

(4) Psychosis is produced by all of the amphetamine-type stimulants. Rarely seen as a hypersensitivity reaction, it often occurs following intake of several hundred mg. per day for one to two days in previously nonpsychotic persons, and more often in prepsychotic persons.

(a) There is a large intersubject variability in the dose and the duration of stimulant intake necessary to produce psychosis. Psychosis occurs sooner with consecutive episodes of stimulant abuse until it ultimately develops following the initial dose.

(b) Development of psychosis is characterized by serial stages of euphoria (peaking about 15 minutes after I.V. injection and lasting up to 10–12 hours), depression and hypochondriasis (peaking at about 14 hours and lasting up to 50 hours), social withdrawal, personality disintegration, controllable paranoid ideation, then abrupt onset of florid psychosis.

(c) Amphetamine-type psychosis is characterized by extreme agitation, paranoid ideation, ideas of reference, auditory, visual, and tactile hallucinations (which may lead to attempts to remove parasites thought to be under the skin) but no significant intellectual disorganization. It is a direct result of drug toxicity rather than food or sleep deprivation. It is distinguished from true psychosis by the presence of a clear sensorium, dissipation within a few days of drug discontinuation, the predominance of auditory and visual hallucinations, and the presence of amphetamine or similar compound in the urine.

(d) These agitated psychotic patients represent the stereotyped "crazed drug addict" and can be physical management problems.

(5) Anorexia may result in malnourishment and extreme hunger when drug use is discontinued.

(6) Physical dependence and withdrawal are not significant. Some symptoms seen upon discontinuation of chronic drug intake include psychological depression and suicidal ideations (which may lead to continued drug use to treat same), marked fatigue, excessive eating, various body and muscle aches and pains, and abdominal pain and cramps.

(7) Psychological dependence may develop to all dosage regimens taken by all routes of administration. This is defined as frequent or excessive drug use with the compulsion to obtain and take the drugs. It results in a disruption of the normal behavioral routine when drug use is discontinued.

(8) Tolerance develops to the cardiovascular effects more rapidly than to the behavioral effects. Tolerance does develop to the acute lethal effects, such as anorexia and euphoria after one to two days of frequent large intravenous doses or after four to eight weeks of oral therapeutic doses. Tolerance dissipates within days of drug discontinuation.

b. Cardiovascular System

(Discussed above under complications)

c. Urogenital-Sexual

(1) Chronic drug use may increase menstrual flow, duration, and cramping.

(2) Effects on sex drive and function are inconsistent but produce increased libido more often than decreased, delayed ejaculation and orgasm, inhibited orgasm, and perhaps potentiate preexisting sexual tendencies (both inhibitions and overt perversity).

d. Other

(1) Pulmonary—pneumonia, emboli, and lung abscesses.

(2) Cutaneous signs may include dry

mucous membranes; foul breath; skin infections and ulcers; shiny, delicate skin which is slow to heal; and fragile, brittle nails.

(3) Muscle and joint pain following high intravenous doses.

(4) Jaw grinding may be observed during drug use, resulting in worn teeth. This can usually be stopped by conscious control.

(5) Rarely, one may see periods of drug use ("speed run") alternating with drug abstinence ("crashing"). During the speed run, high doses of drugs are used intravenously for their euphoric effects. The drug doses are rapidly increased during the run, and the person is extremely active and does not eat or sleep. During drug abstinence there is excessive sleeping and eating and usually depression.

2. Treatment

a. Treat as for acute intoxication, above.

b. Achieve drug-free environment, which may be difficult because of the psychological dependence and the depression and fatigue of drug withdrawal. This may require hospitalization to achieve lack of drug availability and use.

c. Sudden drug withdrawal should produce no physical harm to the patient, but gradual withdrawal will minimize ensuing depression with suicidal ideation.

d. Establish verbal contact to reassure patient and reduce potential for depression to overwhelm patient. Talk-down procedures are useful during psychotic episodes.

e. Consider up to three to four days of therapy with dopamine-blocking antipsychotics to manage the psychosis.

f. Consider phasing in tricyclic antidepressants as the neuroleptics are phased out. A one- to two-month course of therapy may be useful.

g. Bed rest for fatigue, exhaustion, with sleep p.r.n.

h. Correct existing nutritional deficiencies.

i. Begin treatment of personality problems, inadequate coping mechanisms, and drug misuse by beginning psycho, social, or group therapy (which may include "exspeed freaks"). Continued treatment of underlying emotional problems and restructuring of life-style is necessary to achieve drug-free behavior.

3. Prognosis

a. When drug is discontinued, psychosis and hallucinations usually abate in 1–2 days. Delusional thought processes, confusion, and memory loss decrease over 7–10 days. Apathy, irritation, and depression may peak in a few weeks and last up to 2–4 months. Recovery is usually complete. Persistence of paranoia beyond 3–4 days suggests the presence of organic paranoid schizophrenia.

b. Because of psychological dependence, a high percentage of patients relapse to previous pattern of drug use.

c. Withdrawal following chronic use can uncover underlying depression or precipitate a depressive state.

d. There is no evidence of permanent intellectual impairment.

4. Complications

a. Teratogenicity. The incidence of malformations is not different from the normal population for amphetamines, phenmetrazine, ephedrine, and diethylpropion. An elevated incidence has been seen with phenylephrine and phenylpropanolamine. Malformations reported as possibly resulting from amphetamine include congenital heart disease if exposure is in second month of pregnancy (more likely when there is a family history), biliary atresia, and urogenital system defects. Diaphragmatic hernia has been reported in offspring of mothers taking phenmetrazine.

b. Profound neonatal withdrawal does not occur although minor complications in offspring of chronic amphetamine abusers have been reported.

II. COCAINE

Cocaine is a rapidly acting drug. It is unlikely that a patient will be brought into treatment before peak drug effects have passed unless the cocaine was administered in a medical setting. Aside from its local anesthetic effects, the actions and toxicity of cocaine are very similar to the amphetamines. Cocaine is currently a much abused drug, being used mainly in social gatherings by those who can afford to purchase it.

A. ACUTE INTOXICATION

1. Clinical Features and Diagnosis

At low doses the effects are similar to those of amphetamine, but of shorter duration.

a. Systolic and diastolic hypertension and tachycardia are seen which are dose-dependent.

b. Central nervous system toxicity progresses from cortical stimulation (euphoria) to motor stimulation (increased activity) to lower brain center stimulation (convulsions).

c. Two sequences of events have been seen in fatalities. The more common is fainting, collapse, cyanotic cold skin, terminated by depressed circulation and respiration. The less common is delirium, followed by convulsions, tachycardia, rapid dyspneic respiration, and terminal respiratory arrest.

d. The drug is too short acting for any laboratory tests to be of diagnostic value in time to treat the patient. Diagnosis depends on known instance of cocaine use immediately prior to onset of intoxication although, if applied intranasally, some can be recovered from nasal passages up to three hours.

e. The drug is illicitly used most frequently by snorting (intranasal insufflation) but also by injection, inhalation of fumes, or by smoking, orally and topically. Snorting produces peak behaviorial effects in 3–5 minutes and peak blood levels in 10–15 minutes. Cocaine is well absorbed when taken orally.

2. Treatment (Requires Immediate Attention)

a. Support vital functions (see Chap. 1).

b. Prevent absorption. If oral, gastric lavage; if topically onto nasal mucosa, wash the nasal passages; if intramuscular or intravenous, apply ice to the site of injection. Empty the urinary bladder to prevent reabsorption from that site.

c. Monitor the body temperature and correct as for amphetamine.

d. Minimize sensory stimulation as for amphetamine.

e. Intravenous propranolol, 1 mg. per minute up to 6 mg., has been suggested for hypertension, tachycardia, and tachypnea, but it will not influence the nausea, vomiting, or euphoria.

f. For acute anxiety administer 10–40 mg. of oral diazepam.

3. Complications

a. Purchased cocaine frequently contains lidocaine or procaine.

b. The effects of norepinephrine, adrenergics, other psychostimulants, monoamine oxidase inhibitors, tricyclic antidepressants, reserpine, methyldopa, and dopamine are all potentiated by cocaine.

c. Cholinesterase inhibitors interfere with cocaine metabolism.

d. Several deaths have occurred during attempts to smuggle cocaine in condoms which were swallowed, then ruptured in the gut.

4. Prognosis

Recovery is likely if the patient survives one to two hours.

B. CHRONIC INTOXICATION

1. Clinical Features and Diagnosis

a. Psychological dependence may develop but physical dependence does not.

The tolerance to cocaine is not clinically significant.

b. Physical exhaustion and mental confusion secondary to insomnia may be present.

c. Rebound nasal congestion and chronic nosebleeds may develop. Nasal septal perforation is seldom, if ever, seen.

d. A paranoid psychosis, as discussed under amphetamine, is rarely seen.

2. Treatment

a. Benzodiazepines (1.5 times normal dose) for anxiety and nutrition for anemia; refer to amphetamines for depression. Nothing is required for the nasal congestion.

b. Follow-up psychiatric care as discussed under Amphetamine and Related Drugs.

III. STRYCHNINE

Strychnine is used primarily as a rodenticide but is also a component of certain tonics and cathartic tablets despite the lack of evidence of therapeutic efficacy.

The mechanism of action is an increase in the level of neuronal excitability by selectively blocking postsynaptic inhibition. It acts as a competitive antagonist of the inhibitory transmitter at postsynaptic sites. This produces excitation of many portions of the nervous system and, in larger doses, convulsions.

The predominant clinical effect is that of a tonic extensor convulsion pattern. Reduction of reciprocal inhibition of antagonistic muscles occurs and, therefore, the pattern of convulsion is determined by the most powerful muscle acting on a given joint.

A. Clinical Features

1. Central Nervous System

a. Mild. Stiffness of face and neck muscles.

b. Moderate. Coordinated extensor muscle thrust provoked by sensory stimuli, e.g., sound or movement.

c. Severe. Tetanic convulsions with hyperextension of the entire body (opisthotonus). Frequency and severity increased by sensory stimulation.

2. Respiratory System

Arrest due to contraction of the diaphragm, thoracic, and abdominal muscles. Death occurs secondary to hypoxia.

B. Treatment

1. Quiet environment.
2. Prevent absorption.

a. Emesis. This is generally impractical because the drug is absorbed rapidly within 15–20 minutes following ingestion.

b. Gastric lavage. Effective in removing residual drug in stomach when convulsions are controlled. To prevent aspiration secondary to coma or development of convulsions, lavage should be preceded by endotracheal intubation. Following lavage, activated charcoal and a cathartic, e.g., sodium sulfate, should be administered.

3. Convulsions. Diazepam, 10 mg. I.V. Repeat as needed.

4. Respiratory depression. Endotracheal intubation with mechanical support if ventilation not adequately maintained by control of convulsions.

5. Osmotic acid diuresis to promote urinary secretion of questionable value.

6. If the above therapeutic methods are unsuccessful, curarization may be used but this requires concomitant endotracheal intubation and mechanical ventilation.

IV. PSYCHOTOMIMETICS

A. Hallucinogens

The drugs in this group include LSD (lysergic acid diethylamide), psilocybin, mescaline, amphetamine derivatives (STP,

MDA, DOM), phencyclidine (PCP), harmine, ibogaine, and bufotenine.

1. Clinical Features

a. General

Nausea, vomiting, hypersensitivity to environmental stimuli, disorientation, anxiety, psychotic reactions, hallucinations, ataxia, hypertension (occasionally hypotension), hyperthermia, mydriasis, hyperreflexia, convulsions.

b. Specific

(1) LSD and PCP. Respiratory depression, coma, and death occur more frequently than with the other hallucinogens.

(2) PCP. Nystagmus commonly associated with hypertension, agitation, or coma. Also cerebellar dysfunction and potentiation of the effects of amphetamines, phenothiazines, and sedatives.

2. Treatment

a. General

(1) Place patient in a quiet environment to minimize sensory stimuli.

(2) Supportive. For respiratory depression, hyperpyrexia, etc. See Chapter 1.

(3) Convulsions. Administer diazepam orally or parenterally.

b. Specific (PCP)

(1) Gastric suctioning accompanied by osmotic diuresis and reduction in urinary pH $\leq$ 5 by oral or intravenous administration of ammonium chloride.

(2) To acidify through the gastric tube, deliver 2.75 mEq./kg. ammonium chloride in 60 ml. of saline solution every 6 hours until the desired urine pH is achieved. For parenteral acidification, administer 2.75 mEq./kg. of ammonium chloride as a 1–2% solution in saline intravenously with repeated monitoring of blood pH, blood gases, BUN, blood ammonia and electrolytes.

(3) To assist in removing remaining body stores of PCP, acidify urine for 10 days to 2 weeks with cranberry juice.

B. VOLATILES

These chemicals include a variety of solvents present in various glues, lacquers, enamel, brake fluids, lighter fluid, polish removers, paints, cleaning fluids, aerosols, and other agents.

All of the volatiles have a depressant effect on the central nervous system. They do not usually cause coma because of ease in titrating the dose used to get "high." However, coma may occur.

These substances usually enter the body by inhalation but may be absorbed through the skin.

1. Clinical Features

a. Euphoria, excitement, giddiness followed by central nervous system depression. The depression is characterized by confusion, lethargy, disorientation, bizarre behavior, delirium, and visual hallucinations. In addition there may also be photophobia, irritation of the eyes, diplopia, tinnitus, nausea, diarrhea, pains in the chest, head, and neck, cramps in the hands, muscular incoordination, slurred speech, blurred vision, nystagmus, seizures, tremors, paresthesias, and respiratory depression. Mucosal blisters may occur in the mouth and nose.

The most serious acute effect is the development of cardiac arrhythmias, e.g., ventricular fibrillation, which most frequently occurs from exposure to the fluorinated hydrocarbons. The characteristic pattern is inhalation of a solvent followed by a period of hyperactivity with subsequent collapse and death.

b. Hepatic, renal, and bone marrow function may be severely affected by the use of these agents. Complications generally develop 24 or more hours after use.

2. Treatment

Patients presenting in coma should be admitted immediately to an intensive care unit for prompt diagnosis and treatment of cardiac arrythmias.

C. CANNABIS (MARIJUANA)

The major active ingredient is delta-9-tetrahydrocannabinol. The psychoactive effects include euphoria and impairment of concentrating ability without interfering with retrieval of memorized information.

1. Clinical Features

a. Nausea, anxiety, paranoid ideation, disorientation, various perceptual alterations.

b. Following intravenous administration this drug has in rare cases led to gastrointeritis, hepatitis, renal failure, stupor, and death.

2. Treatment

Treatment is supportive (see Chap. 1).

BIBLIOGRAPHY

Baldessarini, R. J.: Pharmacology of amphetamines. Pediatrics, *49*:694, 1972.

Espelin, D. E., and Done, A. K.: Amphetamine poisoning. N. Engl. J. Med., *278*:1361, 1968.

Farber, S. J., and Huertas, V. E.: Intravenously injected marijuana syndrome. Arch. Intern. Med., *136*:337, 1976.

Haddad, L. M.: Management of hallucinogen abuse. Am. Fam. Physician, *14*:82, 1976.

Jaffe, R. B., and Koschmann, E. B.: Intravenous drug abuse: pulmonary, cardiac, and vascular complications. Am. J. Roentg. Radium Ther., *109*:107, 1970.

Klock, J. C., Boerner, U., and Becker, C. E.: Coma, hyperthermia, and bleeding associated with massive LSD overdose: a report of 8 cases. Clin. Toxicol., *8*:191, 1975.

Maron, B. J., Krupp, J. R., and Pune, B.: Strychnine poisoning successfully treated with diazepam. J. Pediatr., *78*:697, 1971.

Petersen, R. C., and Stillman, R. C. (eds.): Phencyclidine (PCP) Abuse: An Appraisal. National Institute on Drug Abuse Research Monograph 21, August 1978.

Richter, R. W.: Medical Aspects of Drug Abuse. Hagerstown, Md., Harper & Row, 1975.

7. AUTONOMIC DRUGS

Edward C. Conradi, M.D., and T. Douglas Cowart, Pharm.D.

Several pharmacological classes exert toxic effects that are mediated through their activity on the autonomic nervous system. In this chapter the discussion is mainly devoted to those drugs primarily classified as autonomic agents: antimuscarinic, parasympathomimetic, ganglionic stimulants and blockers, sympathomimetic and sympatholytic. The toxicity of ergot alkaloids, neuromuscular blocking drugs, and xanthines will also be included. Although antihistamines, antidepressants, antihypertensives, and stimulants also exert significant autonomic activity, their toxicity is reviewed in detail elsewhere in this book.

I. ANTIMUSCARINIC DRUGS

The antimuscarinic agents include the naturally occurring belladonna alkaloids and their synthetic structural analogs (Table 7-1). These atropinelike antimuscarinic agents are available as prescription and nonprescription products to treat parkinsonism, gastrointestinal hypermotility, the common cold, asthma, insomnia, and enuresis, and to produce mydriasis and cycloplegia. Other major uses of these drugs are as preanesthetic adjuncts and for bradyarrhythmias associated with various forms of heart disease. Plants of the Solanaceae family, indigenous to many parts of the United States, also contain atropine and scopolamine.

These drugs are competitive antagonists of acetylcholine at the postganglionic cholinergic receptor. The anticholinesterase drugs may reverse the competitive blockade produced by the antimuscarinics by inhibiting cholinesterase and increasing the concentration of acetylcholine at the synaptic cleft. Physostigmine crosses into the CNS and may antagonize both the central and peripheral effects of the antimuscarinics; however, neostigmine, itself a quaternary amine, is ineffective in reversing centrally mediated effects.

A. CLINICAL FEATURES

From 1970 through 1974, two-thirds of poisonings occurred in children under 5 years of age. Common sources of intoxication are opthalamic drugs (2 drops of 1% atropine contain approximately 1 mg. of atropine), proprietary sleep aids containing scopolamine, and inhalation of smoke containing asthamador. The fatal dose of atropine in adults is estimated to be 1 gm; however, doses of 10 mg. usually produce severe distress. In young children, fatalities are reported after as little as 10 mg. The ingestion of jimson weed, henbane, or deadly nightshade may be fatal since parts of these plants contain as much as 1% of the toxic alkaloid. The onset of symptoms may be quite rapid after ingestion. The peripheral manifestations of intoxication are mydriasis, decreased bowel sounds, urinary retention and urgency, tachycardia, hyperpyrexia, blurred vision, a dry and burning mouth, extreme thirst, difficulty in swallowing, photophobia, hypertension, and a dry skin with a red and flushed appearance. Central nervous system manifestations are: delirium, characterized by incoherent speech; fear and anxiety; and visual and auditory hallucinations, often with poorly coordinated movements of a grasping or picking nature. Central nervous system excitation is more common in young children and infants, and in severe cases, may lead to seizures and coma with respiratory depression and death. Intoxication with scopolamine often produces more CNS depression and less persistent peripheral effects than does atropine. During recov-

Table 7-1. **Characteristics of the Major Classes of Anticholinergic Drugs**

Class A: Naturally Occurring and Semisynthetic Derivatives
1. Action is primarily at muscarinic sites with no appreciable ganglionic or neuromuscular blocking activity
2. These drugs may readily cross into the CNS and produce stimulation or depression
3. Duration of action somewhat shorter than other classes
4. Well absorbed by the oral route
    Examples: atropine, scopolamine, homatropine

Class B: Synthetic Derivatives With Anticholinergic Activity
1. May produce varying degrees of ganglionic blockade
2. Variably absorbed after oral administration
3. Lower incidence of CNS related toxicity than other classes
4. May produce some degree of neuromuscular blockade, hampering respiration
5. Metabolic fate generally unknown
    Examples: propantheline bromide (Probanthine), anisotropine
    methylbromide (Valpin), glycopyrrolate (Robinul)

Class C: Synthetic Derivatives With Mixed Activity (Tertiary Amines)
1. May possess "antispasmodic activity" or a local anesthetic effect in addition to anticholinergic activity
2. May produce CNS toxicity as do the naturally occurring agents
    Examples: dicyclomine HCl (Bentyl), oxyphencyclimine HCl (Dactil), adiphenine HCl (Trasentine)

ery from intoxication, the symptoms usually dissipate within 24–32 hours, leaving the patient with a retrograde amnesia spanning the period of intoxication. Cycloplegia and mydriasis may persist in varying degrees for many days. (Table 7-2).

B. TREATMENT

For supportive therapy, refer to Chapter 1.

1. Assess respiration and review vital signs for tachycardia, arrhythmias, hyperpyrexia, and hypertension or hypotension. Consider catheterization if bladder distention is evident.

2. If signs of intoxication are severe, physostigmine salicylate (Antilirium) may be used in an effort to reverse central and peripheral signs of toxicity. Physostigmine may be hazardous in patients with asthma, coronary insufficiency, peptic ulcer, epilepsy, or obstruction of the G.I. or G.U. tract. In adults and teens an 0.5-mg. test dose may be given very slowly (3–5 minutes) intravenously or intramuscularly. This may be followed by a 1–2 mg. dose given in the same manner if there is no response to the initial dose. If there is no response within 10 minutes, a second dose of 1–2 mg. may be given, and repeated if life-threatening symptoms recur. Children may be given a 50-µg./kg. test dose and 0.5 mg. every 5 minutes until a response is obtained or a 2-mg. cumulative dose is reached. If life-threatening symptoms recur, the 0.5–1-mg. dose may be repeated. Subcutaneous injection is also an effective route of administration. The full onset of effect of physostigmine varies from 3–8 minutes by the various routes. The duration of the effect of one dose is variable between 30 and 60 minutes; therefore dosage may need to be repeated several times if there is still evidence of intoxication (effects seldom last more than 1 hour). Physostigmine may produe toxic parasympathomimetic effects if given in excessive dosage. This drug must be administered cautiously with continuous observation of the patient (atropine should be available).

3. If there is a question of the presence of antimuscarinic intoxication, a methacholine (Mecholyl) test may be helpful. The failure of a subcutaneous dose of 10–25 mg. for adults or 0.1–0.4 mg./kg. for children to elicit flushing, sweating, sali-

Table 7-2. **Anticholinergic Intoxication: Clinical Features**

Adults (71 cases)	Manifestation	Children (48 cases)
79%	Pupils widely dilated and poorly reactive	88%
55%	Flushed facies; dry mucous membranes	90%
44%	Tachycardia (greater than 100 per min.)	65%
66%	Incoherence, confusion, or disorientation	56%
39%	Restlessness, hyperactivity, or agitation	58%
52%	Auditory or visual hallucinations	27%
35%	Ataxia or motor incoordination	48%
37%	Picking, plucking, grasping, or gathering movements	44%
25%	Hyperreflexia, twitching, or increased muscle tone	35%
23%	Apprehension, fear, or paranoid ideation	14%
34%	Somnolence or coma	16%
14%	"Toxic delirium"	40%
18%	Giddiness, labile or inappropriate effect	13%
14%	Dysarthria or slurred speech	14%
18%	Fever greater than 100°F	25%
18%	Complaint of thirst or dry mouth	14%
20%	Complaint of blindness or blurred vision	13%
35%	Return to normal sensorium in 24 hours	40%
18%	Retrograde amnesia	13%

Infrequent manifestations (less than 10% of cases)

Seizures, convulsions, vomiting, rash, urinary retention, abdominal distress, paralytic ileus, constipation, abnormal CSF, leukocytosis, pyuria

(Shader, R I., and Greenblatt, D. J.: Belladonna alkaloids and synthetic anticholinergics: uses and toxicity. *In* Shader, R. I. (ed): Psychiatric Complications of Medical Drugs. New York, Raven Press, 1972)

vation, rhinorrhea, abdominal distress, and bradycardia indicates that an atropinelike substance is the source of intoxication. If these symptoms are elicited with methacholine, they will be of very short duration and may be reversed with atropine if necessary.

4. Phenothiazine analogs should never be used as sedatives since they have significant anticholinergic effects. Sedation, antianxiety, and anticonvulsant effects may be achieved with parenteral diazepam: 5–10 mg. for adults; 0.04–0.2 mg./kg. for children. Although the risk of respiratory depression and adverse cardiovascular effects are lower with diazepam than other agents, the patient must be watched carefully. Diazepam must be injected slowly if given by the I.V. route.

5. If marked hyperpyrexia has been present, there may be some liver damage. Clotting and liver functions should be monitored.

6. Hemodialysis or peritoneal dialysis are of questionable value in the removal of these drugs from the body.

7. Forced diuresis may be beneficial in speeding the elimination of atropine.

II. GANGLIONIC-STIMULATING DRUGS

Agents used to stimulate the autonomic ganglia are rarely used in medical practice today. Nicotine is the most important member of this group and the most toxic.

A. NICOTINE

This is an alkaloidal liquid in both free and salt forms and is found in pesticides and tobacco. The nicotine content of cigarettes and cigars varies from 6 to 40 mg., but smoke contains only about one-half of the total nicotine content, the rest being volatilized. The total absorption from smoking is normally only a few milligrams. After oral ingestion of tobacco, nicotine is slowly absorbed and usually causes nausea and emesis before a toxic dose can be absorbed; however, fatalities have been reported in children from intoxication with tobacco products. The lethal dose of nicotine in adults is 40–60 mg. (0.6–0.9 mg./kg.). Industrial intoxication with concentrated (40%) insecticides has been fatal. Nicotine is readily absorbed topically. Nicotine blood levels of 1 mg./100 ml. have been associated with fatalities.

1. Clinical Features

Symptoms appear rapidly after exposure and are secondary to an initial stimulation of autonomic ganglia, followed by a blockade of autonomic transmission and a noncompetitive neuromuscular blockade. Symptoms and signs consist of nausea, vomiting and G.I. burning sensation, salivation, severe abdominal pain, diarrhea, confusion, hypertension, and weakness. Early in the intoxication there may be an intense respiratory stimulation with deep rapid breathing. The breath may bear a tobaccolike odor from the alkaloid. Initially, bradycardia, miosis, and hypertension are usually noted due to intense cholinergic and adrenergic stimulation. Later in intoxication, tachycardia, mydriasis, and hypotension may develop due to ganglionic blockade. CNS excitation with tremors that may progress to convulsions is seen with severe overdoses. Late in the intoxication, paralysis of the respiratory muscles produces respiratory failure and death.

2. Treatment

Immediate emergency measures are imperative to avoid rapid absorption. Death may occur within 5 minutes.

a. Emesis should be induced, syrup of ipecac, 30 ml. P.O.

b. Lavage stomach with a solution of potassium permanganate, 1:10,000, to oxidize any remaining nicotine.

c. Activated charcoal should be given immediately after emesis and lavage.

d. Large doses of atropine are often required to control the symptoms of parasympathetic excitation (abdominal pain, salivation, and bradycardia).

e. Phenoxybenzamine (Regitine) may be used to control the symptoms of excessive sympathetic stimulation (hypertension).

f. If the contact was topical, the area should be washed with soap and water. Use gloves to avoid contact.

g. Respiratory assistance if necessary.

h. Diazepam is useful in controlling seizures. Adults: 5–10 mg., children: 0.04–0.3 mg./kg. Diazepam must be given slowly I.V.

i. The urine may be acidified to a pH of 5.5 or less to reduce reabsorption and hasten excretion of nicotine by the kidneys.

III. GANGLIONIC-BLOCKING DRUGS

The ganglionic-blocking drugs, mecamylamine hydrochloride (Inversine), pentolinium tartrate (Ansolysen), and trimethaphan camsylate (Arfonad), rarely present as toxicological agents. Overdosage with these agents effectively blocks autonomic transmission at the ganglia level.

A. Clinical Features

Intoxication characteristically produces hypotension with severe orthostasis and syncope and a mixture of anticholinergic and sympatholytic symptoms, the most prominent being mydriasis and difficulty in accommodation, dry mouth, inability to void and absence of bowel sounds. Mecamylamine is the only agent of the group capable of crossing into the CNS and may cause disturbing central effects such as confusion, delirium, tremors, or seizures.

With chronic use, delayed gastric emptying time may allow accumulation of several dosages in the stomach before release into the small bowel where rapid absorption may cause hypotension. Acute pneumonitis has occurred in patients taking hexamethonium and mecamylamine for long periods of time.

B. TREATMENT

1. If hypotension is severe the patient should be treated appropriately with volume expansion and sympathomimetic amines. Sympathomimetic agents should be used very cautiously in patients who have chronically ingested these agents since there may be a supersensitivity of the peripheral vasculature to catecholamines. Duration of action of the oral ganglionic-blocking drugs is 6–12 hours and acute toxicity should be of short duration. Trimethaphan toxicity is terminated by cessation of the infusion. Trimethaphan may cause histamine release and should not be used in asthmatics.

2. Efforts to reduce absorption of the drug from the G.I. tract may be important if there are depressed bowel sounds.

3. Excretion of mecamylamine is increased in acid urine.

IV. PARASYMPATHOMIMETIC AGENTS

Drugs in this class are used medicinally in the treatment of myasthenia gravis, glaucoma, atony of bladder and G.I. tract, and paroxysmal supraventricular tachycardia. Certain genera of mushrooms (*Inocybie* and *Amanita*) contain muscarine, which plays an important role in their toxicity. There are three classes of compounds with parasympathomimetic effect:

1. Agents directly stimulating acetylcholine receptors:
   a. Acetylcholine synthetic analogs (bethanecol; choline esters)
   b. Cholinomimetic alkaloids (pilocarpine)
2. Agents blocking acetylcholinesterase and allowing for an increase in acetylcholine at nicotinic and muscarinic sites:
   a. Reversible anticholinesterase inhibitors (physostigmine, edrophonium)
   b. Irreversible anticholinesterase inhibitors (phospholine and organophosphate insecticides)
3. Ganglionic stimulants (nicotine, lobeline)

The toxic effects depend on the specific class of parasympathomimetic drug. The choline esters (acetylcholine, methacholine, carbachol, and bethanechol) exert varying degrees of muscarinic and nicotinic effects. Bethanecol is almost void of nicotinic (ganglionic) effect.

The cholinomimetic alkaloids chiefly affect the muscarinic receptors; agents blocking the enzyme acetylcholinesterase (physostigmine, neostigmine) produce their effects at muscarinic receptors, autonomic ganglia, and at the neuromuscular junction.

The muscarinic action of these drugs can be blocked by atropine, the nicotinic action at autonomic ganglia by trimethaphan (Arfonad) and the stimulatory effects at the neuromuscular junction by competitive neuromuscular blockers like curare. The anticholinesterase agents may produce an initial stimulation of autonomic ganglia and CNS sites and then induce a subsequent depression of these sites; therefore, treatment with ganglionic and neuromuscular blockers is usually unnecessary.

A. CLINICAL FEATURES

Respiratory difficulty secondary to acute exposure is often the principal manifestation of toxicity. Copious secretions and poor ventilatory effort due to extreme muscular weakness may complicate the problem. The patient may present in pulmonary edema. Hyperactive bowel sounds with involuntary defecation and urination, miotic pupils, blurring of vision, bronchoconstriction, and bradycardia are common. Confusion, anxiety, tremor, and seizures may occur.

B. TREATMENT

For supportive therapy, refer to Chapter 1.

1. Atropine should be given to block the direct action of these agents or the indirect increase in acetylcholine. Large doses are often required. An initial injection of 1–2 mg. I.V. slowly for adults and 0.02–0.04 mg./kg. for children should be administered. In the severely poisoned patient, there may be only minimal effects. This dose should be repeated as often as necessary (every 3 to 10 minutes) to relieve symptoms and maintain a slight degree of atropinism. Atropine has no effect on the neuromuscular junction and does not reverse neuromuscular blockade. Patients should be carefully watched for a reversal of cholinergic symptoms and progression to anticholinergic symptoms if large doses of atropine are continued.

2. For severe poisoning due to one of the reversible anticholinesterase agents (neostigmine, physostigmine), administer pralidoxime (Protopam) I.V. in a dosage of 1–2 gm. at a rate of no more than 500 mg. per minute in adults or 25–50 mg./kg. in children. The rate should be no more than 250 mg. per minute. This may improve muscular strength. Effects at other autonomic sites are variable. There may be some benefit on the CNS manifestations of intoxication even though the drug poorly crosses into the CNS. The clinical efficacy of pralidoxime administration for nonorganophosphate anticholinesterase intoxications has been well established. If repeated injections of pralidoxime are necessary, continuous infusion of 0.25–0.5 gm. per hour in adults may give a more prolonged effect. Administration of pralidoxime to the myasthenic patient may return the patient from the cholinergic to the myasthenic state and severe myasthenic crisis.

3. Morphine, theophylline, and phenothiazines should not be given to the patient poisoned with an anticholinesterase in order to relieve signs of pulmonary edema.

4. It is unknown if dialysis (hemo- or peritoneal) is effective in removing anticholinesterase drugs.

5. Epinephrine may be useful in controlling bronchoconstriction and bradycardia.

6. The toxic effect with the choline esters and edrophonium is of short duration, whereas intoxication with neostigmine, pyridostigmine, and physostigmine may persist for several hours.

7. With continuous monitoring and respiratory care, the prognosis is good.

V. SYMPATHOMIMETIC AGENTS

These agents stimulate alpha, beta, beta$_2$, and dopaminergic receptors and produce characteristic toxicity depending on their general structure. Agents with alpha activity are most useful as vasoconstrictors; beta stimulants, as bronchodilators and cardiac stimulants. Beta receptor stimulants may be further divided into beta$_1$, with principally cardiac effects, and beta$_2$, with mostly bronchiolar effects. Their pharmacological effects are specifically blocked by alpha or beta blocking agents. Catecholamines are poorly absorbed after oral ingestion because they are metabolized in the gut. All of these agents are well absorbed after injection, inhalation, or application to mucous membranes.

A. CLINICAL FEATURES

These include nervousness and anxiety, tremulousness, mydriasis, headache, hypotonic bowel sounds, cardiac rhythm disturbances, hypertension, angina, and convulsions. Toxic effects of these drugs may be potentiated by monoamine oxidase inhibitors, halogenated hydrocarbon anesthetics, guanethidine, and reserpine. An acute syndrome of pulmonary edema which may progress to shock lung has been reported to occur with acute intoxication with both the catecholamine and noncatecholamine sympathomimetic agents. Chronic use may produce cardiovascular injury and psychic depression.

L-Dopa overdosage may present as nausea, vomiting, arrhythmias, and dyskinesia. Hypotension or hypertension may be present. Dopamine, a metabolite of L-dopa, is thought to be responsible for most of these pharmacological effects through stimulation of alpha, beta, or dopaminergic receptors. Emesis may result from dopamine's ability to stimulate central emetic centers.

Inadvertent overdosage with the predominately beta$_2$ stimulant drug, terbutaline, may produce significant toxic cardiac effects.

B. TREATMENT

1. Control hypertension with parenteral phentolamine methanesulfonate (Regitine) given slowly I.V. to carefully titrate the pressure down. Nitroprusside or diazoxide may also be used.
2. Tachycardia should be treated with propranolol, 0.025–0.10 mg./kg., given slowly at no greater than 1 mg. per minute (1–3 mg. usual initial adult dose). Propranolol may cause severe bronchospasm and should not be used in asthmatics.
3. If arrhythmias are persistent, lidocaine may be used as a bolus dose of approximately 1 mg./kg. followed by an intravenous drip of 1 to 4 mg./kg. per minute.
4. Chlorpromazine is useful in controlling psychotic behavior and moderate hypertension at a dose of 0.5–1 mg./kg. I.M. (Dilute 25 mg. to 1 mg./ml. for I.V. use and give at a rate of no greater than 1 mg. per minute.)

5. Tissue necrosis from intramuscular or subcutaneous administration of sympathomimetics may be prevented by local infiltration of phentolamine methanesulfonate (Regitine).
6. Seizures may be controlled with diazepam, 0.04–0.3 mg./kg. for children, and 5–10 mg. for adults, given slowly I.V. push.
7. Pyridoxine, 10–20 mg. I.M. or slow I.V., may significantly reduce dystonia in patients with parkinsonism within one hour; however, its effect on the cardiovascular toxicity of L-dopa is unknown.

VI. ALPHA AND BETA SYMPATHETIC BLOCKING DRUGS

A. ALPHA-BLOCKING DRUGS

These agents are principally used in the treatment of hypertensive disease, peripheral vascular disease, and pheochromocytoma. Rarely do they present as acute intoxicants. They act at the alpha receptor either competitively (phentolamine and tolazoline) or noncompetitively (phenoxybenzamine), and produce a blockade of the alpha receptor-mediated effects of sympathomimetics, resulting in a loss of vasomotor control.

1. Clinical Features

The principal effects seen with administration of these agents are hypotension and cardiac stimulation. The cardiac stimulation is largely reflex with phenoxybenzamine; however, with both tolazoline and phentolamine there are also direct sympathomimetic effects. These latter two agents also produce parasympathomimetic and histaminic effects that may be associated with their toxicity. Gastrointestinal stimulation, CNS stimulation, and nausea occur after large, rapidly administered parenteral doses of phenoxybenzamine, and tiredness and lethargy may accompany chronic intoxication.

2. Treatment

a. Do not use epinephrine to treat hypotension caused by these drugs; the vasodilatory effects of epinephrine will be potentiated by the alpha blockade. Alpha stimulants such as norepinephrine should be cautiously administered.

b. Toxic reactions to phentolamine and to tolazoline are of short duration and treatment is discontinuation of the drug and the maintenance of the supine position. Hypotensive reactions to dibenamine may take up to a week to completely clear.

c. The electrocardiogram should be monitored carefully in intoxication with phentolamine and tolazoline since cardiac arrhythmias and angina have been reported to occur with these agents.

B. BETA-BLOCKING DRUGS (PROPRANOLOL)

The principal use of these agents is in the management of hypertensive cardiovascular disease and angina. Drugs in this class all competitively block beta-adrenergic receptors producing a decrease in A-V conduction, bradycardia, negative inotropism, decrease in blood pressure, and inhibition of glycogenolysis in response to beta-adrenergic stimulation.

1. Clinical Features

Large overdoses of these drugs have been sustained by healthy individuals without mortality; however, even relatively small doses may produce serious cardiac decompensation in those patients with congestive heart failure or conduction abnormalities. Bronchospasm may be produced in asthmatics with therapeutic doses. The intravenous route of administration may be fatal in patients with these diseases. The patient with intrinsic heart disease may present in a hypotensive state with severe bradycardia or heart block and distended neck veins; pulmonary edema may be present secondary to the heart failure. Nightmares and hallucinations have been reported in patients on chronic therapy.

2. Treatment

a. Patients should be placed on a cardiac monitor. Blood pressure and blood sugar should be evaluated frequently.

b. Atropine may increase heart rate at a dose of 0.4–1 mg. I.V. for adults and 0.01 mg./kg. (maximum 0.4 mg./kg.) for children I.V.

Bradycardia also may be treated with I.V. administration of isoproterenol at an initial rate of 1–5 μg./kg. per minute in adults and children. Since there is competitive beta blockade, relatively large doses (30–40 μg./kg. per minute) may be needed. Blood pressure must be carefully monitored with isoproterenol (Isuprel) infusion since it may produce unacceptable vasodilation. Epinephrine may be a useful alternative if Isuprel is unsatisfactory in establishing improved circulatory dynamics.

c. Bronchospasm may be relieved with isoproterenol as outlined above, or with terbutaline, 0.25 mg. S.C. Oral inhalation of beta stimulants or I.V. aminophyllin may also be useful.

d. Glucagon may be effective for bradycardia and A-V conduction defects and produce a positive inotropic effect. It does not appear that the beta-receptor blocking drugs block the stimulatory action of glucagon on the heart. A 50-μg./kg. bolus dose may produce effects lasting approximately 15 minutes. Continuous infusion of glucagon may be helpful in prolonging any beneficial effect (1–5 mg. per hour in adults). Glucagon can produce nausea, which is treated with antiemetics. Hypokalemia and hypoglycemia may occur with prolonged use. Combined use of glucagon, aminophyllin, and isoproterenol may be useful in severe circulatory failure.

e. Abrupt withdrawal of propranolol may cause severe rebound phenomena in

Table 7-3. **A Summary of the Toxicity of Clinically Useful Ergot Preparations**

Drug	Toxicity
Ergotamine tartrate (Gynergen)	Highly active vasoconstrictor and adrenergic blocker useful in symptomatic treatment of migraine. Most common agent implicated in cases of ergotism. Poor efficacy as an oxytocic when given orally.
Ergonovine maleate (Ergotrate)	Highly efficacious as oxytocic.
Methylergonovine (Methergine)	Possess significant vasoconstrictive and vascular toxicity.
Methysergide maleate (Sansert)	Has produced retroperitoneal and cardiac fibrosis with prolonged use. Less potential for vasoconstriction and damage with short duration of therapy.
Dihydroergotamine mesylate (DHE-45)	Parenteral agent retaining significant vasoconstrictive activity after dihydrogenation.
Dihydrogenated amino acid alkaloids of ergot (Hydergine)	Almost negligible vasoconstrictor properties, but retains oxytocic activity.

patients with preexisting heart disease. After an overdose in these patients, therapy should be tapered over 1 week.

VII. ERGOT ALKALOIDS

Ergot is a product of the fungus, *Claviceps purpurea,* which grows principally on rye grain. Contaminated grain has produced severe intoxication and death for centuries. Modern inspection practices protect consumers from grains contaminated with this fungus, with the last serious outbreak reported in France in 1951.

Poisoning with the ergot alkaloids is usually associated with the chronic or acute administration of the antimigraine drugs, ergotrate or methysergide, or the postpartum oxytocics, ergonovine and methylergonovine.

Fatalities have occurred in infants after ingestion of 12 mg. of ergotamine tartrate. Toxic reactions have been reported with therapeutic doses suggesting a sensitivity to these drugs in some individuals. Therefore, children and adults ingesting small amounts of these agents either accidentally or intentionally should be carefully observed. Patients with hepatic disease, renal disease, or febrile illnesses may

be more susceptible to the toxic effects of ergot. The natural and amino acid alkaloids are much more toxic than the dihydrogenated derivatives (Hydergine), which possess very little vasoconstrictor activity. The actual incidence of ergot intoxication has been estimated at less than 0.01% of patients taking ergot preparations. Side effects such as nausea, vomiting, and abdominal or leg pain may occur in 10% of patients receiving ergot preparations by the oral route and as high as 20% of those receiving parenteral therapy.

There are three broad classes of ergot alkaloids. The prototypes of each of these classes are ergotamine, dihydroergotamine, and ergonovine. These agents, along with methysergide, are the ergot alkaloids commonly used in therapy. The pharmacologic effects of these agents are complex and consist of vasoconstriction, oxytocic activity, and alpha adrenergic blockade (Table 7-3). The vasoconstrictor and oxytocic effects are commonly responsible for the toxicity associated with these agents. Other common pharmacologic effects are an increase in blood pressure with bradycardia or tachycardia, a direct central emetic effect, diarrhea, and dizziness. In some patients disturbing side effects may include exacerbation or production of angina and paresthesias of the extremities, with weakness and muscle pains. Any of these symptoms call for reduction or discontinuation of ergot-containing medication. Rebound headaches for up to a week after discontinuation of the drug may occur.

Retroperitoneal, cardiac, and pulmonary fibrosis have been associated with chronic methysergide therapy.

Absorption of the ergot alkaloids is poor from the G.I. tract with the exception of the amine alkaloids. Sublingual administration may produce slightly greater pharmacological effects since the liver, a principal site of metabolism of ergot, is bypassed.

A. CLINICAL FEATURES

Signs and symptoms depend on the specific ergot preparation producing the intoxication, since ergot produces a broad range of pharmacological effects (see Table 7-3). Combination products are also commonly prescribed containing caffeine or a barbiturate that may play an important part in the overall clinical presentation.

Chronic intoxication, occurring over several weeks, often manifests itself as increasing numbness and tingling of the extremities, with or without cyanosis, coldness of the extremities, and often an exacerbation of headache. Confusion, hemiplegia, abdominal pain, angina, renal artery spasm, ophthalmic artery spasm, and myocardial infarction have also been reported with ergot intoxication.

Acute intoxication may occur during chronic ingestion with nausea, vomiting, absence of pulses in extremities with peripheral cyanosis, uterine ischemia, abortion, or convulsions. Albuminuria and cerebral edema have also been reported. The endothelial damage and poor blood flow induced by the ergot alkaloids may give rise to multiple thrombi. Neurological manifestations of ergot intoxication include headache, vertigo, psychotic disturbances, convulsions, and coma.

B. TREATMENT

Discontinuation of the ergot therapy, and in severe cases vasodilation, is mandatory if there is cyanosis and pulses are absent.

1. Papaverine, tolazoline, hydralazine, and methacholine have all been given to the patient poisoned with ergot with varying success. Treatment with a direct-acting vasodilator such as nitroprusside has been reported to be effective in reversing peripheral ischemia within 3–6 hours after beginning the infusion and would appear to be a rational approach to reversing the vasoconstriction. Nitroprusside is given initially at a dose of 0.5 μg./kg. per minute. Dosage is then adjusted according to blood pressure and peripheral cyanosis and pulses. Most recently, sodium nitroprusside has been shown to be the agent of choice in the management of severe ergotamine-induced peripheral ischemia. Sodium nicotinate has also been reported effective in the treatment of ergotamine-induced vasospasm, but it is not as readily available as nitroprusside (Nipride).

2. Abdominal pain may respond to atropine (adults 0.5 mg.; children 0.01 mg./kg.). Nausea is relieved with a phenothiazine antiemetic.

3. A continuous heparin infusion and low molecular weight dextran (Dextran 40) are of possible benefit in reducing thrombus formation and improving microvascular flow in ischemic areas. Vascular intimal damage is probably necessary for the production of thrombosis and tissue necrosis.

4. Caution should be advised in assessing blood pressure since there may be severe arterial spasm, making it difficult to obtain an accurate measurement. Treat hypertension with dopamine or isoproterenol which increase cardiac output and decrease peripheral resistance. The alpha stimulant catecholamines should be

avoided since they may decrease peripheral blood flow to already ischemic areas.

5. Hypothermia and hyperthermia have been reported and may require treatment (refer to Chap. 1).

6. Diazepam is useful in controlling convulsions (children, 0.04–0.1 mg./kg.; adults, 5–10 mg. I.V. by slow push).

VIII. THEOPHYLLINE AND OTHER XANTHINES

Caffeine and theobromine have toxic effects very similar to the most widely used member of this class, theophylline.

Theophylline and its salts are available alone or as combination products usually containing ephedrine or a sedative. Although widely used as a bronchodilator, theophylline is also used in the treatment of congestive heart failure. The salts of theophylline contain different percentages of the parent compound. Dyphylline is a structural analog of theophylline.

Theophylline salts are absorbed rapidly after oral administration, reaching peak plasma concentrations 1–2 hours after a dose. Hydroalcoholic solutions containing theophylline are more rapidly absorbed, reaching peak concentration 0.5–1 hour after a dose. Rectal administration of suppositories produces its peak concentration 2–4 hours after a dose. Theophylline is metabolized by the liver to methyluric acids or to methylxanthines with only about 10% of the drug excreted unchanged in the urine. Hepatic dysfunction and congestive heart failure prolong the half-life of theophylline which in adults is 3–10 hours with a mean of 5 hours and which in children is 2–7 hours with a mean of 3 hours. Some accumulation of the drug usually occurs with chronic administration.

Theophylline acts to inhibit the enzyme phosphodiesterase and thereby causes an increase in the concentration of 3'5' cyclic AMP. Calcium flux may also be affected by theophylline. The therapeutic effects include bronchodilation, CNS stimulation, increased cardiac inotropism, vasoconstriction in cerebral circulation, increase or decrease in blood pressure, increased gastric secretion, increased basal metabolic rate, and a slight diuresis.

The toxicity of theophylline is closely related to plasma levels, and plasma theophylline concentrations of over 20 μg./ ml. are considered toxic. Rapid I.V. injection of aminophylline may produce exceedingly high plasma levels which may be responsible for episodes of cardiac arrhythmias, headache, precordial pain, and sudden death. Intravenous theophylline may be dangerous in patients who have had a recent myocardial infarction. Currently recommended I.V. and oral doses may produce toxic theophylline levels, and therefore plasma theophylline concentrations should be monitored in all patients receiving this drug. Ephedrine and theophylline may produce enhanced toxicity if given together. Rectal suppositories containing theophylline have produced fatalities in children.

A. CLINICAL FEATURES

Overdosage with theophylline-containing products usually occurs after chronic administration, although acute overdoses have been reported. The toxic effects include nervousness and irritability and nausea and vomiting with often severe abdominal cramps. Vomitus may be bloody, and severe thirst may be present. Arrhythmias can occur. Seizures may be preceded by these symptoms, although there have been sudden seizures with no premonitory signs. Seizures may be prolonged and difficult to control.

B. TREATMENT

1. Diazepam may be useful in controlling seizures (0.04–0.2 mg./kg. in children; 5–10 mg. in adults).

2. Respiratory assistance should be available.

IX. NEUROMUSCULAR BLOCKING DRUGS

The toxicities of the depolarizing and the competitive neuromuscular blocking agents are related to their ability to paralyze respiratory muscles and produce apnea. These agents may also produce undesired effects through stimulation or blockade of the autonomic nervous system. Certain members of this group are known to cause the release of histamine. All of the neuromuscular blocking drugs used clinically are devoid of central nervous system effects and are not absorbed by the oral route.

Poisoning rarely occurs with these drugs and is usually due to inadvertent clinical overdosage or injudicious use. Consequently, the occasional adverse reaction associated with these drugs deserves more attention than their more severe toxicity.

The neuromuscular blockers are divided into depolarizing (succinylcholine) and competitive (D-tubocurarine) agents. Succinylcholine mimics the action of acetylcholine at the neuromuscular junction and in a dose of 10–30 mg. causes a transient muscular fasciculation that progresses to relaxation within about 1 minute. The duration of action of a single dose varies from 2 to 5 minutes. A dose of 6–9 mg. D-tubocurarine produces neuromuscular blockade and muscle relaxation within 3–5 minutes and lasts for 20–30 minutes.

The cholinesterase inhibitors, neostigmine (1–3 mg. I.V.) and edrophonium (10 mg. I.V.), may be used to reverse the effect of competitive neuromuscular blockers by allowing acetylcholine to accumulate at the myoneural junction and reestablish neuromuscular transmission. These drugs may aggravate certain side effects of the neuromuscular blockers, such as hypotension and bronchospasm, through their cholinomimetic properties. Atropine must always be given with these cholinesterase inhibitors to block their muscarinic effects. Edrophonium has a short duration of action, and a repeat dose is often necessary. The administration of anticholinesterase drugs is contraindicated when succinylcholine has been given since they block acetylcholinesterase, the enzyme responsible for the degradation of both acetylcholine and succinylcholine.

CLINICAL FEATURES AND TREATMENT

There have been numerous adverse reactions associated with the use of succinylcholine which may limit its use in particular patients. Patients with decreased plasma cholinesterase, i.e., congenital deficiency, liver disease, malnutrition, exposure to organophosphorus compounds, and hyperpyrexia, may experience prolonged apnea. Likewise, patients with oat cell carcinoma of the lung, renal failure, porphyria, familial periodic paralysis, and thyroid disorders may also experience prolonged drug effect.

Cardiovascular toxicity may be produced by succinylcholine through its ability to stimulate the autonomic ganglia (vagal and sympathetic) innervating the heart and the production of severe hyperkalemia. Hyperkalemia and subsequent cardiovascular complications may occur more commonly in patients who have experienced massive trauma or severe neurological disturbances.

Several seemingly unrelated drugs are known to alter the clinical response obtained with the neuromuscular blockers. Magnesium, quinidine, aminoglycosides, polymyxins, and tetracyclines may all produce additive neuromuscular blockade with both competitive and depolarizing agents. There is some suggestion that calcium may antagonize the additive effects of these drugs. The phenothiazine promazine has been noted to produce prolonged apnea in a patient following an infusion of succinylcholine. Phenothiazine analogs are known to possess varying degrees of anticholinesterase activity, which may explain this effect.

Other adverse effects have followed the administration of succinylcholine. Muscle pain, myoglobinuria, and bronchospasm are reported. Succinylcholine has been associated with the malignant hyperpyrexia syndrome in which the fatality rate approaches 70%. Most reports of this syndrome describe the combined use of succinylcholine with halothane and nitrous oxide. Therapy consists of cooling the patient, administration of 100% oxygen with hyperventilation, as well as efforts to control the acidosis and bleeding disorders which may be present. A familial incidence is reported, suggesting the use of other forms of anesthesia for those with a familial history of this syndrome.

D-Tubocurarine and the other competitive blocking agents may produce severe adverse reactions which are often related to their propensity for causing histamine release. High doses of D-Tubocurarine may also produce some ganglionic blockade. After the injection of large doses of D-Tubocurarine there may be a fall in blood pressure which is related to the combined effects of histamine, ganglionic blockade, and sympathetic release. The use of potent inhalational anesthetics with competitive neuromuscular blockers yields a synergistic effect that often requires as much as a 50% reduction in the dose of the neuromuscular-blocking agent.

BIBLIOGRAPHY

Anderson, P. K., Christensen, K. N., and Hole, P.: Sodium nitroprusside and epidural blockade in the treatment of ergotism. N. Engl. J. Med., *296:*1271, 1977.

Brooks, N. H.: Circulatory collapse after oral oxprenolol. Br. Med. J., *4:*24, 1975.

Carliner, N. H., et al.: Sodium nitroprusside treatment of ergotamine induced ischemia. J.A.M.A., *227:*308, 1974.

Cumming, G., Harding, L. K., Prowser, K.: Treatment and recovery after massive overdose of physostigmine. Lancet, *2:*147, 1968.

Fernandez, G., et al.: Cholinesterase inhibition by phenothiazine and non-phenothiazine antihistaminics: analysis of its postulated role in synergizing organophosphate toxicity. Toxicol. Appl. Pharmacol., *31:*179, 1975.

Hoehn, M., and Rutledge, C. O.: Acute overdose with levodopa: clinical and biochemical consequences. Neurology, *25:*792–794, 1975.

Jameson, H. D.: Pyridoxine for levodopa induced dystonia. Journal of the American Medical Association, *211:*1700, 1970.

Jenne, J. W., et al.: Pharmacokinetics of theophylline: application to adjustment of the clinical dose of aminophylline. Clin. Pharmacol. Ther. *13:*349, 1971.

Karhunen, P., and Hartels, G.: Suicidal attempt with practolol. Br. Med. J., *2:*178, 1973.

Merhoff, C. G., and Porter, J. M.: Ergot intoxication: historical review and description of unusual clinical manifestations. Ann. Surg., *180:*773, 1974.

Moore, H. W.: Acute nicotine poisoning: opinion case of the month. J. S.C. Med. Assoc., *58:*445, 1962.

Oberst, B. B., and McIntyre, R. A.: Acute nicotine poisoning: case report. Pediatrics, *11:*338, 1953.

Parmley, W. W.: The role of glucagon in cardiac therapy. N. Engl. J. Med., *285:*801, 1971.

Shader, R. I., and Greenblatt, D. J.: Belladonna alkaloids and synthetic anticholinergics: uses and toxicity. *In* Shader, R. I. (ed.): Psychiatric Complications of Medicinal Drugs. pp. 103–147. New York, Raven Press, 1972.

Snyder, B. D.: Physostigmine: antidote for anticholinergic poisoning. Minn. Med., *58:*456, 1975.

Weinberger, M. W., et al.: Intravenous aminophylline dosage: use of serum theophylline measurement for guidance. Journal of the American Medical Association, *235:*2110, 1976.

8. CARDIOVASCULAR DRUGS

W. Fraser Bremner, M.B., Ch.B., Ph.D.

This chapter deals with drugs that exert a primary therapeutic effect on the cardiovascular system. They are classified into nine functional groups.

1. Cardiac glycosides and other inotropic agents
2. Antiarrhythmic drugs
3. Vasodilator drugs used in angina, claudication, cardiac failure, cerebral arteriosclerosis
4. Diuretic drugs and potassium chloride
5. Antihypertensive agents
6. Beta blocking agents
7. Anticoagulant and antiplatelet drugs
8. Hypolipidemic agents
9. Miscellaneous drugs such as ergonovine maleate and saralasin

I. CARDIAC GLYCOSIDES AND OTHER INOTROPIC AGENTS

Cardiac glycosides, particularly digoxin, deserve emphasis in view of their widespread use. Digoxin was the eighth most frequently prescribed drug by American clinicians in 1976 (Gosselin Survey, 1976). Glycosides remain the drugs of choice in the control of the rate of ventricular response in atrial fibrillation or flutter: this they do both indirectly by vagal stimulation and by a direct effect on atrioventricular nodal cells to increase the degree of atrioventricular block. Some patients require unduly high doses of glycosides for adequate slowing of the ventricular response, or the addition of propranolol. Glycosides are used in treating cardiac failure, both right and left ventricular, by virtue of their positive inotropic effect. They increase the rate of myocardial oxygen consumption, and theoretical considerations and experimental data suggest they may carry some risk in failure due to myocardial infarction. They are potential-ly arrhythmogenic though in some situations suppress arrhythmias.* Patient compliance, particularly in the elderly, is often poor or haphazard. Glycosides are, however, the only effective oral inotropic agents for long-term use.

The advent of a sensitive and specific digoxin radioimmunoassay technique has been of assistance in tailoring dosage to patient requirements and in confirming excessive dosage or detecting potential at-risk candidates for digoxin toxicity. Optimum serum levels are in the range of 0.5 to 2.5 ng./ml., with toxic levels being in general over 3.0 ng./ml. There is, however, a wide overlap. These values, it should be noted, relate to the plateau phase of serum drug levels; i.e., 6–8 hours after an oral or 3–4 hours after an intravenous dose. Also, it should be remembered that commercially available radioimmunoassay kits have relatively low precision and variable accuracy.

A. DIGITALIS INTOXICATION: CLINICAL FEATURES

Digitalis intoxication is one of the commonest adverse drug effects, which serves to emphasize the narrow zone between therapeutic and toxic levels. Toxicity is prone to occur in renal failure, in the elderly (due to the reduced skeletal mass which takes up digoxin plus the frequent minor renal insufficiency found in such individuals), in individuals with untreated hypothyroidism, and in those who are ill, particularly if hypokalemic or hypoxic.

Serum levels are lowered in thyrotoxicosis or if the hypolipidemic resins cholestyramine and colestipol are being given

---

*For example, in congestive cardiac failure due to improvement in function.

simultaneously. Administration of large doses of digoxin may lead to toxic effects if thyrotoxicosis is treated or hypolipidemic drugs are withdrawn. Propranolol may potentiate digitalis-induced nodal slowing and precipitate heart block. Quinidine can displace digoxin from its binding sites and coincidental administration may precipitate digoxin toxicity.

1. Noncardiac Symptoms and Signs

Fatigue and undue muscular weakness

Anorexia, nausea, vomiting, diarrhea

Mental confusion, restlessness, insomnia, apathy, drowsiness, hallucinations, frank psychosis

Blurred vision, difficulty in reading, photophobia, scintillation scotomata, problems with red green colors

---

Many of these may occur as a result of underlying disease whether it be cardiac, gastrointestinal, or senile dementia. Loss of appetite in the elderly may be due solely to digoxin. Often, the only indication of toxicity is a cardiac arrhythmia.

2. Cardiac Symptoms and Signs

Digitalis can induce every arrhythmia, and clinical manifestations may vary from none to palpitation and dyspnea, syncope, and death. The commonest arrhythmias are ventricular, particularly bigeminy, supraventricular, paroxysmal atrial tachycardia with block, and nodal, particularly junctional tachycardia or heart block. A regular ventricular rhythm in the presence of atrial fibrillation suggests toxicity. In children where accidental poisoning is not uncommon, nodal and atrial ectopics are the commonest presenting findings. Ventricular ectopics and gastrointestinal upsets are uncommon in children.

Such arrhythmias may also occur due to the underlying cardiac disease, and a trial of drug withdrawal may be necessary to differentiate. Arrhythmias that are rarely due to digoxin toxicity include parasystole, multifocal atrial tachycardia, atrial flutter/fibrillation with a rapid rate, and Mobitz Type II A-V block.

B. TREATMENT OF DIGITALIS INTOXICATION

There is no specific antidote, and the slow renal excretion means that the toxic effects may be prolonged. Current treatment involves stopping the drug and reversing potentiating factors such as hypokalemia (often due to coincidental diuretic administration), or hypoxia. Serum potassium should be measured and, ideally, renal function should be assessed prior to administration of potassium chloride orally, 20–40 mEq. four times daily, or intravenously into a peripheral vein, 40 mEq. over 2 hours. Close monitoring with intravenous administration is essential. A-V block is a contraindication to potassium chloride administration as the potassium may worsen the degree of block. Some authorities recommend potassium administration even if serum levels are normal because intracellular levels may be low due to glycoside action on the membrane sodium-potassium ATP-ase pump. Cardiac rhythm should be monitored particularly since changing arrhythmias are common. Potassium therapy alone will often promptly suppress the arrhythmias. Lidocaine is the drug of first choice in suppressing digitalis-induced ventricular arrhythmias if they do not respond to potassium. Lidocaine does not suppress A-V conduction and does not cause hypotension. It is relatively ineffective in abolishing junctional tachycardias. A 50–100-mg. bolus is given intravenously and therapeutic levels maintained with 2–4 mg. per minute I.V. infusion.

Diphenylhydantoin is also used for ventricular arrhythmias and does not suppress A-V conduction. Fifty milligrams is given each minute up to 5 mg./kg., followed by 100 mg. orally six hourly. The parenteral preparation is made up in diluent and should not be mixed with other solutions.

Procainamide and quinidine can be used for ventricular arrhythmias or atrial tachycardias, but they potentiate A-V block and may depress myocardial contractility or cause hypotension.

Propranolol, 1–2 mg. I.V., is effective in abolishing ventricular or atrial arrhythmias, but may produce bronchospasm, asystole, or exacerbate cardiac failure.

Cardioversion may precipitate ventricular tachycardia or fibrillation in digitalis toxicity and is a last resort.

Bradyarrhythmias may respond to I.V. atropine (0.6–1.2 mg.) or may require ventricular pacing.

The use of sequestering agents such as cholestyramine has been advocated to remove unabsorbed digoxin from the bowels. Hemoperfusion against activated charcoal may have some value in the very ill.

1. Massive Digitalis Overdosage (Digitalis Poisoning)

This is surprisingly uncommon when one considers the vast number of prescriptions for digoxin issued annually. It is nearly always due to self-poisoning.

Clinically, the spectrum at presentation varies from someone who is relatively well with perhaps some nausea or an arrhythmia to hypotensive collapse with intractable vomiting. Mortality is high, perhaps 20–30%, and the clinical course is unpredictable. Mandatory measurements include continuous cardiac monitoring and frequent assay of serum potassium levels. The latter is essential because hyperkalemia is not uncommon (particularly if vomiting is not marked) and may cause cardiac arrest, especially if more potassium is given inadvertently.

Vomiting may be eased with prochlorperazine, but the large amount of digoxin left in the lower bowel has to be dealt with either by administration of cholestyramine or by purging with a saline cathartic (with monitoring of serum electrolytes and BUN), or both. Gastric lavage may be indicated in the early stages. A ventricular pacemaker may be inserted to deal with bradyarrhythmias, but can induce ventricular tachycardia or fibrillation. Antiarrhythmic drugs are usually required for tachyarrhythmias, but may require the use of rotation to avoid the side effects of large doses of individual drugs. Hemoperfusion through activated charcoal should be considered. Some cardiology centers have available antidigoxin antibody for use in such patients under a trial protocol. These fragments will complex with digoxin and are small enough to be passed through the kidney glomeruli, thereby facilitating excretion of the glycoside. The address of physicians participating in this particular study can be obtained from designated poison control centers in the United States. Patients who would be considered for such therapy would have very high levels of ingestion or life-threatening complications of digitalis poisoning. Cardioversion and the use of inotropes are dangerous.

C. Other Inotropes

Dopamine has assumed a prominent place as the parenteral inotrope in the treatment of frank or impending cardiogenic shock or severe cardiac failure. It is often used in conjunction with vasodilator therapy. It has chronotropic and inotropic effects plus a unique capacity to dilate the renal and splanchnic vascular beds. These vessels possess specific dopaminergic receptors. The drug has a short half-life, being metabolized by monoamine oxidase (MAO). Patients on MAO inhibitors are at high risk if given dopamine. The starting dose, if considered essential, should be ∼10% of the normal dose, which is 2–5 μg./kg./minute, increasing by 5–10 μg./kg./minute increments every five minutes or so to a maximum of 50 μg./kg./minute or until toxicity appears. Ventricular ectopic activity is a warning of impending ventricular tachycardia. Close patient monitoring (rate, rhythm, blood pressure) is essential. Ideally, filling pressure and cardiac output should be measured. Arrhythmia usually only requires cessation of or reduction in infusion rates. The drug may exacerbate or precipitate angina or produce or extend an area of infarction. If hypertension is severe, the short-acting alpha blocker, phentolamine, may be used cautiously. Ventricular tachycardia or fibrillation may require electroversion, but these arrhythmias are often terminal events in a dying patient rather than the direct effects of the drug. The drug is contraindicated in subjects with pheochromocytoma.

Dobutamine, a synthetic cardioactive sympathomimetic amine, is safer than dopamine because it produces less chronotropic (tachycardia) effect for the equivalent inotropic effect. However, it has been on the clinical scene for a shorter time. Toxic effects include headache, nausea, angina, tachycardia, hypertension, and tachyarrhythmia. The usual dose is 2.5–10 μg./kg./minute up to 40 μg./kg./minute, and toxicity usually clears promptly with cessation or reduction of dosage (half-life is two minutes in humans). This drug may largely supersede dopamine, though the latter is a more proficient renal vasodilator.

Aminophyline, used primarily as a bronchodilator in asthma or left ventricular failure, is a potent cardiac stimulant, and may provoke tachyarrhythmias, particularly if given rapidly by the intravenous route. Seizure and vascular collapse may occur. There is no specific antidote and treatment is supportive.

Glucagon has cardiac chronotropic and inotropic effects, is theoretically attractive since it has little arrhythmogenicity, but its effects have been variable and disappointing. It is recommended only for treatment of hypoglycemic states.

Levarterenol, the most potent pressor agent known, may be used in an infusion in hypotensive states and as a cardiac stimulant in a cardiac arrest. Headache may be a precursor of serious toxicity. The drug can produce marked reflex bradycardia. It is contraindicated in patients on monoamine oxidase inhibitors or in those requiring general anesthesia, due to its arrhythmogenic capacity. Reduced blood volume should be corrected prior to use of levarterenol. Extravasation at the site of infusion may cause tissue necrosis. Gangrene of the leg has occurred with administration into an ankle vein. Large doses of levarterenol will also induce hypoglycemia. Large or repeated doses of levarterenol or other sympathomimetic amines can cause damage to the myocardium with marked deposition of calcium. Myocarditis has also been reported.

Treatment involves cessation of therapy. Phentolamine may be used for severe hypertension or for vasospasm at the infusion site. Phentolamine, 5–10 mg. in 10 ml. saline, is infiltrated into the area that is blanched and cold, to induce hyperemia.

Epinephrine may be used in the cardiac arrest situation to restore cardiac rhythm. The drug is rapidly metabolized by COMT and MAO. Toxic effects are largely related to production of tachyarrhythmias; ventricular fibrillation is particularly prone to develop if the patient is anesthetized prior to injection. The drug may produce severe acute hypertension with resultant cerebral vascular catastrophe. The drug can also exacerbate angina. Treatment is usually supportive since the drug's actions are short lived. Hypertension can be counteracted with phentolamine or short-acting vasodilators such as the nitrites.

Isoproterenol has potent inotropic and chronotropic effects but can lower blood pressure if given in large doses. With normal doses, increasing cardiac output is sufficient to maintain or raise the systolic pressure. The drug is primarily used as a bronchodilator but it has some value as a cardiac stimulant. It has been used in cardiogenic shock or in myocardial infarction and in septicemic shock. Oral isoproterenol has been used as a treatment for chronic heart block particularly in elderly subjects where mechanical pacemaking is considered contraindicated. The drug carries risks in this situation and its effects are unpredictable particularly in regard to induction of tachyarrhythmias. Present-day pacemakers are reliable and can be inserted under a local anesthetic. This would appear to be a preferable approach to problems of heart block. The drug is metabolized by the same route as epinephrine and its effects are short lived. Toxic effects are mainly those of cardiac arrhythmia and exacerbation of angina. Treatment is usually supportive.

II. THE ANTIARRHYTHMIC DRUGS

A. LIDOCAINE HCL

Lidocaine HCl, the most frequently used parenteral antiarrhythmic, is used to treat ventricular tachycardia and, on a prophylactic basis, ventricular premature beats. It is the safest drug routinely used. The drug may be given as a rapid intravenous bolus of 50–100 mg. As prophylaxis a loading dose of 1 mg./kg. is given intravenously followed by a continuous infusion of 1–4 mg. per minute. The drug is rapidly metabolized in the liver. Toxicity is primarily due to central nervous system stimulation, and ranges from dizziness, apprehension, blurred or double vision, through muscle fasciculation and tremor to frank convulsions. There are occasional reports of hypotension, accelerated ventricular rhythm, bradycardia, sinus arrest, heart block, pacemaker Wenckebach, and subsequent cardiac arrest. Allergic reactions are rare.

Excretion of lidocaine is primarily by way of hepatic metabolism. Patients in congestive cardiac failure or with severe liver impairment are particularly prone to develop high plasma levels and subsequent toxicity. The threshold for toxic neurological effects is variable. Giddiness, drowsiness, paresthesia, and mood change may occur at levels above 3–5 μg./ml. Between 6 and 10 μg./ml., speech disturbances, confusion, nausea, and frank psychosis may occur. Sweating and muscle fasciculation, particularly of the eyelids, tend to occur at this level. Focal and major seizures with respiratory arrest and coma occur at still higher levels. Patients may progress directly to frank seizures without any obvious preliminary evidence of toxicity. Neurological upset may occur at lower levels of plasma lidocaine, probably as a result of accumulation of its metabolites which are considered to exert part of the toxic side effects. Occasionally, if rapidly given, doses of lidocaine produce bradycardia and hypotension from peripheral vasodilatation and myocardial depression. In sick sinus patients the drug may produce sinus arrest, particularly if given in combination with other antiarrhythmic therapy. Treatment is essentially supportive.

Recurrent convulsions may require diazepam or, if the patient is anesthetized at the time, succinylcholine may be used as a muscle relaxant.

B. PROCAINAMIDE HCL

Procainamide HCl has a wider spectrum of antiarrhythmic effects, being used to treat ventricular and supraventricular arrhythmias. The drug is given intravenously as 100-mg. boluses every five minutes up to 1 gm. total dose until the arrhythmias are abolished, or until toxic effects appear. The drug is available for oral use. The dose is 250–500 mg. every three to four hours. Continuous intravenous infusion of 2–4 mg. per minute may also be used. Absorption from the gastrointestinal tract is rapid and almost complete. Plasma concentration peaks at about one hour after oral administration but this peak may be prolonged up to five hours in cases of severe cardiac failure. Metabolism is mainly by hepatic acetylation with some plasma hydrolysis. Patients may be categorized into fast and slow acetylators. Slow acetylators will have longer and more prolonged procainamide levels at the same dose. The major metabolite of procainamide is *N*-acetyl procainamide, which has antiarrhythmic effects similar to the parent compound. This metabolite has a half-life twice that of procainamide. Procainamide HCl is much more likely than lidocaine to cause depression of cardiac impulse formation and transmission, particularly in the presence of myocardial damage. It may induce cardiac asystole or ventricular fibrillation and induce or worsen A-V block. Pacemaker Wenckebach (progressive increase in the spike to QRS interval) has been recorded in an overdose. Hypotension may occur, particularly if other antiarrhythmic drugs such as propranolol have been administered. Excessive oral dosage has been noted to produce hypotension, reduction in renal function, and junctional tachycardia. Toxic effects on the heart usually occur at high plasma concentrations of the drug. Severe hypotension and shock due to peripheral vasodilatation or reduction in myocardial contractility or a combination of both may occur. They are, however, uncommon if procainamide is administered according to the above dosage schedule. Cardiac toxicity may be manifested by prolongation of the Q-T interval and of the QRS complex. Ventricular arrhythmias subsequently are prone to develop. Syncope is less of a problem with this drug than with quinidine. Cardiac toxicity may be reversed with molar sodium lactate.

High doses given orally tend to induce anorexia, nausea, and vomiting. Dizziness, altered mental mood, and frank hallucinations have been reported. Leukopenia and frank agranulocytosis may also occur.

This drug is particularly likely to produce unexplained fever, usually 14 days after initiation of therapy. The fever is usually remittant with one or more daily spikes. It may be associated with rigors. Fever remits with withdrawal of the drug.

A significant fraction of an administered dose of procainamide is excreted by way of the kidneys. Toxicity is more likely in the presence of renal insufficiency or cardiac failure.

The drug is notorious for inducing a syndrome that may be indistinguishable from systemic lupus erythematosus. A pleuritic rub may occur due to pulmonary involvement and this may be mistakenly treated as pulmonary embolus. Joint involvement, pleural effusions, skin lesions, pericarditis, Coomb's positive anemia, thrombocytopenia, pyrexia, and myalgia have all been reported. The ANF titer is usually positive. Acute hypersensitivity reactions have been reported, as has agranulocytosis with repeated dosage. The kidney tends to be spared. Rhythm disorders may require treatment, e.g., pacing for heart block, lidocaine for ventricular tachycardia, and a pressor agent for hypotension. The lupuslike syndrome usually regresses with discontinuation of therapy but may require steroid therapy.

An increase in antinuclear factor titer is the rule rather than the exception during procainamide therapy. The lupuslike syndrome is more common among slow acetylators of the drug but does occur among fast acetylators. Fast and slow acetylators may be easily differentiated by administration of INH and a measurement of the degree of acetylation obtained from a urine sample.

Pericardial tamponade and constrictive pericarditis have been reported as rare complications of procainamide-induced lupus syndrome.

C. QUINIDINE SULFATE

This antiarrhythmic is given in oral form. Parenteral preparations are available but little used due to their high risks. About 95% of an oral dose of quinidine is absorbed with 70% bound to plasma protein. Peak plasma levels are reached one to two hours after ingestion. The drug is largely metabolized by hepatic hydroxylation. Normal plasma half-time is five to seven hours. Maximal effects are seen within 1–3 hours and persist for some six to eight hours or longer. Therapeutic plasma concentration is 3–6 mg./liter. Most of the drug and its metabolites leave the body by way of urine.

Quinidine in toxic doses may produce cinchonism, which is manifest as tinnitus, temporary deafness, headache, and blurred vision. This may progress to diplopia, photophobia, vertigo, delirium and frank psychosis. Gastrointestinal side effects are common with this drug. Diarrhea is a frequent problem. Vomiting and colic also occur. This appears to be a local irritant effect and is reduced in frequency when quinidine is administered as the polygalacturonate. The sulfate may become available as a slow preparation in the future. The diarrhea may be offset by concurrent use of aluminum hydroxide.

Hypersensitivity reactions are frequent. Drug fever, urticaria rash, and exfoliative dermatitis have all been reported. Platelet-quinidine complexes, to which circulating antibody responds, cause platelet agglutination and lysis with purpura. Hemolytic anemia, bone marrow hypoplasia, and agranulocytosis have been reported. These effects are not known to be antibody-related.

Dose-related toxicity is particularly common in patients with reduced glomerular filtration rates. This occurs not only in renal insufficiency but also in congestive cardiac failure. There is prolongation of the Q-Tc interval, widening of the QRS complex, and lengthening of the PR interval as atrial ventricular conduction is impaired. Notching of the T waves with loss of amplitude is common as is ST-segment depression and T-wave inversion. In severe toxicity, P waves widen, atrial rate slows, and intraatrial block develops lead-ing to atrial standstill. At very high levels (greater than 20 μg./ml.), the QRS complexes are markedly widened and progress to ventricular tachycardia and fibrillation. On occasion, malignant arrhythmias have been reported to respond to DC countershock, isoprenaline, or propranolol. Instances of sudden death have been reported. These deaths can occur without toxic drug levels. Elderly patients seem particularly prone to quinidine syncope from ventricular tachycardia or flutter. This frequently occurs with conduction system damage (sick sinus syndrome). The ventricular tachycardia may show *torsade de pointes* (undulation in the amplitude of the QRS complexes).

Molar sodium lactate is a specific antagonist for the toxic effects of quinidine. In cases of intractable ventricular tachycardia, overdrive pacing may be effective.

Parenteral administration of quinidine is rarely used except in intractable cases of dysrhythmia. Idiosyncrasy, malignant cardiac arrhythmias, and cardiovascular collapse are particularly common with this approach.

Quinidine has the capacity to displace digoxin from its binding sites on body proteins and may thereby elevate levels into the toxic range.

D. DISOPYRAMIDE

This drug has similar pharmacological properties to quinidine. It has a myocardial depressant effect which is largely offset by its anticholinergic action. Common adverse effects of oral doses of 200–800 mg. a day are dry mouth, abdominal pain and bloating, constipation, and vomiting. Visual disturbances are also common. Skin rashes with spotty erythema and photosensitization have been reported. Urinary retention occurs, particularly with intravenous therapy. Hypotension has been reported and has been sufficiently severe to cause circulatory arrest in several patients. The drug produces a dose-related increase in Q-Tc interval.

The QRS complex widens, particularly if it is initially prolonged.

Syncopal episodes due to ventricular tachycardia with fluctuating QRS amplitudes (*torsade de pointes*) have been described. Ventricular fibrillation has also been reported.

Plasma levels between 2 and 10 μg./ml. produce an increase in the PR, QRS, and Q-T intervals of the ECG. The greatest prolongation occurs in the PR interval.

Gross overdose causes death with cardiac arrhythmia, pulmonary edema, and respiratory arrest.

Supportive measures include emesis or lavage, cardiorespiratory support, physostigmine as anticholinergic antagonist, and hemodialysis.

E. DIPHENYLHYDANTOIN

This drug is used as a second-line antiarrhythmic medication. Some consider it of particular value in cases of digitalis toxicity because it does not depress A-V nodal conduction at therapeutic levels. It may also augment A-V conduction in atrial flutter, and this is hazardous. The drug appears to be of greater hazard in elderly patients. Fatalities from ventricular fibrillation, intractable shock, and heart block and respiratory arrest have been reported. Patients have required temporary pacemaking when this drug has been given in cases of atrial fibrillation and myocardial infarction with induced slow nodal rhythm. Sinoatrial arrest has also been reported.

Hypotension is a problem due to peripheral vasodilatation as well as myocardial depression. These effects are usually short-lived and generally clear without any therapeutic intervention apart from stopping the drug.

The drug is supplied with a particular diluent, propylene glycol, which is prone to induce local irritation and phlebitis at injection sites.

Adverse effects of this compound are well known in the context of its use as an anticonvulsant. Side effects are generally dose related. They are uncommon in the therapeutic range of 5–20 μg./ml. Nystagmus occurs at levels above this, cerebellar ataxia commonly at levels of 30 μg./ml., and mental slowing at levels above 40 μg./ml. Patients with a genetic deficiency of the parahydroxylation enzyme system that metabolizes the drug are prone to develop toxic side effects at therapeutic levels. This parahydroxylation system can also be depressed by drugs such as warfarin and antituberculous agents. Barbiturates and uremia augment the parahydroxylation process and may lower therapeutic levels to the subtherapeutic range. Drug hypersensitivity with induction of hepatitis has been recorded. The drug is prone to cause lymphadenopathy with chronic therapy. Megaloblastic anemia with low serum folate levels develops in a fair proportion of patients on long-term therapy.

Gingival hyperplasia is another well-known side effect of the drug.

F. VERAPAMIL

It is useful for the treatment of arrhythmias. It is particularly effective in the treatment of supraventricular tachycardia. It is effective in hypertensive emergencies because of its vasodilator properties. It is also useful clinically in the management of angina pectoris. The drug is well absorbed orally but undergoes extensive biotransformation with less than one-fifth available in its original form after first pass. Peak levels occur at 30–120 minutes. Action following intravenous administration is particularly rapid.

By virtue of its action on calcium transport, the drug selectively slows A-V nodal conduction. The commonest ECG effect of the drug is prolongation of the PR interval. The drug also suppresses S-A nodal activity and may be hazardous in patients with S-A node disease. The drug probably suppresses reentry tachyarrhythmias through its ability to depress conduction of slow calcium currents in damaged cardiac fibers.

Following an oral dose of 80 mg. of verapamil, maximal plasma levels reach 30–80 ng./ml. 30–45 minutes after ingestion.

The clinical features of toxicity are stupor, hypotension, shock, bradycardia with A-V dissociation, abdominal distention, liver enlargement, and contracted nonreacting pupils.

In 27 patients treated with the drug for supraventicular tachycardia, the systolic blood pressure fell in all. Isoprenaline was found to be useful in restoring circulation in those who recovered. The drug may induce ectopic activity.

Intravenous calcium gluconate is recorded as antagonizing verapamil-induced heart block and hypotension.

G. Mexiletine

This is a new antiarrhythmic drug that is effective against ventricular arrhythmias. It is available in parenteral and oral forms. Toxic effects include bradycardia and hypotension which have been reported at drug levels within the therapeutic range. Lidocaine administration appears to potentiate the toxic effects of this drug. It also causes nausea and vomiting, drowsiness, confusion, dizziness, dysarthria, diplopia, nystagmus, ataxia, tremor, paresthesias, and seizures.

Therapeutic levels of the drug occur with plasma levels between 0.5 and 2 mM./ml. Toxicity occurs above 3 mM./ml. The mean half-life is 18.5 hours.

This drug is virtually completely absorbed following oral administration with peak plasma concentrations occurring some 3 hours later in healthy volunteers. Absorption is delayed and incomplete in the context of myocardial infarction and if narcotic analgesics are used. Daily

doses of 600–1000 mg. are usually required to maintain plasma concentration in the therapeutic range of 1–2 μg./ml. The drug is rapidly taken up and distributed to the body tissues, and is more rapidly excreted if the urine is acidic. It is primarily metabolized by oxidative and reductive processes.

H. Aprindine

This drug is available only on special prescription and should be used only for resistant dysrythmia as a drug of last resort. It causes agranulcytosis that may be fatal.

Neurological toxicity includes tremor of the fingers followed by dizziness, ataxia, hallucinations, memory upset and seizures. Cholestatic jaundice is reported. The margin between therapeutic and toxic levels is small.

I. Bretylium Tosylate

This drug is used to treat refractory ventricular tachycardia. It is the only available drug that will chemically cardiovert ventricular fibrillation. It has a useful positive inotropic effect.

Oral absorption is variable and incomplete. Parenteral routes are necessary; 500 mg. is given as 2-$\times$-5-ml. I.M. injections or over 10 minutes as a 50 ml. infusion. Bolus administration has a rapid onset of action. The drug accumulates in adrenergic neurons and cardiac fibers. Most eventually passes out unchanged in the urine.

Side effects include orthostatic hypotension due to peripheral sympathetic blockade, nausea, vomiting, parotid pain, and swelling.

Treatment involves stopping the drug and supportive measures.

J. Amiodarone

This drug may be useful in patients with drug-resistant tachyarrhythmias, including atrial fibrillation and WPW syndrome.

The drug is a general myocardial depressant. The usual dose is 200 mg. t.i.d. The drug can cause nausea, rashes, corneal deposits (usually without visual impairment and reversible with cessation of therapy), hypothyroidism (possibly due to release of iodine by metabolic degradation), photodermatitis, melanodermatitis (due to crystal deposition), Parkinsonian-type tremor, and neuropathy.

Treatment of toxic effects involves stopping the drug and treating complications.

K. NIFEDIPINE

This is a calcium-blocking drug of the verapamil class. It is said to be more effective than verapamil in the treatment of coronary artery spasm.

For treatment of toxic effects, see verapamil.

L. ETHMOZIN

This new drug is of some value in treating paroxysmal atrial and ventricular tachycardia. It suppresses ventricular ectopic beats. The drug is well absorbed.

The reported side effects are nausea, vomiting, vertigo, hypotension, and dimmed vision.

M. TOCAINIDE

This is an oral analog of lidocaine. It is rapidly and almost completely absorbed. Oral doses of 400–600 mg. give therapeutic levels of over 6 μg./ml. Peak serum levels occur 60–90 minutes after an oral dose. Forty percent is excreted in the urine; 60% is degraded in the liver.

The drug has a wider spectrum of antiarrhythmic efficacy than lidocaine.

Side effects include anorexia, nausea, vomiting, and constipation. Neurological effects are twitching, dizziness, visual and aural upset, paresthesia, and altered mood. It may elevate ANF titers.

Treatment of complications is to discontinue the drug.

III. VASODILATOR DRUGS

A. NITRITES AND NITRATES

These drugs are used primarily for the alleviation of anginal symptoms. This group includes nitroglycerin and the longer-acting nitrates. Amylnitrite may be given by inhalation but its effects are extremely rapid and very potent. It commonly produces a pounding headache and syncope. It is extremely difficult to control its effects, and it is probably unwise to use this drug for this purpose. Nitroglycerin's widespread use attests to its safety. The main problems are headache, hypotension, occasional nausea and vomiting, rashes, and idiosyncratic reactions. As the drug's effects are short-lived, supportive therapy is usually all that is required. In case of syncope, laying the patient flat and elevating the legs is adequate. It should be noted that nitroglycerin tablets deteriorate unless kept in sealed containers. Condition of the tablets should be considered before increasing a patient's dosage schedule where therapy appears ineffective. Nitrites and nitrates disappear rapidly from the bloodstream, being metabolized by various pathways to ammonia and glycerol.

Tolerance has been reported with nitroglycerin administration.

The action of such drugs is to relax smooth muscle by a nonspecific effect independent of muscle innervation.

Headache due to these agents indicates a rise in intracranial pressure, but the risks from this seem to be largely theoretical rather than practical. Recent studies suggest that nitroglycerin may cause hypoxemia by blocking the lungs' capacity to vasoconstrict in response to alveolar hypoxia and shift perfusion to better ventilated areas. Whether this is of any practical consequence clinically remains to be shown. Long-acting vasodilators such as isosorbide dinitrate have the same side effects as the shorter-acting nitrates but the side effects are not as severe.

Use of glyceryl trinitrate in the first 24 hours following myocardial infarction is probably contraindicated as the vascular responses may be unpredictable. Patients have been reported to develop severe arterial hypotension and bradycardia. These circulatory changes are usually reversed by stopping the drug, elevation of the legs, and administration of atropine. These effects are a result of increased vasovagal activity facilitated by excessive venodilatation induced by the trinitrate.

High doses of nitrite convert hemoglobin to methemoglobin. Occasionally this can be severe enough to be fatal. Treatment involves administration of methylene blue in low doses, methylene blue acting as an electron acceptor in a transfer of electrons from reduced nucleotides to methemoglobin.

Long-acting nitrates available include erythrityl tetranitrate, pentherythritol tetranitrate, mannitol hexanitrate, and isosorbide dinitrate. The last drug is frequently used in relatively high dosage to provide prolonged relief from pain in severe unstable or variant angina. The side effects are the same as those of the short-acting nitrates. Nitropaste, a topical nitroglycerin application, has the same side effects as the oral preparation.

B. Vasodilator Drugs Used in Cardiac Unloading Therapy

1. Sodium Nitroprusside

The recent marketing of stable preparations of this compound has resulted in its widespread use as a vasodilator and cardiac unloading agent. The drug is extremely potent, is administered intravenously, and acts as a metabolic poison on the cytochrome respiratory chain with consequent vasodilatation. Toxicity of the drug is due to its metabolism to cyanide. The cyanide is detoxified to thiocynate,

but the capacity for this is limited and intoxication with sodium nitroprusside presents clinically as cyanide intoxication.

Four distinct responses to sodium nitroprusside are described:

1. Constant response to a low dose (less than 10 μg./kg./minute). This is the commonest reaction
2. A constant response to high dosage
3. Tachyphylaxis to sodium nitroprusside appearing some 30–60 minutes after commencement, with increasing doses of nitroprusside required to maintain hypotension of the same level
4. A definite resistance to the drug with inability to obtain a hypotensive effect even at high doses

Each of the last three types of reactions has a high risk of intoxication. Tachyphylaxis may be related to lack of endogenous thiosulfate and/or deficiency in the enzyme system. Measurement of thiocyanate levels, which should not exceed 5–10 mg.%, has been used to warn of impending intoxication. The presence of a metabolic acidosis means that intoxication is already present. Antidotes are hydroxycobalamin, which forms cynacobalamin and is largely excreted, and thiosulfate, especially in the case of tachyphylaxis.

Controlled administration at low doses appears fairly safe. Switching over to another antihypertensive agent can produce severe interactions. Administration of clonidine following a course of nitroprusside and the use of methyldopa during a nitroprusside infusion have been reported to induce severe hypotension.

Tachyphylaxis probably indicates that a certain cyanide level has been reached beyond which continued infusion will produce no further hypotension. Tachyphylaxis is mainly seen in young and relatively healthy patients, especially men. Prolonged use of nitroprusside interferes with iodine uptake by the thyroid and may lead to hypothyroidism. Nitroprusside is a potent inhibitor of platelet function. Excessive infusion of the drug causes sweating, nausea, vomiting, anxiety at rest, and muscle twitching. The inability to maintain hypotension at the desired level should be regarded as a symptom of impending cyanide intoxication. Death from cyanide poisoning is preceded by an increase in the respiratory rate, bradycardia, ectopic beats, metabolic acidosis, and finally cardiac arrest. Inhibition of oxidative enzymes produces anaerobic glycolysis and tissue anoxemia. As the drug's effect is short-lived, cessation of drug therapy is usually adequate to prevent impending catastrophe. Manifestations of toxicity from sodium nitroprusside have included fatigue, nausea, disorientation, psychotic behavior and muscle spasm from accumulation of thiocyanate.

2. Hydralazine

This drug has a direct effect on vascular smooth muscle, causing relaxation. It is used as a cardiac unloading agent, particularly when maintenance therapy is required, and as a antihypertensive agent. The drug is well absorbed from the gastrointestinal tract and blood levels peak three to four hours after oral administration. The drug is metabolized by hydrolyzation, conjugation, and acetylation. A small fraction is passed in the urine unchanged, and renal insufficiency may potentiate its effects. The drug produces tachycardia, but in doses up to 300 mg./day this is usually not significant.

Side effects include headache, palpitations, nausea, vomiting, diarrhea, nasal congestion, lacrimation, and abdominal cramps. Fever, skin eruptions, and an induced pyridoxine deficiency with peripheral neuropathy are dose-related and are more common in slow acetylators. The main problem relates to occurrence of a lupuslike syndrome, which may occur in perhaps 10–20% of cases. Most such cases are slow acetylators, and the acetylator

phenotype can be established simply by determining T½ of INH. Some 90% of such cases have a positive LE cell test or elevated ANF antibody titers, which often parallel the severity of the disease. Other autoimmune tests may become positive. Bone marrow depression and hemolytic anemia have been reported in association with administration of this drug.

The lupuslike syndrome is more common with high doses or prolonged administration of this drug.

Treatment of toxicity involves cessation of the drug, administration of fluid if the patient is also on a diuretic, and use of a pressor agent if hypotension is severe and will not respond to lying the patient down and elevating the legs. The lupuslike syndrome usually clears with cessation of therapy but may on occasion require long-term steroid administration. For the possible presenting symptoms of this syndrome, see procainamide.

Like other vasodilators the drug may promote fluid retention.

C. PERIPHERAL VASODILATORS

These drugs in general are of little proven value but nevertheless are widely prescribed.

1. Phenoxybenzamine Hydrochloride

This is sometimes effective when vasospasm is a problem (Raynaud's disease). Toxic effects include orthostatic hypotension, reflex tachycardia, nausea, vomiting, diarrhea, miosis, and nasal congestion. Impairment of sexual function is also a problem.

2. Papaverine Hydrochloride

Toxic effects of papaverine include nausea, abdominal discomfort, constipation, malaise, drowsiness, headache, diarrhea, and flushing. Abnormal liver function tests, jaundice, and eosinophilia have been reported.

3. Cyclandelate

This may cause flushing, headache, and tachycardia. Gastrointestinal upset is uncommon. The main problem is severe hypotension due to vasodilatation.

4. Azapetine

This causes nausea, vomiting, dizziness, orthostatic hypotension, and syncope. Tachycardia, dry mouth, and anorexia have also occurred. The drug is contraindicated in the presence of angina. Niacin and nicotinyl alcohol cause flushing of the face and neck, nausea, vomiting, diarrhea, and rashes.

5. Tolazoline

Toxic effects of tolazoline include nausea, gastric discomfort, tachycardia, flushing, and piloerection.

6. Isoxsuprine

This is a direct-acting stimulant and has been used to treat peripheral and cerebral vascular disorders. Toxic effects include tachycardia, hypotension, nausea, vomiting, and dizziness.

7. Nylidrin

This is a beta-adrenergic stimulator. It may cause nervousness, palpitations, tachycardia, and hypertension. It is contraindicated in the presence of angina. Flushing may occur.

8. Hydergine

This drug is a combination of three ergot alkaloids and is occasionally used as a vasodilator and hypotensive agent. It can be used orally or by infusion. It causes nasal stuffiness, orthostatic hypotension, abdominal discomfort, flushing, and rashes. It is also reported to cause sinus bradycardia.

9. Meclofenoxate

This drug has been promoted as a cerebral vascular vasodilator. Several trials have suggested an increased incidence of death among patients receiving this drug by development of cardiac arrythmias.

10. Praxilene (Naftidrofuryl Oxalate)

This drug is used as a vasodilator and appears to induce thrombophlebitis if given intravenously. Minor side effects include headache, nausea, abdominal discomfort, diarrhea, insomnia, and vertigo. High doses produce seizures.

11. Nicergoline

This drug is said to be an alpha-adrenoreceptor blocker. Reported side effects include nausea and abdominal discomfort, and hypertension and sweating.

12. Indoramin

This drug is an alpha-adrenoreceptor blocking agent. It has a minimal negative chronotropic effect. Main side effects are sedation and tiredness. Other side effects include weakness, dizziness, dry mouth, nasal congestion, and nausea. Headache and depression have also been recorded, and weight gain due to edema is not uncommon.

13. Oxpentifylline

This drug is a methylxanthine derivative that appears to improve blood flow in peripheral vascular disease. It reduces whole blood viscosity. Vascular fibrinogen levels are reduced and fibrinolytic activity augmented. It appears efficacious in diabetics.

Side effects include nausea and vomiting, particularly on an empty stomach, as well as abdominal cramps and diarrhea. The drug may possibly interfere with control of diabetes by increasing insulin release from the pancreas. The drug has hypotensive effects and may potentiate antihypertensive drugs. Exacerbation of angina has been reported. Interference with sleep has also been noted.

14. Xanthinol Niacinate

The drug xanthinol niacinate has been used both intravenously and orally to augment the vascular flow in peripheral vascular disease.

The adverse effects are those of methylxanthines and nicotinic acid. They include digestive upset, rash, and alteration in plasma bilirubin levels.

IV. DIURETICS AND POTASSIUM CHLORIDE

Diuretics are commonly used drugs for excess fluid retention and edema.

Hypokalemia is a common side effect of most diuretics, particularly the thiazides. Unfortunately, the fall in serum potassium relates poorly to changes in total body potassium, and effects of long-term diuretic treatment on serum and body potassium are controversial. It is generally felt the people who are hypokalemic on diuretic therapy are more prone to develop arrhythmias during acute myocardial infarction whether they are on digitalis or not. On the basis of this, some authorities advocate routine potassium replacement.

Potassium-sparing diuretics are often used as a means of obviating hypokalemia. If supplementary potassium is also given, this can be dangerous due to the production of hyperkalemia.

Diuretic-induced hyponatremia has occasionally been reported.

Other adverse effects that are common, particularly with sulfonamide diuretics, are elevation of blood sugar level and glycosuria. Usually this is not a significant problem but in some diabetics adjustment of diabetic therapy may be required.

Diuretics may impair renal handling of uric acid and induce hyperuricemia. This, if asymptomatic, requires no therapy, but if there is a history of gout or if frank gout develops then the diuretic should be stopped. If the diuretic is still required, then standard treatment of the acute attack of gout with long-term allopurinol subsequently should be instituted. An acute attack usually responds to phenylbutazone or colchicine. Hypercalcemia

has been reported on occasion in conjunction with diuretic therapy, but the exact relationship of this to the diuretic (usually furosemide) is obscure.

A. CLINICAL FEATURES AND TREATMENT

1. Furosemide

This potent diuretic may occasionally cause such a profound diuresis as to induce vascular collapse. Treatment is by replacement of fluid and salt.

If high doses are given by rapid intravenous injection deafness may result.

There is some evidence that nephrotoxic effects of cephalosporins may be potentiated by furosemide.

Bullous pemphigoid skin lesions have been reported in patients receiving high and normal doses of furosemide. The condition mimics porphyria cutanea tarda.

2. Spironolactone

This can cause gynecomastia. It has been shown to interact with both the biosynthesis and the peripheral action of androgens. It may cause menstrual disturbances. A relation between use of this drug and breast cancer has been suggested but there is no good evidence to confirm this.

3. Chlorthalidone

This has been reported as causing transient myopia and retinal edema.

4. Bumetanide

This potent diuretic causes hyperuricemia and arthritis fairly frequently. Myalgia is not uncommon and may be severe. It can be used when furosemide ototoxicity has occurred.

5. Metolazone

This drug appears to have similar side effects to other diuretics, namely, hypokalemia, hyperuricemia, and hyperglycemia.

6. Ethacrynic Acid

This diuretic commonly causes nausea, vomiting, anorexia, and diarrhea. Hypokalemia and hyponatremia with metabolic alkalosis occur with prolonged usage. Gastrointestinal hemorrhage has been reported following intravenous administration. Large doses have caused vertigo tinnitus and reversible and permanent deafness. The last toxic effect is more frequent in patients with impaired renal function. Rashes, agranulocytosis, and thrombocytopenia have been reported.

7. Triamterene

This diuretic acts directly on tubular transport by inhibiting reabsorption of sodium and chloride. Potassium excretion is not affected. Toxic effects include nausea, vomiting, diarrhea, headache, and rash. It tends to produce hyperkalemia particularly in patients with congestive failure, hepatic cirrhosis or renal disease. This drug has been reported to produce megaloblastic anemia in patients with alcoholic cirrhosis of the liver. Therapy consists of parenteral folate administration.

Minor elevation in plasma cholesterol and triglyceride levels have been reported with diuretic therapy. The significance of these changes in regard to atherosclerosis is unknown. A relationship between the use of diuretics during pregnancy and the occurrence of neonatal hypoglycemia has been suggested. Evidence is still inconclusive, but such reports do emphasize the need for caution in administering any drugs during pregnancy. Diuretics frequently induce secondary hyperaldosteronism. Further problems may occur when a patient stops diuretic therapy after long-term treatment. Occurrence of edema shortly after such discontinuation has been reported mainly in younger women on diuretics for obesity and idiopathic edema. Do not restart the diuretic. No treatment is necessary.

8. Aldactazide

Aldactazide is a combination of spironolactone and hydrochlorothiazide.

9. Dyazide

Dyazide combines triamterene and hydrochlorothiazide. Combinations are used to achieve diuresis without hypokalemia and also to treat hypertension. Toxic effects are those of the individual drugs.

10. Potassium Chloride

This medication is currently available both as an oral liquid, tablet, and slow-release preparation and as an intravenous preparation. Hyperkalemia may result from rapid excess intravenous administration or from oral administration, particularly in renal insufficiency or with the concomitant use of a potassium-sparing diuretic such as spironolactone. Cardiac arrhythmias, heart block, or cardiac arrest usually in asystole may occur. ECG classically shows tall, peaked T waves. As levels rise, the QRS complex widens progressively; the P wave widens and disappears.

Oral administration may be extremely irritating with diarrhea, nausea, and vomiting. Occasional perforation and stricture have been reported subsequent to oral ingestion. Treatment of hyperkalemia involves administration of hypertonic dextrose solution and insulin, 10 units per 20 gm. of dextrose. Cation exchange resins in the sodium phase may be administered orally to sequester potassium. Hemodialysis and peritoneal dialysis are alternative modes of therapy.

Hyperkalemia has been reported in patients on combined diuretic and potassium chloride therapy. There also have been reports of severe hyperkalemia in a few such patients who have also been on antihypertensive therapy, usually beta blockade. It is suggested that very high serum potassium levels may be produced as a result of subsequent hypotension or possibly by a direct effect due to beta blockers.

V. ANTIHYPERTENSIVE AGENTS

Hydralazine and sodium nitroprusside have been discussed under vasodilator drugs.

A. PRAZOSIN

This drug acts directly to block arterial alpha-adrenergic receptors. However, there is some doubt about its long-term efficacy.

The most dramatic side effect is the first-dose orthostatic hypotensive reaction manifested as sudden syncope following an initial 2-mg. dose. It still occurs though less frequently following the currently recommended lower doses. This effect is less common with the capsule form than the tablet used in Britain. This may be due to a difference in bioavailability. Combination with a beta blocker appears to potentiate this toxic effect, and it may occur even after 0.25 mg. Currently, treatment involves changing to another agent or administering prazosin at bedtime. Orthostatic faintness and dizziness also have been described on long-term treatment with the drug. The drug produces restlessness, sleep disturbances, mental depression, pruritis, epigastric discomfort, anorexia, and diarrhea.

An interaction between prazosin and glycerol trinitrate causing syncope has been reported.

B. ADRENERGIC NEURON-BLOCKING AGENTS

These drugs are little used today except in cases resistant to other therapy. They can induce orthostatic hypotension that may be severe and incapacitating. They also cause sexual dysfunction. Tiredness, weakness, sedation, and depression are common side effects. Withdrawal of therapy may be related to acute elevations of blood pressure or cardiac arrhythmias.

C. TRIMETAPHAN

This short-acting drug is used in hypertensive crises. Its adverse effects include constipation, paralytic ileus, urinary retention, and allergic phenomena due to histamine release.

Vasodilators and quinidine may increase the hypotensive effect by additional peripheral vasodilatation.

D. LABETALOL

This is a new compound that has been shown to have both alpha- and beta-adrenoceptor-blocking properties. It can be used orally or intravenously. Intravenous medication produces a rapid fall in blood pressure and on occasion nausea, faintness, and sweating.

E. MINOXIDIL

This drug acts directly on arterial smooth muscle and is a potent vasodilator. Oral administration produces maximum blood levels in about an hour. The half-life averages 4.2 hours. The hypotensive effect sometimes requires repeated doses. The drug produces a reflex tachycardia. It causes fluid retention that may precipitate or worsen cardiac failure. This tends to make control of the hypertension more difficult. It nearly always requires combined administration with a diuretic. Palpitation is a common complaint and the tachycardia is dose-related. A beta blocker will reduce this effect. The main side effect is hypertrichosis; women in particular complain about hirsutism. Treatment is discontinuation of the drug.

F. DIAZOXIDE

This drug is a nondiuretic benzothiazide. It is usually given as a bolus injection to obtain maximal hypotensive effect which may last for 2 to 24 hours and is partly related to serum levels of the drug. The hypotensive effect is increased by keeping the head raised; the postural effect is marked. There is a concomitant tachycardia and increase in cardiac output that may exacerbate angina. Potentially serious ECG changes are not uncommon when the drug is used. Use of a beta blocker has been advocated to combat the tachycardia, but this combination may produce severe and long-lasting hypotension. Cerebral vascular problems may ensue.

A further problem is that the drug is prone to cause salt and water retention. Repeated use usually requires diuretic therapy.

The drug inhibits ureteric and gastrointestinal activity and may stop uterine contractions if given to parturient women. The drug can cause hyperglycemia with direct effect on pancreatic beta cells reducing insulin secretion. Continued use with a diuretic has been reported to result in marked hyperglycemia, and some cases of hyperglycemic coma and keto acidosis have been reported. Hyperosmolar nonketotic coma also has been reported.

Other side effects are peculiar taste sensations, nausea and vomiting, low back pain, constipation, and a burning sensation at the injection site. Hematological abnormalities include neutrocytopenia, thrombocytopenia, and eosinophilia. The drug crosses the placenta and may upset fetal carbohydrate metabolism. Children of mothers treated over longer periods with the drug have been noted to have small areas of localized alopecia.

Acute pancreatitis has been reported.

Concurrent use of a thiazide diuretic will augment the hypotensive hyperglycemic and hyperuricemic effects of the drug.

Diazoxide displaces warfarin from plasma albumin, and changes in dosage in anticoagulant may be required. The drug may cause hypertrichosis.

Prolonged use in children has produced accelerated bone maturation.

G. CLONIDINE

This antihypertensive agent produces an initial pressor response by direct stimulation of alpha-adrenergic receptors followed by a prolonged and persistent fall due to a direct central neural effect which inhibits efferent outflow from the sympathetic centers. An effective hypotensive effect is usually apparent one hour following oral administration with maximal response at two to four hours. The half-life is increased in patients with renal insufficiency.

The major toxic effect of this drug occurs when the drug is discontinued or several doses are omitted. Within 24 hours there is severe hypertension, tachycardia, sweating, uncontrollable tremor, and headache. If the drug has to be withdrawn it should be tapered off, but this may not prevent rebound hypertension. The hypertensive effect upon withdrawal may be treated with sodium nitroprusside or beta blockers. It appears that the elevated pressure is due to sudden release of catecholamines from their terminals where they have been stored as a result of the stimulation of inhibitory alpha receptors.

The initial pressor response can be abolished by prior administration of tolazine.

Clonidine also causes sedation which can be dangerous in drivers, vivid dreams and nightmares, and increased intraocular pressure and dilatation of the pupil. It may potentiate the effects of alcohol, sedatives, and central nervous system depressants. High doses combined with high doses of propranolol may worsen the central nervous system side effects.

Other side effects include dry mouth, headache, and constipation. The side effects may be minimized by taking clonidine at bedtime.

H. RESERPINE

Rauwolfia alkaloids deplete stores of catecholamines and trihydroxytryptamine in many organs including brain, heart, blood vessels, and adrenal medulla. Besides its amine-depleting action, the drug has other peripheral vasodilatory effects that occur in sympathectomized human extremities. Side effects are particularly common with high doses and in patients who are also receiving barbiturates. The major side effect is depression, which may reach suicidal levels. Because it is often insidious, it is frequently missed. The drug is a central sedative, and drowsiness, weakness, lethargy, fatigue, and headache have been noted. Undue anxiety and inability to concentrate are frequent early signs of impending toxicity.

Several reports suggest that reserpine may be linked with an increased incidence of breast cancer. The majority of the studies have been negative suggesting the relationship may be largely coincidental.

The hypotensive effects of reserpine are increased by concurrent administration of diuretics, vasodilators, or alcohol. Reserpine and tricyclic antidepressants are mutually antagonistic. The drug may predispose to cardiac arrhythmias if given in conjunction with digitalis.

Treatment consists of withdrawal of the drug. In the case of severe depression close observation or admission to the hospital is indicated until mood returns to normal.

I. METHYLDOPA

This drug inhibits dopa decarboxylase and depletes tissue stores of biogenic amines, particularly norepinephrine. The drug is converted in the body to alpha methylnorepinephrine, which may act as a false transmitter and so prevent uptake of norepinephrine by tissues. Some 50% of an oral dose is absorbed. The drug is rapidly excreted in the urine, and there is a small degree of conjugation and degradation. The drug interferes with standard chemical assays for catecholamines.

Methyldopa can cause fever, sedation, sleep disturbances, mental depression, and impotence. Several cases of drug-related hepatotoxicity confirmed by a diagnostic challenge have been reported. This hypersensitivity reaction may be serious and potentially fatal, and necessitates immediate withdrawal of the drug. Hemolytic anemia and elevated rheumatoid and antinuclear factor titers have been reported. These abnormalities have been reported in patients recently commenced upon the drug but more commonly following long-term therapy. Up tp 30% of patients on methyldopa for more than six months develop a positive Coomb's test. This is particularly the case with high-dosage regimens. However, only up to 3% of these cases develop frank hemolytic anemia.

Several skin reactions, commonly seborrheic, nummular eczema and nodular or lichen planus type, have been reported. They respond to withdrawal of the drug. Diuretics and alcohol increase the hypotensive effect of the drug.

Treatment involves withdrawal of the drug. In regard to milder side effects hypotensive therapy may be adequate on a low dose if a beta blocker is added to the therapy regimen. Most problems clear quickly but the Coomb's test may be positive for months along with other of the antoimmune phenomena. However, chronic hepatitis may develop and persist. Readministration of methyldopa to a patient showing signs of liver dysfunction is particularly dangerous.

Inability to maintain an erection, ejaculation problems, and decreased libido are common problems with the drug and are often not reported by the patients. They should be inquired after when the drug is prescribed.

J. GUANETHIDINE SULFATE

This agent acts by depleting norepinephrine stores. Maximal hypotensive effect is not apparent until two to three days after initial administration. It persists frequently for over a week after withdrawal of the drug. The drug causes fluid retention and frequently requires concomitant diuretic therapy.

The main adverse effects are orthostatic hyotension and exertional hypotension.

Use of this drug in patients with pheochromocytoma may be fatal due to accelerated hypertension due to the release of endogenous amines. Bradycardia, diarrhea, and retrograde ejaculation also occur.

VI. BETA BLOCKING DRUGS

The widespread use of these drugs emphasizes the importance of recognizing toxic side effects. They are often taken continuously for years and careful monitoring is essential to detect unwanted side effects, particularly of late onset. Practolol is a classic example of this problem: recognition of its severe ocular and abdominal toxic effects was delayed because they were not related to the drug.

Propranolol, the earliest available beta blocker, has been in clinical use for some 13 years. It is effective as an antianginal agent, an antihypertensive compound, and an antiarrhythmic. More recently oxprenolol has been released. It is generally difficult to assess the efficacy of such compounds in regard to individual patients. There is a placebo effect with virtually every drug and so symptomatic improvement is not necessarily an indication of efficacy of a particular compound. It is not practicable to challenge individual patients with sympathomimetic compounds and measure dose-related responses to evaluate individual requirements of beta blocking drugs. The resting pulse rate is occasionally used as a guide to the required propranolol doses but it is a relatively crude indication of the adequacy of beta blockage. Fortunately, most of the toxic effects are noted in the early stages of administration.

The blood level of propranolol associated with suppression of ventricular ectopic beats is similar to that which relieves symptoms of angina pectoris, 30–85 ng./ml. The drug is metabolized by the liver to 4-hydroxypropranolol, which is pharmacologically active. This conversion occurs with both oral and intravenous administration. The plasma half-life of propranolol varies between 2 hours 20 minutes and 5 hours. The peak blood levels are roughly 1–2 hours after oral administration. The excretion is largely by way of the kidneys.

The rebound phenomenon, consisting of an exacerbation of angina or frank infarction following abrupt withdrawal of propranolol, has been described. Initially, the frequency of this occurrence was considered high but experience of withdrawal of beta blockers, particularly prior to bypass surgery suggests it is in fact fairly uncommon. It appears to occur most frequently in those who had severe symptoms prior to therapy and may represent the recurrence of symptoms in a high-risk group. However, withdrawal should be gradual and treatment should be reinitiated if pain, particularly at rest, becomes severe. Many patients have been subjected to anesthesia and bypass surgery while on beta blockers.

The major toxic effects of propranolol and all beta blockers include precipitation of cardiac failure, presumably due to blockade of sympathetic stimulation in patients dependent upon a relative tachycardia or inotropy for preservation of an adequate cardiac output. (This generally occurs with initiation of beta blocker therapy and does not appear to be dose-related.) Acute bronchospasm (commonest in asthmatics), cold extremities (due to the unbalanced peripheral alpha vasoconstriction), severe hallucinations, and nightmares also occur. Cardioselective blockers such as atenolol or metopolol are less likely to cause bronchospasm and do not inhibit the bronchodilatory effect of isoproterenol. Hypoglycemia may occur, particularly in diabetics, but is generally not a problem if blood sugar is monitored and the dose readjusted. Fetal hypoglycemia and bradycardia are definite risks in pregnant mothers given beta blockers.

Propranolol may occasionally cause a paradoxical rise in blood pressure particularly in pheochromocytoma if alpha blockade is inadequate, in diabetics having hypoglycemic episodes, and in patients with mental disorders. Intravenous phentolamine and oral phenoxybenzamine have been used to treat these hypertensive episodes. Propranolol rarely causes heart block unless given in conjunction with other antiarrhythmic therapy. However, it may induce S-A or A-V block in patients with sick sinus syndrome.

Some beta blockers are partial agonists and are described as having intrinsic sympathomimetic activity. This is said to offer some protection against myocardial depression.

Metoprolol, currently available as an antihypertensive, is a cardioselective beta blocker. It may eventually be prescribed for angina. It would appear to offer a greater degree of safety in regard to acute bronchospasm compared to propranolol.

Massive propanolol overdosage usually produces severe circulatory depression in patients with poor left ventricular function. Therapy consists of large doses of atropine and beta agonists. Glucagon and calcium have also been suggested.

Propranolol appears to potentiate the adverse effects of alcohol on performance, particularly in tasks requiring attention. It has been shown to have little effect on tremor following alcohol withdrawal. Propranolol antagonizes some of the effects of smoking marijuana; in particular the increase in heart rate and arterial pressure. Impairment of the ability to learn is opposed and the characteristic "high" is reduced.

Beta-adrenergic blocking drugs may produce cold hands and feet and Raynaud's phenomenon. Beta blockers should be used with caution in patients with peripheral vascular disease.

Propranolol has been shown to produce a dose-dependent reduction in respiratory sensitivity to carbon dioxide rebreathing in normal subjects. This is considered to be a central effect, and this might produce serious consequences if the drug were given to a patient with incipient respiratory failure.

There are theoretical considerations, supported by some clinical observations, which suggest that beta blockers may be contraindicated in the syndrome of variant angina. Beta blockade may leave the alpha receptors unopposed in the coronary arteries and potentiate the degree of coronary artery spasm that is postulated to underlie variant (Prinzmetal's) angina. Therapy with trinitrin and/or verapamil seems to be safer in the first instance.

VII. ANTICOAGULANT AND PLATELET-INHIBITING DRUGS

A. HEPARIN

Heparin is a naturally occurring mucopolysaccharide present in liver, lung, and intestines. In conjunction with an alpha-2-globulin it is an antagonist of the thrombin-activated Factors IX and X and prevents fibrin formation. It has to be given by intramuscular, subcutaneous, or intravenous routes. The drug disappears exponentially from the circulation at a rate dependent upon the dose. It is metabolized by a liver enzyme, heparinase. A breakdown product, uroheparin, has some antithrombic activity and appears in the urine. A significant fraction of nonmetabolized heparin may appear in the urine. The major toxic effect of this drug is hemorrhage. Commonly this presents as hematuria or rectal blood loss. Bleeding into the wall of the small bowel and more commonly into the large bowel may occur and mimic carcinoma. Acute adrenal insufficiency due to hemorrhage has been reported as has bleeding into the abdominal wall. Severe and massive retroperitoneal hemorrhage occurs. Bleeding is prone to occur where there is already a lesion predisposed to bleeding, such as a peptic ulcer or carcinoma. It may occur at sites of infection or inflammation and may produce or convert pericarditis into tamponade. Bleeding following lumbar puncture in patients on heparin has produced quadriplegia.

Other toxic effects of heparin include thrombocytopenia which appears to have an autoimmune basis and which may precipitate micro- and macrothrombosis with diffuse intravascular coagulation.

Treatment of bleeding due to heparin involves cessation of the drug. Its effect is short-lived, and withdrawal may be adequate in cases of mild bleeding. However, where bleeding is severe, protamine sulfate, 1 mg. for 1 mg. of heparin up to a maximum of 50 mg. over a 10-minute period, should be given. The amount given depends on the interval after the administration of heparin; only 0.5 mg. of protomine is required to antagonize each 1 mg. of heparin 30 minutes after administration. Administration of excess protamine can cause hypotension and allergic reactions and should be avoided.

Heparin causes elevation of SGOT and SGPT, and this may lead to diagnostic problems. Long-term heparin therapy may produce alopecia and osteoporosis.

B. ORAL ANTICOAGULANTS

Two main groups are available: coumarins and indanediones. The latter (e.g., phenprocoumon) are little used because they produce hypersensitivity reactions. These compounds act by reducing the amounts of the coagulation factors that require vitamin K for their synthesis (Factors II, VII, IX, and X). Proteins are produced that are antigenically similar to these factors but that lack their normal procoagulant activity. Factor VII has the shortest half-life of the vitamin-K-dependent factors, and so plasma levels of this factor fall first during warfarin therapy. This produces a prolonged prothrombin time. It is considered that diminished levels of the other factors may in fact be more important for the antithrombotic effect.

The major problem related to the use of warfarin is hemorrhage. Hematuria is the most common manifestation. Deaths due to hemorrhage have largely been the result of intracerebral bleeding. The second most common cause of bleeding is from an unsuspected peptic ulcer.

Prevention is the best defense against toxic effects. Risk of hemorrhage can be minimized by following certain general principles. Uncooperative patients and those of limited intelligence are unsuitable for long-term therapy, as are patients with significant hepatic or renal disease. Severe uncontrolled hypertension, recent major head trauma, or bleeding diathesis are major contraindications. Peptic ulcer, particularly if symptomatic, usually contraindicates therapy.

The most important cause of excessive prolongation of the prothrombin time is a drug interaction. The patient should be warned about the dangers of aspirin-containing analgesics. An analgesic such as paracetamol and a hypnotic such as nitrazepam can be prescribed if required because they are not known to interact with warfarin. The list of drugs that interact with warfarin is long and a standard reference should be consulted.

Another major side effect appears to be hepatitis.

Coumadin derivatives cross the placenta and enter the breast milk of nursing mothers. The drug causes fetal abnormalities. Three types of fetal warfarin syndrome have been described. The first group are fetuses exposed during the first trimester only who develop teratogenic effects. The major abnormality is chondrodysplasia punctata (Conradi-Hunermann syndrome). The second group are those exposed for a month during the second and third trimesters, and show anomalous growth (microcephaly, optic atrophy, etc.). The third group are fetuses exposed throughout pregnancy, and develop severe nasal hypoplasia, stippled epiphyses, optic atrophy, microcephaly, and mental retardation.

The onset of action of oral anticoagulants is slow. If hemorrhage occurs, it is often prolonged. Therapy consists of stopping the drug, transfusion, and administration of large doses of vitamin K_1.

C. Thrombolytic Drugs

The drugs in current use are streptokinase, streptodornase, and urokinase. The main toxic effect of these drugs is severe hemorrhage. Streptokinase produces systemic plasmacytosis due to induction of an immune complex syndrome. This is also the probable cause of the pyrexia that occurs with the use of this drug. Streptodornase is rarely used nowadays.

1. Urokinase

This beta globulin activates plasminogen. The drug has the theoretical advantage of a greater preferential affinity for gel-phase plasminogen within a thrombus than for soluble-phase plasminogen, suggesting that infusion of urokinase should cause less systemic hyperplasminemia and risk of hemorrhage. It does not cause allergic reactions or stimulate antibody formation.

2. Streptokinase

Purified preparations of streptokinase are now available. The drug has a plasma half-life of less than 30 minutes. Immune antibodies to streptokinase occur in all individuals, probably as a result of previous streptococcal infection, but the actual concentration is extremely variable. Streptokinase therapy, therefore, should begin with an antibody-neutralizing dose followed by a maintenance dose that produces the required level of thrombolytic activity.

Like other streptococcal proteins it can act as an antigen in humans with subsequent allergic phenomena. Its use may produce pyrogenic reactions, though these are much less common now that the drug has been further purified. It activates plasminogen bound within a thrombus and also circulating plasminogen.

Allergic manifestations of streptokinase infusion include bronchospasm, chills, and pyrexia. They are particularly common if the initial dose of streptokinase is given too rapidly. Late pyrexia (at 48 hours) is not infrequent. Its mechanism is unknown. Treatment involves withdrawal of the drug and administration of steroids.

The major toxic effect is hemorrhage which may be severe. Of the many procedures available to monitor these drugs the most useful is a well-standardized thrombin clotting time which reflects the degree of hyperplasminemia. Plasmin impairs hemostasis by causing proteolysis of plasma fibrinogen and of clotting Factors V and VIII. The fibrin degradation products that it produces impair fibrin polymerization, compete with the clotting action of thrombin, and interfere with platelet function.

Therapy involves stopping the drug. This should be considered even when bleeding is not obvious if the hematocrit has fallen inexplicably. Both drugs are rapidly cleared from the circulation and these may suffice. Blood transfusion may be necessary as well as administration of a fibrinolytic inhibitor such as aminocaproic acid (EACA) or tranexamic acid (AMCA). Reconstituted lyophilized plasma is effective but stored plasma is not. In an emergency 5 gm. of EACA can be given intravenously over 30 minutes followed by an additional gram by infusion. Because of the interval between the administration of these compounds and correction of the streptokinase- or urokinase-induced coagulation defect, bleeding may continue into body cavities to produce large clots that are rich in inhibitor and resistant to lysis.

3. Fibrinolytic Inhibitors—EACA

EACA is available for both intravenous and oral administration. The drug is rapidly excreted by the kidneys. The clearance is about 75% of that of creatinine. The drug is well absorbed from the gastrointestinal tract. Peak plasma levels occur two hours after an oral dose. A single intravenous dose has a duration of action of about three hours.

A continuous infusion is necessary to maintain sustained plasma levels. A loading dose of 0.1 gm./kg. is recommended to rapidly produce a significant inhibitory plasma level. This may be followed by continuous infusion of 1 gm. per hour.

Toxic, dose-related effects are common with EACA and include nasal stuffiness, abdominal pain, nausea, headache, diarrhea, dizziness, and, rarely, arrhythmias and hypotension. The latter two effects are common with rapid intravenous infusion. Abnormal elevations of muscle enzyme levels and myoglobinuria have been reported with high-dose therapy. Reports of cardiac and hepatic necrosis have been reported.

The drug is hazardous in cases of hematuria because it tends to produce renal or ureteric clots. This complication has been fatal. Renal cortical necrosis has been reported. It has been suggested that the drug should be combined with low-dose heparin therapy to reduce thrombotic side effects.

4. Ancrod (Viper Venom)

This defibrinating agent has been used to treat thrombotic problems. It is a foreign protein and may only be given for one short course. It will lose its efficacy after several days of therapy. It can produce hematomata at the site of injection. Severe hemorrhage occurs with surgical wounds in totally defibrinated patients. The dose of ancrod is usually adjusted to produce only partial defibrination.

Allergic reactions are potentially seri-

ous. The venom alters red cell membranes and may worsen hemolysis in patients with renal microangiopathy.

D. PLATELET-INHIBITING DRUGS

1. Aspirin

This drug inhibits the platelet release reaction induced by stimuli such as antigen-antibody complexes, adrenalin, collagin, and thrombin. The drug inhibits synthesis of cyclic endoperoxides and thromboxane A2 from platelet membrane arachidonic acid. These are potent stimuli of the platelet release action and of platelet aggregation. The drug acetylates the platelet enzyme cyclo-oxygenase. In normal subjects 300 mg. of aspirin will prolong the bleeding time for up to 5 days. The platelets affected by the drug are inactivated, though their survival time is not reduced. The drug has been used as an antithrombotic agent in doses of 300–1500 mg. per day. The drug also inhibits prostaglandin synthesis by the arterial vessel wall. The toxic effects of this drug are dealt with elsewhere in this text.

2. Dipyridamole

This drug inhibits primary and secondary ADP-induced platelet aggregation and in high concentrations inhibits the platelet release reaction induced by collagen, adrenalin, and thrombin. Its effect is partly by way of stimulation of the adenyl cyclase enzyme system and inhibition of phosphodiesterase activity with a consequent increase in platelet cyclic AMP levels. In patients with thrombotic diseases, 400 mg. of the drug daily prolongs shortened platelet survival. Side effects at this level of dosage seem mild and include nausea, vomiting, diarrhea, and headache.

3. Sulfinpyrazone

Sulfinpyrazone is a nonsteroidal antiinflammatory drug that is related to phenylbutazone. It inhibits the platelet release reaction induced by collagen and adrenalin, and it inhibits adherence of platelets to subendothelial structures. The drug appears to inhibit platelet prostaglandin synthesis. An antithrombotic effect is produced with 600 to 800 mg. a day of the drug.

The drug has antiinflammatory and uricosuric effects. It is well absorbed after oral administration and is almost completely bound to plasma proteins. Some half of the oral administered dose appears in the urine in 24 hours; 90% is eliminated unchanged and the rest is metabolized.

The side effects of the drug include gastrointestinal upset which is reduced when the drug is taken in divided doses with meals. Hypersensitivity reactions include rash and fever.

VIII. HYPOLIPIDEMIC DRUGS

A. BILE ACID SEQUESTRANTS

Drugs in this group (cholestyramine, colestipol) are not absorbed and sequester bile acid and cholesterol in the gut. The liver increases the output of bile acid to meet the loss with decline of blood and body pools of cholesterol.

Many patients find these medications unpleasant to take, particularly over a long period. They cause dyspeptic symptoms which may be mild, such as flatulence, or more severe, particularly in the presence of active ulceration. They may cause constipation and diarrhea. There is a clinical impression that diarrhea is commonest among children and constipation among adults. These toxic effects need not necessitate cessation of therapy but can be dealt with by adding some dried prune and figs to the diet to deal with constipation or by the use of antidiarrheal compounds in the case of diarrhea. Hemorrhoids may be a problem.

These drugs will sequester anionic materials in the gut and will interfere with antibiotic absorption or with fat-soluble vitamin absorption. It is advisable to screen children for the possibility of vitamin deficiency or to give them prophylactic courses of fat-soluble vitamins.

B. CLOFIBRATE

This drug lowers blood lipid levels by its effect on the liver and on the peripheral metabolism of lipid. Its main action is to reduce triglycerides with a smaller reduction in cholesterol levels. The drug is given in doses of 2 gm. a day. Further increase produces little additional lipid-lowering effects.

Acute adverse effects with this drug are uncommon. The drug has been reported to cause myalgia, stiffness, weakness, and malaise, particularly in patients with nephrotic syndrome. There is evidence that administration of the drug to patients with hypothyroidism may produce a similar syndrome.

The drug displaces certain drugs from albumin. This can effect anticoagulants and require a change in dosage schedule. The drug enhances the response of diabetics to sulfonylurea therapy and necessitates a dose adjustment.

Treatment of toxic effects involves stopping the drug and treating the complication that has developed. Some of the alterations in bile secretion the drug produces may be reversed by using chenodeoxycholic acid.

C. GEMFIBROZIL

This is a clofibrate analog that has very similar effects on lipid levels, the dose is 800–1600 mg. per day. Side effects are uncommon but include dyspepsia, abdominal discomfort, nausea, and occasional allergic skin reactions. The drug has not been reported to produce the muscular syndrome of clofibrate, but clinical experience is scanty. The drug has been shown to decrease platelet adhesiveness, and care in prescribing anticoagulants is advisable.

D. NICOTINIC ACID

This drug has hepatic and peripheral metabolic effects on lipid handling by the body. It reduces both triglyceride and cholesterol levels.

Adverse effects are severe flushing and pruritis. This occurs within one to two hours after a dose and often clears after a few weeks on therapy.

Nausea, vomiting and diarrhea are not infrequent but tend to be transient. The main toxic effect is hepatotoxicity with abnormal liver function. Less commonly, the drug produces hyperglycemia. Nicotinic acid may precipitate acute gout in patients with preexisting hyperuricemia.

E. NEOMYCIN

This antibiotic increases fecal bile acid and neutral sterol excretion by forming insoluble complexes with sterols. It commonly produces diarrhea. Ototoxicity and nephrotoxicity have been reported. The drug can be hazardous in patients with reduced renal function.

F. D-THYROXIN

The sodium salt of the D-isomer of thyroxin decreases plasma cholesterol by 15 to 25% in hypercholesterolemic patients. The drug appears to accelerate low density lipoprotein (LDL) metabolism. It has fewer of the metabolic effects associated with the L-isomer. The drug can produce cardiotoxicity, including frequent ventricular ectopic beats. Myocardial infarctions were commoner in patients treated with the preparation. Other effects include glucose intolerance, abnormal liver function, and leukopenia. The drug is contraindicated in patients with proven or suspect ischemic heart disease.

G. BETA-SITOSTEROL

This vegetable sterol forms complexes with cholesterol or competitively inhibits absorption of cholesterol. Because patient variability in terms of response to this therapy is marked, the drug is not much used. It may produce diarrhea and nausea since it has a mild laxative effect. This problem may be relieved by restriction of roughage in the diet.

IX. MISCELLANEOUS DRUGS

A. ERGONOVINE MALEATE

This drug is an ergot alkaloid that is considered to be highly specific as a provocative test for coronary artery spasm. The drug is given in increasing increments up to 0.4–0.8 mg. The test is usually performed at the time of angiography, and spasm is confirmed by the angiographic appearance or ECG alterations. The test is not without risk, and myocardial infarction has been reported following use of this drug. Prolonged chest pain, bradycardia, and hypotension may occur. In addition, side effects of ergot alkaloids may be experienced: nausea, vomiting, abdominal cramps and muscle spasms.

The test should be performed only if rapid-acting vasodilators are at hand. Usually trinitrin is adequate given sublingually but it may be required intravenously. Inhalation of amylnitrate may also be used. Treatment otherwise is directed to complications of the use of this drug.

B. SARALASIN

This drug is a specific antagonist of the pressor effect of angiotension on vascular smooth muscle. It is usually used as a diagnostic agent for detecting angiotension-mediated hypertension. The drug requires prior sodium depletion because hypervolemia blunts the blood pressure response. Hypotensive shock has been reported following its use. Severe rebound hypertension has been reported following infusion of the drug. Hypertension with bradycardia, ectopics, sweating, and severe headache have occured in a patient studied with the drug who was later found to have a pheochromocytoma. Sodium nitroprusside is used to treat the hypertensive effects.

C. CARDIOVASCULAR DRUG INTERACTIONS

For a detailed discussion of interactions in this area, the reader is referred to Brater and Morrelli (1977).

BIBLIOGRAPHY

Anderson, J. L., and Mason, J. W.: Successful treatment by overdrive pacing of recurrent quinidine syncope due to ventricular tachycardia. Am. J. Med., *64:*715, 1978.

Brater, D. C., and Morrelli, H. F.: Cardiovascular drug interactions. Annu. Rev. Pharmacol. Toxicol., *17:*293, 1977.

Bremner, W. F., Third, J. L. H. C., and Lawrie, T. D. V.: Massive digoxin ingestion: report of a case and review of currently available therapies. Br. Heart J., *39:* 688, 1977.

Coffman, J. D.: Vasodilator drugs in peripheral vascular disease. N. Eng. J. Med., *300:*713, 1979.

Cottrell, J. E., Casthely, P., Brodie, J. D., Patel, K., Klein, A., and Turndorf, H.: Prevention of nitroprusside-induced cyanide toxicity with hydroxycobalamin. N. Eng. J. Med., *298:*809, 1978.

Furhoff, A. K.: Adverse reactions with methyldopa: a decade's reports. Acta Med. Scand., *203:*425, 1978.

Geltner, D., Chajek, T., Rubinger, D., and Levi, I. S.: Quinidine hypersensitivity and liver involvement: a survey of 32 patients. Gastroenterology, *70:*650, 1976.

Greiss, L., Tremblay, N. A. G., and Davies, D. W.: The toxicity of sodium nitroprusside. Can. Anesth. Soc. J., *23:*480, 1976.

Harty, R. F.: Sclerosing peritonitis and propranolol. Ann. Intern. Med., *138:*1424, 1978.

Henningsen, N. C., Cederberg, A., Hanson, A., and Johansson, B. W.: Effects of long-term treatment with procainamide. Acta Med. Scand., *198:*475, 1975.

Horn, J. R., and Hughes, M. L.: Disopyramide and dialysability. Lancet, 2214, 1978.

Humphrey, S. H., and Nash, D. A.: Lactic acidosis complicating sodium nitroprusside therapy. Ann. Intern. Med., *88:*58, 1978.

Koch-Weser, J.: Brethylium. N. Eng. J. Med., *300:*473, 1978.

Lloyd, B. L., and Smith, T. W.: Contrasting rates of reversal of digoxin toxicity by digoxin specific IgG and Fab fragments. Circulation, *58:*280, 1978.

McCrum, I. D., and Guidry, J. R.: Procainamide-induced psychosis. J.A.M.A., *240:*1265, 1978.

Nawar, T.: Hyperkalemia and overdosage of antihypertensive agents. Lancet, *1:*717, 1978.

Perkins, C. M.: Serious verapamil poisoning: treatment with intravenous calcium gluconate. Br. Med. J., *1:*112, 1978.

Romankiewicz, J. A., Reidenberg, M., Drayer, D., and Franklin, J. E.: The noninterference of aluminum hydroxide gel with quinidine sulfate absorption: an approach to control quinidine-induced diarrhea. Am. Heart. J., *46:*518, 1978.

Singh, B. N.: Side effect antiarrhythmic drugs. Pharmacol. Ther. [C], *2:*151, 1977.

Sonnenblick, E. H., Frishman, W. H., and Lejemtel, T. H.: Dobutamine: a new synthetic cardioactive sympathetic amine. N. Eng. J. Med., *300:*17, 1979.

Stockley I. H.: Interactions with oral anticoagulants. Pharmaceut. J., *210:*133, 1973.

Sunder, S. K., and Shah, A.: Constrictive pericarditis in procainamide-induced lupus erythematosus syndrome. Am. J. Cardiol., *36:*960, 1975.

Wheeler, P. J., Puritz, R., Ingram, D. V., and Chamberlain, D. A.: Amiodarone in the treatment of refractory supraventricular and ventricular arrhythmias. Postgrad. Med. J., *55:*1, 1979.

Zipes, D. P., and Troup, P. J.: New antiarrhythmic agents. Am. J. Cardiol., *41:*1005, 1978.

9. ENDOCRINE DRUGS

Richard Kozera, M.D.

Drugs used for treatment of endocrine disorders may be divided into two broad categories: natural or synthetic hormones used in physiological or pharmacological doses and nonhormonal substances used to alter the structure or function of an endocrine organ or system. Untoward effects of the drugs may be manifested by altered endocrine function or by reactions not obviously related to the endocrine system.

I. THYROID

A. THYROID HORMONES (TH):

Generic	Trade Name
Thyroxine (T$_4$)	Synthroid, Letter
Triiodothyronine (T$_3$)	Cytomel
T$_4$/T$_3$ combinations	Euthroid, Liotrix
Thyroglobolin	Proloid
Dessicated thyroid, U.S.P.	

Thyroid hormones may be used as replacement therapy for subjects with hypothyroidism, either primary or secondary, or for control of goiter growth in euthyroid persons. They may also be taken (unwisely) for control of obesity or as pep pills or "uppers."

1. Clinical Features

a. The clinical presentation of subjects taking excessive quantities of thyroid hormone is similar to that of persons with endogenous hyperthyroidism. Prolonged overuse of these drugs leads to suppression of the hypothalamic-pituitary-thyroid axis, making goiter a less common finding. There is no obvious difference in toxic manisfestations of T$_4$ or T$_3$, or their combinations, either synthetic or natural

(dessicated thyroid). Occasionally, patients on usual replacement doses of dessicated thyroid will present with symptoms of hyperthyroidism that may be due to an unusually high content of T$_3$ in that batch of tablets. Subjects acutely ingesting large quantities of thyroxine may have chemical changes that precede clinical manifestations by 24 hours.

b. Presenting signs and symptoms of TH-induced toxicosis include:

Nervousness	Tachycardia
Tiredness	Atrial fibrillation
Irritability	Warm, moist hands
Palpitations	Fine finger tremor
Preference for cold	Lid retraction
Menstrual changes	Lid lag
Weight loss	

c. The clinical presentation depends on both the quantity and duration of excess TH ingestion. Adaptive mechanisms are such that euthyroid subjects on a fixed dose of TH may develop signs and symptoms of TH excess for limited periods of time, revert to a euthyroid status, and develop toxic signs and symptoms again only if the quantity of TH ingested is increased. Hypothyroid subjects may be less tolerant of high doses of TH than euthyroid subjects.

2. Laboratory Diagnosis

a. In all instances of suspected exogenous thyroid hormone-induced thyrotoxicosis, the state of increased concentration of thyroid hormone in the blood must be established, and additional tests must be performed to separate drug-induced from naturally occurring disease.

b. Elevated serum levels of T$_4$ and T$_3$ will establish TH excess in the blood.

Normal ranges vary among laboratories depending on analytical methods used, but in general, normal T_4 values are 5–14 μg./dl.; normal T_3 values, 60–180 ng./dl. These values represent the concentration of total T_4 or T_3 in the serum. Over 99% of T_4 and T_3 is bound to thyroxine-binding globulin (TBG) and is metabolically inactive but in dynamic equilibrium with the metabolically active "free" or "unbound" hormone. Changes in the concentration of free hormone are reflected by directly proportional changes in the bound hormone if the concentration of TBG remains constant.

c. The concentration of TBG is increased in subjects who are pregnant or taking estrogens and is decreased in those taking androgens or large quantities of glucocorticoids and in a few families with a genetic predisposition. Changes in TBG are reflected by directly proportional changes in bound T_4. Serum levels of total T_4 may be high or low, but since there is no change in the concentration of free thyroxine, subjects are euthyroid.

d. The resin T_3 uptake (RT_3U) is inversely proportional to TBG concentration and should be performed whenever an altered concentration of TBG is suspected. Some physicians prefer to perform the RT_3U whenever serum T_4 is determined. Normal value for RT_3U is 25–35%. This may be expressed as a percent of a control value, with normal range of 85–105%, or as a ratio of the test serum to a control serum, with normal values of 0.85–1.05.

e. When an abnormality in TBG concentration is suspected, the free thyroxine index (FTI) provides an accurate reflection of the free thyroxine in the serum:

$$FTI = T_4 \times \frac{RT_3U \text{ in subject}}{RT_3U \text{ in control}}$$

Normal range is 4–15. A similar expression has recently been derived for T_3 but is not yet widely used clinically.

Table 9-1. **Chemical Findings of TH Toxicity**

TH excess	T_4	T_3	RT_3U	FTI
T_4	↑	↑	↑	↑
T_3	N1 or ↓	↑	N1	N1,↓
Dessicated thyroid	↑	↑	↑	↑
Dessicated thyroid	N1	↑	N1	N1
T_4/T_3	↑	↑	↑	↑

T_3 decreases serum T_4 by suppressing T_4 output by the thyroid gland.

f. Table 9-1 summarizes chemical findings in euthyroid subjects made toxic by exogenous TH.

g. Exogenous TH suppresses radioiodine uptake (RAIU) by the thyroid gland. RAIU is increased with endogenous thyrotoxicosis (Graves' disease, toxic nodular goiter). Thyrotoxicosis associated with thyroiditis will show elevated serum TH and may show decreased RAIU, but this diagnosis can be established by the presence of goiter, thyroid pain or tenderness, or antimicrosomal antibodies in the serum. RAIU may be performed at 1 or 4 hours after the dose is administered, rather than the normal 24 hours, providing timely data for early management decisions.

h. Serum studies will not be completed from 24 to 36 hours, so initial treatment will be undertaken on the basis of clinical findings and RAIU data.

3. Treatment

a. Appropriate treatment depends on the severity of the clinical presentation and the presence of underlying disease, particularly cardiovascular disorders, and should not be judged by arbitrary levels of thyroid hormone in the serum.

b. The half-life of T_4 is approximately seven days in the euthyroid and four days in the hyperthyroid state. Half-life of T_3 is about one day and probably shorter in subjects with hyperthyroidism. This gives some idea of how long the clinical syndrome will persist without further ingestion of TH.

c. Subjects without underlying disease

(1) Acute ingestion of large quantities of TH

(a) Gastric lavage, if ingestion within previous four hours.

(b) Admit to hospital for observation. Symptoms and signs may appear at 4–24 hours. Mild symptoms require no treatment, although propranolol, 10–40 mg. P.O. every 6 hours, may be used to relieve annoying symptoms of restlessness and tachycardia.

(c) Severe symptoms may be controlled with propranolol, 10–40 mg. P.O. every 6 hours, or 1–2 mg. I.V. every 1–4 hours. Sedation with diazepam may be helpful. Salicylates should be avoided because of the possibility of dissociating the protein-bound hormone, leading to increased concentration of the active "free" hormone. Reserpine, 2.5 mg. I.M. every 6 hours may be used when propranolol is contraindicated.

(d) Treatment is continued until symptoms are controlled. It is unlikely that intensive therapy would be needed beyond two or three days.

(2) Chronic ingestion of large quantities of TH

(a) Signs and symptoms are usually mild, and withdrawal of TH is all that is necessary. Propranolol, 10–40 mg. P.O. every 6 hours, or mild sedation with diazepam or phenobarbital may be given for alleviation of annoying symptoms.

(b) More severe symptoms are treated as indicated above.

(c) Subjects may develop symptoms suggestive of mild hypothyroidism following discontinuation of TH. Reassurance that the symptoms will clear within a few weeks is all that is usually needed.

d. Subjects with underlying disease

(1) Acute ingestion of large quantities of TH

(a) See above.

(b) Subjects with angina will improve with propranolol, usually administered intravenously, 0.5–2 mg. every 1–4 hours. Subjects with controlled congestive heart failure may be treated with propranolol with careful monitoring for signs of cardiac decompensation. Should these develop, the dose of propranolol may be decreased or terminated and more vigorous treatment instituted for cardiac failure. If the thyrotoxicosis is so severe that treatment other than mild sedation is necessary, plasmapheresis may be performed, which effectively removes enough circulating TH to reduce symptoms.

(c) Subjects with underlying thyroid disease are treated as indicated above.

(d) Patients who may have adrenal insufficiency or who are taking physiological doses of glucocorticoids should receive the equivalent of 200–300 mg. of hydrocortisone for the first 24–48 hours. This may then be rapidly (two to four days) returned to physiological doses of steroids. Patients on pharmacological doses of steroids may require increased amounts to maintain the desired effect because steroids will be cleared from the blood more rapidly in subjects with thyrotoxicosis.

B. IODIDES

1. The ingestion of iodides frequently interferes with laboratory tests of thyroid function but infrequently leads to overt disease. Nevertheless, ingestion of inorganic iodides such as saturated solution of potassium iodide (SSKI) and Lugol's solution, iodides found ubiquitously in proprietary medicines, especially cold remedies, and organic iodides found in x-ray contrast media may cause either hypothyroidism or hyperthyroidism (Jod-Basedow's disease). These problems are more frequently seen in subjects with nodular goiters.

2. Diagnosis is made by history, with laboratory confirmation of deficient or excessive thyroid hormone in the blood.

3. Management is conservative. Iodides are discontinued. Hypothyroidism may be treated with thyroxine 0.1–0.2 mg./day. Symptomatic hyperthyroidism is treated initially with mild sedation or propranolol until the disease process has abated. If hyperthyroidism becomes permanent, standard therapy with thionamides, radio iodine, or surgery is prescribed.

C. RADIOIODINE (^{131}I, ^{123}I)

1. The small amount of iodide administered as radioiodine is extremely small and causes adverse reactions only in those allergic to iodides. In these persons, radionuclide uptake and scan may be performed with ^{99m}Tc (Technetium-99m) pertechnetate.

2. Adverse reaction to the biological effects of radioactivity are not seen in doses of radioiodine (^{131}I or ^{123}I) given for diagnostic uptakes and scans (usually 10–100 μCi.). Larger doses (greater than 5 mCi.) given either for treatment of thyrotoxicosis or ablation of thyroid remnants in thyroid carcinoma may cause radiation thyroiditis or thyroid storm.

   a. Radiation thyroiditis is seen infrequently after treatment of thyrotoxicosis with usual doses of 5 to 10 mCi. The incidence increases with the size of the dose, and is quite common above 20 mCi. The usual symptoms are mild discomfort on swallowing and tenderness to touch, although moderate to severe pain may develop in the area of the thyroid gland. The process is self-limited and usually lasts for a few days to a few weeks. Treatment is symptomatic with nonsalicylate analgesics.

   b. Persons with thyroid ablation receiving radioiodine may be given doses as high as 100 mCi., but because of a reduced mass of functioning, tissue will not transport ("trap") a large percentage of ^{131}I within the thyroid gland, making radiation thyroiditis no more of a clinical problem than in the treatment of thyrotoxicosis.

   c. Therapeutic doses of radioiodine are contraindicated in persons with retrosternal goiter. Such persons may develop increasing dyspnea secondary to tracheal compression from the edema accompanying radiation thyroiditis. This constitutes a medical emergency and may necessitate intubation or tracheostomy.

   d. A few cases of thyroid storm have been reported in thyrotoxic persons treated with radioiodine. Storm may be defined as a potentially life-threatening syndrome which consists of exaggerated manifestations of thyrotoxicosis and temperature above 101°F (38°C). Treatment is with:

   (1) Iodides: Sodium iodide, 1 gm. I.V. per 24 hours or SSKI, 5 drops P.O., 3 times daily.

   (2) Propylthiouracil: 100 mg. every 8 hours P.O., or by nasogastric tube if necessary.

   (3) Propranolol: 20–40 mg. every 4–6 hours, P.O., or 1–2 mg. I.V., every 1–4 hours.

   (4) Hydrocortisone: 300 mg. I.V. given continuously over 24 hours.

   (5) I.V. fluids containing B-complex vitamins and at least 150 gm. glucose per 24 hours.

   Although some authorities treat the syndrome with propranolol alone, it is felt that the entire therapeutic regimen outlined above should be given.

D. THIONAMIDES: PROPYLTHIOURACIL (PTU), METHIMAZOLE (TAPAZOLE)

1. These drugs block thyroid hormone synthesis within the thyroid gland and are used to treat thyrotoxicosis. In usual doses (PTU, 50–300 mg. per day; methimazole 15–30 mg. per day), they may produce goiter. In these or higher doses they may produce hypothyroidism. Occasionally they cause gastrointestinal distress or skin rash, and less commonly they may produce hepatitis or inhibition of myelopoiesis. Both metabolic and other adverse effects are reversible on dis-

continuation of the drug. Subjects sensitive to one drug may be tolerant of the other, but it is inadvisable to substitute one drug for another in patients with major adverse reactions, and only quite cautiously in subjects with minor adverse reactions. Induced hypothyroidism is controlled by decreasing the dose of the thionamide. Addition of thyroid hormone is rarely indicated.

2. Thionamides cross the placenta from mother to fetus, in whom they will commonly induce goiter, and uncommonly hypothyroidism. Both problems are minimized by treating the mother with the smallest dose of thionamide required to control her hypothyroidism. Addition of thyroid hormone to the regimen does not further protect the fetus, since there is little if any transfer of thyroid hormone across the placenta from mother to fetus.

3. Because thionamides are secreted into breast milk, they may cause neonatal goiter or hypothyroidism in infants who are breast feeding. The only acceptable treatment is maternal avoidance of thionamides.

II. CARBOHYDRATE DRUGS

This section deals with substances that cause hypoglycemia or hyperglycemia. Hypoglycemic agents may be categorized into two groups: those which are used in the treatment of diabetes and those which interfere with glucose homeostasis. Hyperglycemic agents include those used in the treatment of organic hypoglycemia and others which promote glycogenolysis or gluconeogenesis or interfere with insulin release or activity. The hypoglycemic agents may present the more serious problems because they are more apt to be taken in suicide gestures or attempts, and because the management of drug-induced hypoglycemia is frequently treated rather casually, ignoring the potential seriousness of the problem.

A. HYPOGLYCEMIA

1. Clinical Features

a. Signs and symptoms of hypoglycemia may be divided into two categories: sympathetic and cerebral (Table 9-2). The former are more closely related to the rate of fall of blood sugar, and the latter to the degree and duration of hypoglycemia.

Selection of a critical level of plasma sugar below which hypoglycemia exists is fraught with hazard and deception. Recent studies have demonstrated that after a 72-hour fast normal women may reach a plasma sugar level 30 mg./dl. and remain completely asymptomatic. It has been suggested that further diagnostic evaluation be carried out in women with blood sugars less than 40 mg./dl. and men with blood sugars less than 60 mg./dl. It is probably still best to use the criteria of Whipple's triad as the clearest indicator of clinically important hypoglycemia:

(1) Cerebral symptoms of hypoglycemia

(2) A low plasma sugar when symptoms occur

(3) Prompt response to glucose (usually given as 25–50 gm. I.V.)

2. Classification

a. Although this section is primarily intended to deal with drug-related hypoglycemia, it must be remembered that the clinical presentation does not define the etiology. This can be determined only by extensive history taking, complete physical examination, and appropriate diagnostic studies. A simple classification which covers the more frequent causes of hypoglycemia is as follows:

Organic
Hyperinsulinism: islet cell tumors, hyperplasia
Hypopituitarism
Adrenocortical hypofunction
Diabetes mellitus

Hepatic disease
Fibrosarcomas
CNS lesions

Reactive
Prediabetic
Postgastrectomy
Idiopathic (functional)

Drug-Induced
See below, B, "Hyperglycemia"

Artificial
Test tube metabolism of glucose, especially if serum is not separated quickly or WBC is high, and no glycolysis inhibitor is added.

3. Initial Treatment

a. Hypoglycemia should be suspected in anyone presenting with the cerebral or sympathetic symptoms listed in Table 9-2.
  b. Draw blood for:
     Plasma sugar (in a tube with inhibitor of glycolysis)
     Cortisol (for pituitary or adrenal insufficiency)
     Growth hormone (for pituitary insufficiency)
     Insulin (for organic hyperinsulinism)
     Drug concentration
  c. Collect urine specimen for toxic screen.
  d. Begin I.V. infusion of D_5W. Administer 50 ml. of 5% dextrose in water I.V. over 3–5 minutes. Repeat in 15 minutes if no response.
  e. For subsequent treatment, see sections below.

4. Hypoglycemic Agents

a. Insulin

(1) Patient-induced insulin hypoglycemia may be accidental or intentional. Almost all diabetics have insulin reaction from time to time and usually present with sympathetic symptoms that are readily recognized by the patient and

Table 9-2. **Symptoms of Hypoglycemia**

Sympathetic	Cerebral
Weakness	Headache
Nervousness	Bizarre behavior
Tremulousness	Visual changes
Anxiety	Confusion
Hunger	Torpor
Sweating	Coma
Palpitations	Convulsions
Tachycardia	

promptly self-treated by ingestion of sugar. Rarely, an accidental overdose may produce severe sympathetic and even cerebral symptoms requiring treatment by a physician. Overdoses of insulin by diabetics are more commonly seen during the adolescent years when prescribed treatment regimens may be abandoned or replaced by experimentation. Patients may become "brittle," swinging from symptomatic hyperglycemia to hypoglycemia.

(2) Rarely, a person will take hundreds or thousands of units of insulin in a suicide gesture or attempt. This differs from the usual case of mild insulin overdose in that the absorption of insulin from the injection site and its subsequent metabolism changes. The hypoglycemia produced is severe and prolonged to many times the usual duration of action of the insulin taken. Several hundred units of regular (crystalline zinc) insulin injected into one site has produced hypoglycemia for several days.

(3) Laboratory studies in patients with insulin-induced hypoglycemia and without other endocrine disease reflect the process of gluconeogenesis and show high serum cortisol (usually above 20 μg./dl.) and growth hormone (usually above 7 ng./dl.) levels. Serum insulin levels will be disproportionately high for the level of blood sugar (greater than 10 $\mu\mu$/ml.).

(a) Patients who have received insulin for more than a few weeks will have circulating antibodies to insulin that interfere with the laboratory measurement of

Table 9-3. Sulfonylureas

Generic	Trade Name	Duration of Action (hours)
Acetohexamide	Dymelor	12–24
Chlorpropamide	Diabenese	60–96
Tolazamide	Tolinase	14–24
Tolbutamide	Orinase	12

serum insulin done by radioimmunoassay. A double antibody method will report a very high level of insulin whereas a method using charcoal separation will report a very low level of insulin. A detailed explanation of this phenomenon is beyond the scope of this chapter, but the clinician must always keep it in mind to avoid incorrect interpretation of lab results.

(b) If the patient presenting with hypoglycemia is a known diabetic who is known to have taken an overdose of insulin, serum insulin, cortisol and growth hormone need not be measured. If he is not known to have taken an overdose of insulin, serum should be obtained for cortisol and growth hormone measurement and other studies that may be indicated by subsequent evaluation.

b. **Sulfonylureas**

(1) The sulfonylureas used in this country are listed in Table 9-3, together with their approximate durations of action. When given acutely, sulfonylureas act directly on the pancreatic beta cells to cause insulin release. When given chronically their mechanism of action is unknown.

(2) Sulfonylurea metabolism and excretion is diagrammed in Figure 9-1. Hepatic or renal impairment may have a profound effect on the intensity and duration of sulfonylurea-induced hypoglycemia. When taken in large doses, as in a suicide attempt, the duration of hypoglycemia is unpredictable and may be several times as long as Figure 9-1 indicates. Such persons may drift in and out of hypoglycemia for several days, even under appropriate medical therapy.

(3) Laboratory evaluation of patients with suspected sulfonylurea hypoglycemia should include blood and urine screening for sulfonylureas in addition to the basic studies obtained on all patients with suspected hypoglycemia. Sugar will be low; cortisol, growth hormone, and insulin will be elevated. Sulfonylurea overdose is at least as common a cause of hyperinsulinemia with hypoglycemia as endogenous organic hypoglycemia, demonstrating the importance of the toxic screen for sulfonylureas in arriving at a correct diagnosis.

(4) Chronic administration of sulfonylurea may be associated with hypoglycemia if the clinical or nutritional status of the patient changes. Long-term toxic effects of the sulfonylureas remain largely undefined. The University Group Diabetes Program (UGDP) has generated data strongly suggesting that at least one sulfonylurea, tolbutamide, given for more than five years, may be cardiotoxic and lead to increased deaths from myocardial infarction. Whether this may be attributed to other sulfonylureas remains an open question.

c. **Phenformin (DBI, Meltrol)**

(1) Phenformin is now available for the treatment of diabetes only under special circumstances. Nevertheless, enough remains available to necessitate awareness of its toxicity. Although it does not cause insulin release, it directly promotes glucose uptake by peripheral tissues and may delay gastrointestinal absorption of nutrients.

(2) In addition to hypoglycemia, phenformin causes lactic acidosis in a small percentage of patients, particularly those with hepatic, renal, cardiovascular, or pulmonary disease.

(3) Laboratory studies, in addition to those listed in section 3, "Initial Treatment," should include serum bicarbonate, serum lactate, arterial blood pH, and P_{CO_2}. Sugar will be low; cortisol and growth hormone, high; insulin, low; bicar-

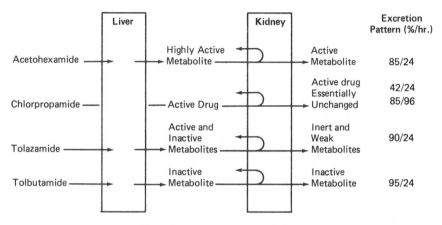

Fig. 9-1. Sulfonylurea metabolism.

bonate, low; lactate, proportionately elevated; pH; and P_{CO_2}, low.

(4) Phenformin is associated with an increased risk of cardiovascular death when taken for several years, according to data generated in the UGDP study.

d. Ethanol

(1) In a large city hospital emergency room, ethanol stands second only to insulin as a cause of hypoglycemia. The induced inhibition of hepatic gluconeogenesis superimposed on acute or chronic starvation can lead to severe and prolonged hypoglycemia, with potentially disastrous consequences, ranging from permanent neurological deficits to death.

(2) As a consequence of ethanol metabolism by the liver, lactic acid production is increased and its utilization decreased. The lactic acidosis may be quite severe and unresponsive to therapy.

(3) Alcoholics who have hypoglycemia do not necessarily have alcoholic hypoglycemia, and not all alcoholics with poor nutrition develop hypoglycemia. It is well, therefore, to always look for other underlying disorders. Hypocortisolism, for example, with its accompanying poor gluconeogenesis will aggravate the inhibitory effect of alcohol on gluconeogenesis.

Thus, persons with this combined problem are quite prone to the development of clinical hypoglycemia.

(4) Laboratory studies are listed in section 3, "Initial Treatment."

e. Other Drugs

(1) A great many other drugs have been reported to cause hypoglycemia, some when given in standard therapeutic doses and others when administered in large amounts.

(2) The following drugs have caused serious hypoglycemia:

Propranolol (Inderal)	Blocks hepatic glycogenolysis
Clonidine (Catapres)	Blocks hepatic glycogenolysis, Blocks catecholamine inhibition of insulin release
Phenotalamine (Regitine)	Blocks catecholamine inhibition of insulin release

Again, it must be emphasized that although these drugs and those listed below have clearly been associated with the development of hypoglycemia in patients, it is an unusual complication.

(3) Drugs causing mild to moderate hypoglycemia include:

Guaneth-idine	Methy-sergide	Reserpine
Leucine	Methyl xanthines (amino-phylline)	Monoamine oxidase inhibitors
Glucagon		
Oxytetra-cycline	Salicylates	Acetami-nophen
Chlorpro-mazine plus	Propoxy-phene	Ethion-amide
Orphen-adrine	Haloperidol	

(4) Hypoglycemia may be produced or enhanced by drug interactions:

(a) Bishydroxycoumarin and sulfonamides inhibit the metabolism of sulfonylurea.

(b) Phenylbutazone prolongs the half-life of hydroxyhexamide, an active metabolite of acetohexamide.

(c) Anabolic steroids and salicylates displace sulfonylureas from their protein-binding sites.

Potentially offending drugs must be searched for in anyone presenting with hypoglycemia of any degree. Mechanisms of action may be largely unknown and the causal relationships established only by withdrawal and rechallenge, but such drugs must be identified and withdrawn from susceptible patients.

5. Treatment

a. Hospitalize the patient with hypoglycemia if:

(1) The cause is unknown.

(2) It is induced by sulfonylureas.

(3) It is caused by severe insulin overdosage.

b. Lavage the stomach to remove any remaining drug.

c. The cornerstone of medical therapy is intravenous glucose: high enough for long enough. After initial therapy with one or two ampules of 50% dextrose in water I.V. (25–50 gm. glucose), a continuous glucose infusion should be begun, using whatever concentration is necessary to maintain the plasma sugar at 100 mg./dl. Usually 5% or 10% dextrose in water is sufficient, in quantities to provide 150–300 gm. glucose for 24 hours. Occasionally higher concentrations of glucose will be required. This should be given into a central vein. If the patient is sufficiently alert and can tolerate food, he may eat, but the I.V. glucose should be continued.

The rate of glucose infusion may be decreased at any rate that will maintain plasma glucose at about 100 mg./dl. The common error is to taper too rapidly. Patients with sulfonylurea, severe insulin, or alcoholic hypoglycemia may, for a few days, suddenly and without warning, drop their blood sugar levels and develop severe sympathetic or cerebral symptoms. It is better, therefore, to err on the side of too much rather than too little glucose. The patient should remain hospitalized until his glucose is stable, and off I.V. glucose therapy for at least 24 hours.

d. Some authors recommend the addition of hydrocortisone hemisuccinate, 100–300 mg. I.V. per day. This probably is unnecessary except in patients with pituitary or adrenal hypofunction.

e. Glucagon, 1 mg. subcutaneously, is occasionally used to correct hypoglycemia, especially in pediatric age groups, but this is a temporizing measure only, and not a substitute for glucose.

f. Diazoxide, which decreases insulin secretion and inhibits peripheral glucose utilization, is not useful in acute treatment of hypoglycemia.

B. HYPERGLYCEMIA

1. As blood sugar concentration rises above the normal range, patients experience a diminution in their cerebral function, which may be obvious or subtle with

vague symptoms of malaise or fatigue. As blood sugar rises into the 200s, an osmotic diuresis and secondary thirst develop. As it continues to rise, these symptoms become more severe, and when high enough to cause a serum osmolality of $\geq$ 340 mOsm./liter stage I.V. coma occurs.

2. Many drugs may cause symptomatic hyperglycemia in an apparently normal population, but persons with diabetes mellitus are at special risk and are more likely to develop severe drug-induced hyperglycemia with ketoacidosis or hyperosmolar coma.

3. Laboratory diagnosis for suspected glucose hyperosmolar coma should include plasma glucose and serum osmolality. For suspected ketoacidosis, laboratory diagnosis should include serum Na, K, Cl, HCO_3; arterial blood gases; and serum and urine ketones.

4. Steroids (glucocorticoids) are the most common causes of drug-induced hyperglycemia. They may precipitate hyperosmolar coma or ketoacidosis. They increase gluconeogenesis, diminish glucose utilization, antagonize the effect of insulin and, at least in prediabetics, diminish the amount of insulin secreted in response to a given stimulus.

5. Diazoxide (Proglycem) is a thiazide that causes sodium retention, diminishes insulin secretion, and inhibits peripheral glucose utilization. Its effectiveness in diminishing insulin secretion makes it particularly useful in treating states of organic hyperinsulinism (e.g., beta-cell adenoma of the pancreas). Its effect on sodium and water retention is easily managed by a thiazide or loop diuretic. On prolonged use, it may cause hirsutism, which no specific regimen will prevent or treat. Excess hair is removed by shaving, a depilatory or electrolysis.

6. Streptozotocin (investigational) is an antibiotic with antitumor properties, and has a cytotoxic effect on the pancreatic beta cell. It has been used in the treatment of functioning islet-cell tumors, especially islet-cell carcinoma. Its most common serious toxicity is renal tubular damage, for which proteinuria is the earliest manifestation. Toxicity is reversible at this point with discontinuation of the drug. Interestingly, streptozotocin has not produced overt clinical diabetes in patients with non-insulin-secreting malignancies.

L-Asparaginase is another antitumor agent which will cause pancreatic destruction.

7. Diuretics, including thiazides and loop diuretics, cause hyperglycemia primarily through induced hypokalemia leading to potassium depletion in the pancreas and consequent interference with insulin release.

8. Other drugs causing hyperglycemia by a variety of mechanisms include:

Diphenylhydantoin (Dilantin)	Epinephrine
Sympathomimetics	Phenothiazines
Oral contraceptive agents	Thyroid hormones

9. Treatment

a. Mild asymptomatic hyperglycemia, with plasma glucose in the 100s, probably needs no specific treatment. Diabetics may require minor adjustment of insulin regimens.

b. Moderate to severe hyperglycemia, almost always symptomatic, may require initiation of insulin therapy if the offending drug cannot be discontinued.

c. Hyperosmolar coma is treated as outlined in section 3 on page 94.

d. Diabetic ketoacidosis is treated according to any standard regimen.

III. ADRENAL/STEROIDS

A. GLUCOCORTICOIDS/ MINERALOCORTICOIDS

Most steroid preparations have both glucocorticoid (GC) or mineralocorticoid

Table 9-4. **Steroid Preparations**

Generic	Proprietary	Relative GC Potency	Relative MC Potency
Hydrocortisone (cortisol)	CORTEF	1	1
Cortisone		0.7	0.7
Prednisone	Deltasone, Meticorten	4	0.7
Prednisolone	Delta-Cortef, Meticortelone	4	0.7
Triamcinolone	Aristocort, Kenalog	3	0
Dexamethasone	Decadron, Gammacorten, Hexadrol	30	2
Methylprednisolone	Medrol	5	0.5
Fludrocortisone	Florinef	10	400

(Liddle, G. W., and Melmon, K. L.: The adrenals. *In* Williams, P. H. (ed.): Textbook of Endocrinology. 5th ed., p. 246. Philadelphia, W. B. Saunders, 1974)

(MC) effects. At doses used for physiological replacement, available preparations will have primarily GC or MC effects, but at pharmacological doses, drugs with primarily GC activity will show a significant amount of MC effect, and vice versa. Steroid preparations in common use are listed in Table 9-4.

For reference, average doses of steroids per day for physiological replacement are: hydrocortisone 30 mg., cortisone, 37.5 mg.; prednisone, 7.5 mg.; fludrocortisone, 0.1 mg (in conjunction with a glucocorticoid).

Persons with steroid toxicity are usually taking pharmacological doses as prescribed by a physician, most commonly for asthma or arthritis. Intentional chronic ingestion of steroids for their euphoric effect is rare. Some persons may embark on a long-term course of steroids for inappropriate reasons, such as to "build them up" or to cure some real or imagined chronic illness. In these instances, the source of the drug may be a friend or relative in a medical or paramedical profession. All such possibilities must be pursued intensively, since the patient or provider may be reluctant to disclose this information.

1. Clinical Features

a. Cushing's syndrome is the well-known presentation of chronic steroid excess, but there are some differences in the manifestations of endogenous and exogenous hypercortisolism (Table 9-5). Effects seen also depend on the glucorticoid/mineralocorticoid potency of the agent taken.

b. Acute ingestion of large quantities of steroids by normal subjects is either inadvertent or just one of a large number of drugs taken in a suicide attempt. It is of little concern because the drug is cleared from the body in a few hours and meta-

Table 9-5. **Hypercortisolism: Clinical Features**

More Common in Endogenous Disease	More Common in Exogenous Disease	Common to Both
Hypertension	Benign intracranial hypertension	Centripetal obesity
Abnormal menses/impotence	Glaucoma	Edema
Hirsutism/virilism	Posterior subcapsular cataract	Poor wound healing
Striae	Aseptic necrosis of bone	Proximal muscle weakness
Purpura	Panniculitis	Osteoporosis/fractures
Plethora	Euphoria	Hyperglycemia
Depression		Hypokalemia
		Metabolic alkalosis

Table 9-6. **Effect of Exogenous Steroids on Body Fluid Levels of Endogenous Steroids**

Exogenous Steroid	Serum Cortisol	Urine-Free Cortisol	17-Hydroxy-steroids	17-Keto-steroids
Hydrocortisone	↑	↑	↑	↓
Cortisone	↑	↑	↑	↓
Other synthetic steroid	↓	↓	↓	↓

bolic effects are slight. Persons with diabetes mellitus in poor control, however, may develop diabetic ketoacidosis or hyperosmolar coma.

2. Laboratory Diagnosis

a. The laboratory provides limited direct evidence for immediate diagnosis of states of GC or MC excess. Ready measurement of serum or urinary levels of steroids other than hydrocortisone is not available in most laboratories. Specialized laboratories have developed methods for the determination of other GC in the blood.

b. Steroid measurements are not indicated in subjects taking prescribed pharmacological doses of steroids. The signs and symptoms that develop are known and predictable consequences of such therapy.

c. Steroid measurements are indicated in (1) subjects not known to be taking steroids who present with clinical features of steroid excess, and (2) subjects with unexplained hypokalemic and, hypochloremic metabolic alkalosis.

Serum may be sampled at any time. A 24-hour urine specimen should be collected for analysis. Serum and urine specimens may be frozen for future measurement of steroids other than hydrocortisone.

d. Pharmacological doses of steroids will suppress the hypothalamic-pituitary-adrenal (HPA) axis, causing diminished production of endogenous hydrocortisone. Cortisone is in physiological equilibrium with hydrocortisone (Table 9-6).

(1) Determination of 17-ketosteroids, while not essential, will help to separate states of exogenous GC excess, in which they are depressed, from states of endoge-

nous GC excess, in which they are normal or elevated.

(2) Measurement of serum ACTH levels is not helpful since it will be suppressed in both exogenous GC excess and GC-producing adrenal adenomas. In addition, ACTH assays are expensive and not readily available.

e. Subjects suspected of steroid toxicity should also have determination of a complete blood count, serum electrolytes, and glucose. Hemoglobin is usually normal. The white blood count may be high as a result of release of the marginated pool seen transiently after acute ingestion of steroids. Sodium is usually normal. Depending on the dose and type of steroid and duration of ingestion, potassium and chloride may be low and bicarbonate high. Glucose may be elevated, especially in subjects with latent diabetes.

3. Treatment

a. GC effects such as centripetal obesity and osteoporosis must be accepted as an inevitable consequence of daily pharmacological doses of steroids. Whenever possible, attempts should be made to reduce these effects and minimize suppression of the HPA axis by employing alternate-day therapy. This and other metabolic effects are reversible or stabilize on discontinuation of the GC.

b. Hypokalemia that is asymptomatic or associated with mild symptoms of nausea or anorexia may be treated by oral administration of potassium chloride, 40–80 mEq. per day. Intravenous potassium chloride is indicated in cases of serious potassium depletion with severe muscle weakness or paralysis, ileus, hypotension, depressed mentation, or cardiac arrhythmia. Although administration of 5–15 mEq. of potassium chloride per hour is usually safe in these patients, it should be accompanied by continuous electrocardiographic monitoring. Treatment is continued until the serum potassium returns to normal. Subsequent potassium chloride may be administered by mouth if possible. As indicated above, these patients will often have a metabolic alkalosis. Should a state of metabolic acidosis exist, much larger doses of potassium chloride will be necessary. An initial dose of 15–20 mEq. per hour I.V. is begun, and may be increased as needed. Larger quantities should be given into a central vein. Under extraordinary circumstances, over 100 mEq. per hour has been given.

c. Hyperosmolar nonketotic coma is manifested by a progressively decreasing state of consciousness to coma that is caused by a progressive increase in plasma osmolality. Steroids have precipitated the syndrome by contributing to increased concentration of glucose in the blood. The diagnosis is established by extreme hyperglycemia and a plasma osmolality of greater than 340 mOsm./liter which may be measured directly or estimated with the following formula:

$$Osm = 2 \ (Na^+ \ mEq./liter) + \frac{glucose \ mg./dl.}{18} + \frac{BUN \ mg./dl.}{2.8}$$

(1) Initial Therapy

(a) Half-normal saline (normal saline if shock intervenes). In addition to usual daily fluid needs, replace one-half the estimated volume deficit in the first 12 hours, the remainder over the next 36 hours.

(b) Insulin, 8 units per hour I.V., until the blood sugar returns to normal.

(c) Potassium 10–15 mEq./liter of fluid if there is no renal failure. Monitor serum potassium, and ECG.

(d) Diabetic ketoacidosis may be precipitated by steroids and is treated according to any standard regimen utilizing subcutaneous or continuous intravenous insulin, fluids, and potassium.

(e) Benign intracranial hypertension (pseudotumor cerebri) may be caused by steroids or steroid withdrawal. In the former case the syndrome may be self-limited and require only symptomatic treatment. There is no good evidence that steroids should be withdrawn. In difficult cases, consult a neurologist. If associated with steroid deficiency, the syndrome responds to physiological doses of steroids.

4. Withdrawal

a. Steroid withdrawal must always be undertaken cautiously. Pharmacological doses of steroids given for longer than a week result in HPA suppression. As the dose administered approaches the physiological replacement dose, HPA suppression takes longer to develop, perhaps as long as a month. Abrupt withdrawal of steroids may lead to mild to moderate symptoms of malaise, fatigue, and arthralgias (steroid withdrawal syndrome), acute adrenocortical insufficiency with nausea, vomiting, hyperthermia, and vascular collapse, or an exacerbation of the underlying disease being treated. A reasonable and conservative approach for withdrawal would be to taper steroid dosage over several days to the physiological range and then taper to discontinuation over several weeks.

b. Permanent HPA suppression from exogenous steroids has not been documented. Full recovery of the HPA axis after prolonged high dose steroid administration may take up to 12 months after discontinuation of steroids. These persons, when subjected to physical illness, trauma, or surgery, should be maintained on steroids until the acute event is over.

B. ANTIADRENAL AGENTS

Four drugs are used to treat states of glucocorticoid excess, three marketed and one investigational. One of these, the anti-

histamine antiserotonin drug cyprohepta-
dine (Periactin), is thought to work by
suppressing pituitary ACTH secretion but
is of doubtful value and has no defined
endocrine toxicity. The other three, mitotane (o,p' DDD, Lysodren), metyrapone
(Metopirone), and aminoglutethimide
(Elipten, investigational), have direct
effects on adrenal steroid metabolism
and produce adrenal insufficiency as a
major toxic effect. They are most commonly used in treatment of Cushing's
syndrome caused by adrenocortical carcinoma but have been used to treat other
causes of Cushing's syndrome. All have
low abuse potential.

1. Clinical Features

Depending on the way the antiadrenal
drug is used, toxicity may be manifested
by signs and symptoms of acute and/or
chronic adrenal insufficiency (Table 9-7).

a. Mitotane is a drug approved and
used for the treatment of adrenocortical
carcinoma and occasionally used to treat
other causes of Cushing's syndrome. It
suppresses steroid production, alters peripheral steroid metabolism, and has an
estrogenlike effect in increasing blood levels of cortisol-binding globulin. Because
of these complex metabolic interactions,
its biochemical effect is best measured by
urinary-free cortisol excretion or a cortisol secretion rate. Its most prominent side
effects are nausea and vomiting, symptoms also seen with adrenal insufficiency.
Treatment includes discontinuing the
drug or lowering its dosage, symptomatic
treatment of nausea and vomiting, and
steroids for adrenal insufficiency as listed
below.

b. Metyrapone is an 11 beta-hydroxy-
lase inhibitor, preventing the conversion
of 11-deoxycortisol to cortisol. Although
primarily used as a diagnostic agent to
determine the integrity of the HPA axis,
it is occasionally used for short periods of
time in the treatment of states of cortisol
excess, especially adrenocortical carcino-

Table 9-7. **Adrenal Insufficiency**

Acute	Chronic	
Hypotension	Weakness	Hypoglycemia
Nausea	Hypotension	Hyperkalemia
Vomiting	Syncope	Hyponatremia
Hyperthermia	Salt-craving	Vomiting
Vascular collapse	Anorexia	Nausea

ma. Its toxicity is that of adrenal insufficiency, but the half-life of the drug is very
short and its metabolic effects dissipate in
a few hours, obviating the need for prolonged treatment.

c. Aminoglutethimide (investigational)
was originally released as an anticonvulsant but was withdrawn when its effect
on steroid metabolism became known. It
interferes with an early step in cortisol
synthesis (cholesterol $\rightarrow \Delta$ 5 pregneno-
lone) and can be used to perform a
"chemical adrenalectomy." The toxicity is
that of adrenal insufficiency.

2. Treatment: Drug-induced Adrenal Insufficiency

a. Discontinue the offending drug.

b. If symptoms are mild, draw blood
for cortisol determination (24-hour urine
for mitotane-treated patients) and treat
with physiological doses of glucocorticoids (cortisol, 30 mg. per day; prednisone, 7.5 mg. per day). Mild symptoms
related to metyrapone toxicity do not
need steroid treatment.

c. If symptoms are moderate to severe,
draw blood for serum cortisol and give
hydrocortisone hemisuccinate, 100 mg.
I.V. over 3 minutes, followed by continuous I.V. drip of 200–300 mg. over 24
hours. Taper dosage as patient stabilizes.
All I.V. fluids should contain glucose and
saline. Five to seven liters may be required over the first 24 hours. If blood
pressure does not respond satisfactorily,
give deoxycorticosterine in oil (DOCA), 5
mg. I.M. Volume expanders and vasopressors may be necessary.

Table 9-8. **Drugs Used in the Treatment of Diabetes Insipidus**

Generic	Proprietary	Usual Duration of Action (hr.)	Route of Administration
Hormone Replacement			
Vasopressin, aqueous	Pitressin	3–6	Subcutaneous
Vasopressin tannate in oil	Pitressin tannate in oil	24–72	Intramuscular
Lysine vasopressin (lypressin)	Diapid	2–6	Intranasal
Desmopressin	DDAVP	10–12	Intranasal
Non-hormonal Potentiators			
Chlorpropamide	Diabenese	24	Oral
Clofibrate	Atromid-S	24	Oral
Thiazide diuretics		24	Oral

IV. POSTERIOR PITUITARY/ ANTIDIURETIC HORMONE

A. VASOPRESSIN

Drugs affecting the body's water balance include those which stimulate or suppress antidiuretic hormone (ADH) release from the posterior pituitary (vasopressin) and those which augment or block the effect of ADH on the renal tubule.

ADH is synthesized in specialized hypothalamic nuclei and travels down neuroaxons to the posterior pituitary where it is stored. It is released in response to volume depletion and increase in plasma tonicity. It acts on the renal tubules to accelerate the rate of water resorption. Lack of ADH produces neurogenic diabetes insipidus. The defect may be complete or partial, with a clinical presentation ranging from severe dehydration and thirst to nothing at all.

Nephrogenic diabetes insipidus involves insensitivity of the renal tubule to vasopressin (Table 9-8), and it may be distinguished from neurogenic diabetes insipidus by evaluation of the response to exogenous vasopressin.

Neurogenic diabetes insipidus is treated either with exogenous vasopressin or drugs which will enhance the effect of remaining endogenous vasopressin.

1. Clinical Features

a. Lypressin irritates the nasal mucosa, and the attendant congestion and edema may lead to lack of absorption, hence ineffectiveness, of the drug.

b. Toxicity of the analogs of vasopressin is a virtual extension of their physiological function: excessive water retention with resulting hemodilution, hyponatremia, and symptoms of water intoxication, which include headache, irritability, nausea, vomiting, confusion, lethargy, coma, convulsions, and death.

2. Laboratory Diagnosis

Laboratory diagnosis includes measurement of serum sodium (or osmolality) and urine for specific gravity (or osmolality). Serum osmolality and sodium will be low with urine osmolality inappropriately high due to the antidiuretic effect of vasopressin on the renal tubule.

Measurement of serum or urinary vasopressin levels is currently not feasible. Immunoassays are available only in a very few research laboratories. Fortunately, neither diagnosis nor management depend on its measurement.

3. Treatment

Management depends on the severity of the symptoms and the duration of action of the drug used.

a. Mild symptoms: mild headache, irritability

(1) If due to short-acting drug, discontinue or change dose.

(2) If due to long-acting drug and serum sodium is greater than 125 mEq./

liter, restrict fluid intake to less than 1,500 ml. per day. Such patients may require hospital admission.

b. Moderate symptoms: headache, muscle weakness, nausea, personality change

(1) Admit to hospital if serum sodium $\geq$ 125 mEq./liter. Restrict fluid intake to less than 1,000 ml. per day.

(2) If serum sodium < 125, see below.

c. Severe symptoms: vomiting → convulsions

(1) Serum sodium almost always < 125 mEq./liter.

(2) Give furosemide, 1 mg./kg. I.V.

(3) Monitor urine volume, sodium, potassium, and serum sodium hourly.

(4) Give 3% sodium chloride with potassium chloride (depending on urinary excretion of potassium). Replace the sodium and potassium lost in the previous hour.

(5) Continue until symptoms are relieved and serum sodium is above 125 mEq./liter.

(6) Subsequent therapy is water restriction only, until serum sodium is > 130 mEq./liter.

B. CHLORPROPAMIDE AND CLOFIBRATE

Chlorpropamide and clofibrate may also cause water intoxication, which is diagnosed and treated as above. Chlorpropamide is more notorious as a cause of hypoglycemia. Clofibrate may cause an acute muscle syndrome, requiring discontinuation of the drug and symptomatic treatment. In high doses it may cause malabsorption with or without diarrhea. Treatment is symptomatic, with discontinuation or lowering of the dose.

C. THIAZIDE DIURETICS

Thiazide diuretics rarely cause water intoxication. The mechanism is due to rapid potassium depletion in certain individuals, in which, together with mild sodium depletion, leads to continuing stimulation of

ADH release. Patients return to normal water balance several days following discontinuation of the drug. Mild to moderate symptoms may be treated by potassium replacement and water restriction. Severe symptoms with serum sodium less than 125 mEq./liter may be treated by infusion of 100 ml. of 5% saline over one hour. Repeat once, if needed, after one to two hours. Other treatment regimens, as outlined above, may be used, with attention given initially to potassium replacement.

D. EXCESS/INAPPROPRIATE ADH SECRETION

1. Certain drugs other than those listed above will cause water retention, dilutional hyponatremia, and the syndrome of water intoxication. It has not been established that they all work by stimulating endogenous ADH, but the pathophysiology is the same as that seen in subjects given excessive amounts of ADH and allowed free access to water. Features fit the criteria for the syndrome of inappropriate secretion of ADH (SIADH), which include:

Hyponatremia/hypoosmolal serum and extracellular fluid

Continued renal excretion of sodium ($\geq$ 25 mEq./day)

Normal renal function

Absence of volume depletion

Absence of obvious edema

Urine osmolality > serum osmolality

---

2. The syndrome is "inappropriate" because there is continuing reabsorption of water by the kidney despite an already expanded extracellular fluid volume, whereas under normal circumstances there would be suppression of ADH with increased free water clearance by the kidney, which would return serum sodium and osmolality to normal. Drugs causing SIADH are listed in Table 9-9.

Table 9-9. **Drugs that Cause SIADH**

Generic	Proprietary	Comment
Tolbutamide	Orinase	Produces SIADH rarely, erratically
Cyclophospha-mide	—	—
Vincristine	Oncovin	SIADH self-limited
Carbamazepine	Tegretol	
Amitriptyline	Elavil	
Thioridazine	Mellaril	
Thiothixine	Navane	
Acetaminophen	Tylenol	

3. Treatment

Principles of treatment of SIADH caused by these drugs are given on page 96. Treatment of SIADH which is not drug-induced follows.

a. Other causes of SIADH include:

Carcinoma: bronchogenic, small intestine, pancreas
Tuberculosis
Pneumonia
CNS disease: trauma, tumors, abscess
Myxedema
Acute intermittent porphyria
Postcardiac bypass

b. The most effective form of treatment is to cure the underlying disease. As a temporizing measure, therapy outlined above (p. 96) may be used. When the underlying cause cannot be treated, drugs may be used which block the effect of ADH on the renal tubule. The two drugs most commonly used are lithium carbonate (Lithane) and demeclocycline (Declomycin). The former is a drug used for the manic-depressive states; the latter is an antibiotic. Both are used therapeutically to take advantage of a toxic effect: the production of nephrogenic diabetes insipidus. Demeclocycline is preferred because it has fewer side effects, chiefly causing nausea and photosensitivity. Lithium carbonate toxicity includes sluggishness, drowsiness, tremor, muscle twitching, gastrointestinal disturbances, goiter, and myxedema. It has been postulated, but not proved, to be a general inhibitor of cAMP-medicated hormone action. Treatment is discontinuation of the drug.

V. CALCIUM/BONE

A. HYPERCALCEMIA

1. Causes of hypercalcemia can be divided into the following four groups:

Neoplasia
Squamous cell carcinoma of the lung
Squamous cell carcinoma of the head and neck
Multiple myeloma
Leukemias, lymphoma

Endocrine
Hyperparathyroidism
Acute adrenal insufficiency
Hyperthyroidism

Drugs
Vitamin D
Vitamin A
Milk-alkali syndrome
Thiazide diuretics
Furosemide

Other
Sarcoid

2. The rapid onset of hypercalcemia with serum levels usually above 13 mg./dl. is predominantly associated with CNS symptoms, including malaise, fatigue, lethargy, confusion, psychosis, torpor, and coma.

3. Hypercalcemia that develops more slowly and is more prolonged may also produce renal and gastrointestinal symptoms which include:

a. Polyuria/polydipsia, secondary to lack of concentrating ability of the renal tubules

b. Flank pain and/or renal colic due to renal stones

c. Epigastric pain, anorexia, nausea, vomiting, constipation, secondary to the hypercalcemia itself

4. Laboratory evaluation of hypercalcemic status should include:

Serum calcium
Serum phosphorus
Serum alkaline phosphatase
Serum electrolytes
Serum parathormone (suppressed in drug-induced hypercalcemia)
Serum vitamin D (if indicated)
Serum vitamin A (if indicated)
Blood count
Urinalysis
Urine calcium (if milk-alkali syndrome suspected)

---

5. Drug-induced Hypercalcemia

a. Vitamin D toxicity is the most important of this group. Increased amounts of calcium and phosphorus are absorbed across the intestinal mucosa, increased calcium is reabsorbed in the proximal renal tubule, and increased osteoclastic activity leads to increased bone resorption. Serum calcium levels increase. Phosphorus may be normal, low, or high. Clinical manifestations are due to hypercalcemia, listed above. In addition there may be ectopic (soft tissue) calcification, especially if the phosphorus is high, and bone changes which range from osteopenia (more common) to osteosclerosis (less common) or combinations of these.

(1) There is probably no acute toxicity that results from the ingestion of single large doses of vitamin D. Toxic manifestations are seen with the continuing ingestion of greater than 50,000 units of vitamin D per day.

(2) The biological effects of vitamin D may last for several weeks after discontinuation of the drug. Careful monitoring of the clinical and laboratory manifestations is mandatory.

(3) Management of vitamin D toxicity includes discontinuation of the drug and treatment of the symptomatic hypercalcemia (below).

b. Acute vitamin A toxicity consists of lethargy, irritability, nausea, vomiting and headache. Chronic toxicity includes anemia, leukopenia, hepatosplenomegaly, and periosteal proliferation, which may be very painful. Rarely, vitamin A toxicity will produce hypercalcemia. All changes except hepatosplenomegaly are reversible on discontinuation of the drug.

c. The milk-alkali syndrome may occasionally be seen with the chronic ingestion of calcium carbonate (milk) and sodium bicarbonate. The chief manifestations are those of chronic hypercalcemia.

(1) Laboratory studies show a mild metabolic alkalosis, and hypercalcemia with hypocalciuria.

(2) Treatment consists of a low-calcium diet. The clinical response is usually rapid.

(3) Because milk and antacids are commonly used to treat peptic ulcer disease, and because peptic ulcer is more common in persons with hyperparathyroidism, care must be taken to exclude coexistent parathyroid disease in patients presenting with the milk-alkali syndrome.

d. Diuretics are associated with hypercalcemia. There is still some controversy concerning whether this occurs only in the presence of hyperparathyroidism, which may be overt or subclinical. Thus, persistence of hypercalcemia must be checked after withdrawal of the diuretic for several weeks.

Both thiazides and furosemides have caused hypercalcemia, which is usually mild and asymptomatic. In our experience, the associated hypercalcemia has not caused symptoms or organ dysfunction if unassociated with hyperparathyroidism. Our practice has been to discontinue the diuretic only if it has been administered for inappropriate reasons, such as weight loss.

e. Treatment

(1) Drugs causing hypercalcemia are withdrawn.

(2) The rapid improvement seen in vitamin A toxicity or milk-alkali syndrome and the mild nature of diuretic-induced hypercalcemia usually precludes the need for further therapy.

(3) Vitamin D toxicity requires prompt treatment in the hospital.

(a) Hydrate adequately: 3 liters/day, oral or I.V. If dehydration, correct estimated deficit over 48 hours.

(b) Decrease calcium and phosphorus intake to less than 800 mg./day.

(c) Give hydrocortisone, oral or parenteral, 100 mg./day, until calcium returns to normal and symptoms clear. This may take as long as two weeks.

6. Drugs Used in the Treatment of Hypercalcemia of Other Causes

a. Severe symptomatic hypercalcemia which needs immediate treatment is most frequently due to neoplastic disease. The clinical presentation is one of CNS dysfunction, and calcium is usually greater than 15 mg./dl. Three drug treatment regimens are commonly employed.

(1) For saline diuresis, about 6 liters of sodium chloride are given over a 24-hour period. Complications are few and primarily include those of water overload which is usually treated with administration of a loop diuretic.

(2) For furosemide diuresis, 80–100 mg. of furosemide are given intravenously every one to two hours. All fluids and electrolytes are replaced intravenously except calcium. Complications include those of fluid or electrolyte imbalance, but these are minimal if there is close and critical monitoring of clinical and laboratory data.

(3) Mithramycin (Mithracin), a cytotoxic agent which suppresses calcium egress from bone, is given as a single 25-µg./kg. bolus intravenously, which may be repeated 24 hours later if calcium response is minimal or absent. In excessive amounts, it may produce hypocalcemia, easily treated with infusion of 500–1000 mg. calcium gluconate over 24 hours. It has hematologic toxicity, causing bone marrow depression, renal toxicity with a rise in BUN and creatinine, and nausea and vomiting. We have not observed these side effects when mithramycin is used as described above.

(4) Intravenous phosphates (IN-PHOS) and sulfates are of limited use. Phosphates, in particular, even when used as prescribed, may cause soft-tissue calcification throughout the body and result in irreversible renal functional impairment (nephrocalcinosis) and pulmonary edema (precipitation of calcium salts in alveolar walls). We prefer other forms of therapy.

b. Prolonged minimal hypercalcemia is sometimes treated with oral phosphates (Fleet's Phospho-Soda) for a total dose of 1–2 gm. of phosphorus per day. The most common toxicity is that of diarrhea, treated by reduction of the dose given. Administration of oral phosphates to persons with severe hypercalcemia could lead to ectopic calcification.

c. Calcitonin (Calcimar), used for the treatment of Paget's disease of bone, has occasionally been used to treat hypercalcemia when other methods have failed. Results have not been encouraging. For toxicity, see below.

B. Hypocalcemia

1. Hypocalcemia is seen in the following disorders:

Hypoparathyroidism (idiopathic; secondary to metastases)
Pseudohypoparathyroidism
Vitamin D deficiency
Malabsorption
Hyperphosphatemia (renal failure)

Hypomagnesemia
Hypoproteinemia
EDTA toxicity
Mithramycin toxicity

2. Treatment of parathyroid hormone deficiency or end organ insensitivity is with vitamin D or dihydrotachysterol (Hytakerol) and calcium salts. Toxicity of dihydrotachysterol is similar to that of vitamin D, but of shorter duration, and has hypercalcemia as its major manifestation. Treatment is outlined above.

3. Mithramycin toxicity is discussed above.

4. EDTA (ethylenediaminetetraacetic acid), an agent which chelates calcium, was much used in the treatment of hypercalcemia but was largely abandoned because its effect was quite transient and, if used excessively, was highly nephrotoxic.

C. BONE

1. Osteoporosis is the loss of mineralized bone. It is seen in states of nitrogen loss, is part of the aging process, and may be related to the menopause. When the bone mass is reduced below a critical point, fractures occur, most commonly of the axial skeleton. Treatment has included a variety of regimens, none of which has been satisfactory. Drugs used have included vitamin D, calcium salts, androgens, estrogens, and fluoride. Fluoride is given as an aqueous sodium fluoride solution, or as pills, with a desired dose of 25 mg. of fluoride daily. Acute toxicity consists of gastrointestinal intolerance, with epigastric discomfort, nausea, and vomiting. Treatment is symptomatic plus discontinuation of the fluoride. Chronic administration produces fluorosis, a condition in which new bone that is formed incorporates the fluoride anion. Although the bone formed is denser, it is also more brittle and more susceptible to fracture. When used in doses of less than 1 mg. per day, toxic effects are not seen.

2. Osteomalacia (rickets) is seen in a variety of settings, including genetic defects, malnutrition, malabsorption, and renal tubular defects. Treatment is with calcium and vitamin D or with vitamin D and phosphates. Phosphates, given in doses of 1–2 gm. of phosphorus daily, is frequently associated with diarrhea. Treatment is reduction of the dose of phosphorus.

3. Paget's disease of bone is a metabolic disorder of unknown cause, associated with an increase in osteoclastic and osteoblastic activity. The radiological appearance is that of areas of osteosclerosis adjacent to areas of osteopenia. The problem may be asymptomatic and merely a radiological finding, or severe with fractures and pain. Two drugs have recently become avilable for treatment.

a. Salmon calcitonin (Calcimar) is given subcutaneously. It is allergenic and may cause pain at the site of injection. Patients may become refractory to the drug because of the development of neutralizing antibodies. Acute toxicity consists of a possible allergic reaction and rather severe nausea, which is usually self-limited. Chronic administration may lead to hypocalcemia, usually treated with lowering of the dose administered. If signs of hypocalcemic tetany develop (Chvostek's or Trousseau's signs, muscle cramps, carpopedal spasm), the patient should be admitted and treated with intravenous infusion calcium gluconate, 500–1000 mg. per day. Usually, such therapy is not required beyond 24 hours.

b. Etidronate (EHDP, Didronel) is an oral diphosphonate that, depending on the dose given, may either reduce the fractures and pain or lead to further demineralization. Usual doses range from 5–10 mg./kg. per day. Acute toxicity includes abdominal cramps and diarrhea and is usually alleviated by administering the drug in divided doses. On theoretical grounds, acute toxicity could produce hypocalcemia, but this has not yet been reported in the literature. Chronic toxicity

Table 9-10. Androgens

Generic	Proprietary	Usual Maintenance Dose, Route
Testosterone enanthate	Delatestryl	200 mg. I.M. every 2 weeks
Testosterone pellets	Oreton	450 mg. s.c. every 4–6 months
Methyltestosterone	Android, Metandren, Oreton	25–50 mg., oral or buccal, daily
Fluoxymesterone	Halotestin	5–10 mg., oral or buccal, daily

is a reflection of the demineralization and is manifested by increasing fractures and pain. Treatment is symptomatic, with discontinuation of the drug.

VI. ANDROGENS/ESTROGENS

A. ANDROGENS/ANABOLIC STEROIDS

1. Androgens are primarily used for replacement therapy in states of male hypogonadism. They are occasionally used to induce growth of sexual hair in females with primary amenorrhea, in chemotherapy of breast cancer, to encourage linear growth in short adolescents with open epiphyses, to masculinize female transsexuals, to stimulate hematopoiesis, and as anabolic agents.

2. Androgens are available in oral, buccal, and parenteral preparations, with representative examples listed in Table 9-10. The parenteral forms of the medication are the most effective, and hence the more desirable.

a. Single large doses cause no clinically important endocrine or nonendocrine effects. Chronic administration of high drug doses can produce toxicity that is an extension of their endocrine effects. These include:

Hirsutism (excessive growth of terminal hair)
Virilism: hirsutism, increase in muscle mass, deepening of the voice, enlargement of the clitoris, acne, and breast atrophy
Small, soft testes
Inhibition of spermatogenesis
Gynecomastia
Erythrocytosis
Hypertension
Premature epiphyseal fusion
Priapism

---

(1) Androgens do not seem to have an adverse effect on prostatic hyperplasia but may stimulate already existing prostatic carcinoma.

(2) On occasion, androgens, particularly methyltestosterone and fluoxymesterone, may cause obstructive jaundice. The disease is mild and reversible on discontinuation of the drug.

(3) Erythrocytosis and hypertension, should they develop, are mild and respond to reduction in drug dosage.

(4) Gynecomastia is usually only mild to moderate and regresses on discontinuation of the drug, but may not disappear altogether.

b. Laboratory studies are not necessary if signs of androgen excess occur in a person known to be taking androgens. Unusual problems arise in persons taking androgens as a "body-builder" and in female transsexuals. Serum and urinary testosterone levels will be high if the drug taken is testosterone and low if it is fluoxymesterone. Serum luteinizing and follicle-stimulating hormones will be low. In transsexuals, history and physical examination, including inspection of the genitalia, suffice. Differentiation of endogenous from exogenous hyperandrogenemia is difficult and relies on careful family and personal history, physical examination, and laboratory diagnosis. Conditions to be considered include congenital virilizing adrenal hyperplasia, virilizing adrenal adenoma, and ovarian neoplasms both primary and metastatic.

c. The only therapy necessary is discontinuation of the drug or modification of its dose.

3. Anabolic steroids include nandrolone (Durabolin), stanozolol (Winstrol), methandrostenolone (Dianabol), oxandrolone (Anavar), and oxymetholone (Anadrol), a potent anabolic and androgenic agent. Their primary effect is to promote positive nitrogen balance, hence their use in nitrogen-wasting states, such as end-stage renal disease, and by athletes. Oxandrolone is also used in the treatment of Type V hyperlipoproteinemia. Oxymetholone is frequently used in states of bone marrow depression for its hematopoietic effect.

a. Toxicity is seen only with chronic administration and includes virilization, hypertension, and erythrocytosis. Treatment is by withdrawal of the drug.

B. ESTROGENS/PROGESTINS

1. Estrogens are available both alone and in combination with progestins. They are used:

a. As contraceptives.

b. As physiological replacement in hypoestrogenic states.

c. To treat irregular menses.

d. To treat hirsutism.

e. To treat dysmenorrhea.

f. To treat metastatic cancer of the prostate.

g. To treat some forms of breast carcinoma.

h. To treat osteoporosis.

i. In the postmenopausal syndrome.

j. By male transsexuals and others wishing more feminine body contours.

2. The three estrogen preparations in common use are:

a. The pill: estrogen/progestin combinations.

b. Conjugated estrogens (Premarin, Ogen).

c. Diethylstilbestrol.

3. As with androgens, estrogen toxicity is an extension of its natural hormonal effect, but it has important nonhormonal effects.

a. Acute ingestion of large quantities of estrogen probably has no important hormonal or nonhormonal effects.

b. Chronic administration of estrogens, in addition to feminization, may cause:

Nausea and vomiting
Hypertension (stimulation of renin-angiotension system)
Venous thromboembolism
Increased varicosities
Migraine
Strokes

---

c. Effects are reversible with discontinuation of the estrogen.

(1) Nausea and vomiting tend to be self-limited.

(2) Hypertension is also self-limited, but estrogens should not be given to persons with preexisting hypertension, and should be discontinued should hypertension develop.

(3) Controversy still exists concerning the relation of estrogens to thromboembolic disease, but they should not be used in persons with a previous history of thromboembolism or in the presence of other conditions, such as chronic obstructive bronchopulmonary disease, which are associated with increased risk of pulmonary embolism.

(4) Migraine is frequently worsened by estrogens and should be considered a contraindication to their use.

(5) Whether estrogens cause strokes is unknown, but they should not be given to patients with hypertension or advanced cerebrovascular disease. Administration to diabetics must be done judiciously, considering the problems of possible acceleration of vascular disease and those of a high-risk pregnancy.

Table 9-11. **Biologic Classification and Clinical Effects of Progestins**

Classification/Animal-Effects	*Clinical Human-Effects*		
	PROGESTATIONAL	ESTROGENIC	ANDROGENIC
True progestogens			
Progesterone	+	−	−
Dydrogesterone	+	−	−
Megestrol acetate	+	−	−
True progestogen with androgenic effects			
Medroxyprogesterone acetate	+	−	−
Norgestrol	+	−	+
Androgens with progestational effects			
Norethindrone	+	−	+
Estrogen with progestational effects			
Norethynodrel	+	+	−

(Adapted from Endgren, R. A.: Comparative effects of new progestogens. *In* Gold, J. J. (ed.): Gynecological Endocrinology. ed. 2, p. 323. Hagerstown, Md., Harper & Row, 1975)

d. Prolonged use of estrogens has been reported to increase the risk of endometrial cancer. The use of diethylstilbestrol during pregnancy is associated with vaginal malignancy in female offspring and must not be used during pregnancy.

4. Progestins are of two types: derivatives of progesterone and derivatives of androgens. In addition to their progestational effects, they may have androgenic, estrogenic, antiestrogenic, or glucocorticoid effects (Table 9-11). Toxicity is related to chronic administration and is similar to that of androgens and estrogens described above. It is treated by avoiding use in high risk groups, and discontinuing the drug if toxicity occurs.

5. Recently, tamoxifen (Nolvadex) has been made available for treatment of certain types of breast cancer. It blocks the peripheral effects of estrogens without causing androgenic effects. Toxic effects are those seen in estrogen-deficient states: hot flashes, nausea, vomiting. Tamoxifen may also lead to hypercalcemia in patients with bone metastases.

VII. HYPOTHALAMIC/ANTERIOR PITUITARY DRUGS

Drugs discussed in this section are used to substitute for, enhance, or suppress substances secreted by the hypothalamus or pituitary. Target organ hormones are discussed in other sections.

A. ANALOGS OF PITUITARY HORMONES

1. Thyrotrophin (TSH, Thytropar) is extracted from bovine pituitary glands and is chiefly used for diagnostic purposes, including separation of primary from secondary hypothyroidism and enhancement of radioiodine uptake by the thyroid for anatomical delineation. Its abuse potential is low.

a. The chief toxic manifestation of acute administration is allergy, e.g. mild erythema to anaphylaxis. Although an uncommon reaction, TSH should not be administered unless epinephrine is readily available.

b. Chronic administration of greater than 10 units daily may induce goiter, which responds to discontinuation of the drug.

2. Corticotropin (ACTH) is available as a purified extract from bovine pituitaries (ACTHar, ACTHar gel) or a synthetic product (Cosyntropin, Cortrosyn), consisting of the first 24 amino acids of naturally occurring ACTH. It is given only parenterally and has both diagnostic and therapeutic uses.

a. Diagnostically it helps in the differentiation of primary and secondary adrenal failure.

b. It is sometimes used therapeutically instead of glucocorticoids, especially in multiple sclerosis.

c. The most important acute toxic manifestation is anaphylaxis. This is seen chiefly with the bovine extract, when administered to persons with hypoadrenal states. Cosyntropin, the synthetic product, is far less antigenic, and in our experience has never been associated with anaphylaxis. Nevertheless, epinephrine should always be immediately available whenever ACTH is administered.

d. Chronic toxicity of ACTH is that of steroid excess. Whereas both chronic glucocorticoid and ACTH administration results in Cushing's syndrome, manifestations attributable to androgen and mineralocorticoid excess (hypertension, acne, increased pigmentation) are more common with ACTH excess.

e. Therapy includes discontinuation of the medication and treatment of the effects of steroid excess. ACTH does not cause the prolonged suppression of the hypothalamic-pituitary-adrenal axis seen with glucocorticoid administration.

B. DRUGS THAT CAUSE RELEASE OF ANTERIOR PITUITARY HORMONES

1. Protirelin (Thyrotrophin-releasing Hormone, TRH, Thypinone) is used diagnostically to help differentiate between hypothalamic, pituitary, and thyroidal forms of hypothyroidism, and to check for complete suppression of TSH secretion from the pituitary caused by states of thyroid hormone excess. It will also stimulate release of prolactin from the pituitary.

a. Because it is used only acutely, toxicity on chronic administration has not been reported.

b. Acute toxicity is chiefly that of hypertension, severe nausea, and flushing. Occasionally, it will cause breast engorge-

ment and galactorrhea, which is self-limited and lasts only a few days. There is no specific treatment indicated. The drug must be administered judiciously to persons who may be unable to tolerate a blood pressure rise of 20–30 mm.Hg.

2. Clomiphene (Clomid) is a nonsteroidal agent chemically related to the estrogen chlorotrianisene (TACE). It is used to induce ovulation by causing the release of pituitary gonadotropins.

a. Toxicity may be seen with a single 5- or 10-day course of therapy and includes hot flashes, mild hair loss, and blurring of vision. These are all reversible with discontinuation of the drug.

b. Rarely, clomiphene will cause ovarian hyperstimulation, with resultant ovarian enlargement, which may occur two or more weeks after the last dose of the drug. This, too, is reversible on discontinuation of the clomiphene. No specific treatment is necessary. Clomiphene should not be administered to women with large ovaries and should not be readministered to females until ovaries return to normal size.

C. HUMAN MENOPAUSAL GONADOTROPINS (MENOTROPINS, PERGONAL)

These are used to induce ovulation in women who do not respond to clomiphene. They are associated with multiple pregnancies and massive ovarian enlargement, which precludes frequent use.

D. HUMAN CHORIONIC GONADOTROPIN

This has limited therapeutic usefulness in the treatment of sterility, cryptorchidism, and delayed puberty. Although a single large dose probably is not associated with important toxicity, chronic administration may cause virilization, formation and rupture of ovarian cysts, and thromboembolism. Changes are reversible with discontinuation of the drug.

E. BROMOCRYPTINE
(5 α-BROMERGOCRYPTINE, PARLODEL)

This is a dopamine receptor agonist which mimics the action of prolactin-inhibiting factor (PIF) in causing suppression of prolactin release from the anterior pituitary. It is useful in treatment of amenorrhea and galactorrhea which is caused by prolactin excess.

1. The drug has been only recently released in the United States, and clinical experience is limited.

2. There are no reports of important toxicity due to ingestion of single large doses of bromocryptine.

3. Chronic administration is associated with numerous side effects, chiefly consisting of nausea, headache, and dizziness. Slight hypotension may occur. Treatment is by reduction of dose or discontinuation of the drug.

BIBLIOGRAPHY

Axelrod, L.: Glucocorticoid therapy. Medicine, *55:* 39, 1976.

Doar, J. W. H.: Metabolic side-effects of oral contraceptives. Clin. Endocrinol. Metab., *2:*503, 1973.

Gold, J. J., ed: Gynecologic Endocrinology. ed. 2. Hagerstown, Md., Harper & Row, 1975.

Hantman, D., et al.: Rapid correction of hyponatremia in the syndrome of inappropriate secretion of antidiuretic hormone. Ann. Intern. Med., *78:*870, 1973.

Schneider, A. B., and Sherwood, L. M.: Pathogenesis and management of hypoparathyroidism and other hypocalcemic disorders. Metabolism, *24:* 871, 1975.

Seltzer, H. S.: Drug-induced hypoglycemia: A review based on 473 cases. Diabetes, *21:*955, 1972.

Sussman, K. E., and Metz, R. J. S.: Diabetes Mellitus. ed. 4. New York, American Diabetes Association, 1975.

Suki, W. N., et al.: Acute treatment of hypercalcemia with furosemide. N. Engl. J. Med., *283:*836, 1970.

Werner, S. C. and Ingbar, S. H.: The Thyroid. ed. 4. Hagerstown, Md., Harper & Row, 1978.

Williams, R. H., ed: Textbook of Endocrinology. ed. 5. Philadelphia, W. B. Saunders, 1974.

10. CATHARTICS

Alastair Connell, M.D.

I. CLASSIFICATION

Laxative classifications are largely traditional and rarely reflect the underlying functional changes produced by the agents. The FDA Panel on Laxatives, Antidiarrheal, Antiemetic and Emetic Products classifies laxatives under:

1. Stimulant or irritant
2. Saline
3. Stool softeners
4. Bulk
5. Lubricant

(FDA Over-the-Counter Drugs, 1975). This classification does not take into account mechanisms of action.

II. STIMULANT OR IRRITANT LAXATIVES

The names *stimulant* or *irritant* are not precise, but included under this heading are:

1. Bile acids, phenolphthalein, castor oil
2. Bisacodyl
3. Oxyphenisatin (now withdrawn in the United States because of its unwanted effect of chronic hepatitis)
4. The anthracene group, e.g., senna, cascara, aloes, rhubarb, and frangulia

Laxatives in this category alter fluid and electrolyte absorption with intestinal fluid accumulation. The materials which have been studied most are castor oil, dihydroxy bile acids, bisacodyl, and oxyphenisatin.

Bile acids alter colonic electrolyte and fluid exchanges and are a factor in the choleretic enteropathy which occurs in patients with ileal resection or dysfunction. Some histological damage in the co-lonic mucosa following perfusion of unconjugated hydroxy bile acids has been recognized, resulting in alteration of colonic mucosal permeability. Dihydroxy bile acids probably exert their effect by stimulating adenylate cyclase activity in the colon and by increasing mucosal cyclic AMP in the small intestine.

Ricinoleic acid (castor oil) and other hydroxy or nonhydroxy fatty acids act on both small and large bowel and have similar effects on fluid absorption, although the evidence that this ricinoleic acid increases mucosal cyclic AMP is less emphatic than it is for dihydroxy bile acids. Ricinoleic acid also effects the basal electrical rhythms of the colon in cats in a way similar to effects of other diarrhea states. Bisacodyl administration also results in net fluid and electrolyte accumulation in the colon and the small intestine. It also stimulates peristalsis and diminishes segmentation. Phenolphthalein, which has a similar chemical structure to bisacodyl, probably acts similarly. Oxyphenisatin is now of historical interest only because it appears to cause chronic liver disease. Some older irritant resins such as podophyllum, colocynth, ipomea, elaterin, gamboge, and jalap act on both the small and large intestine. These highly irritant substances are toxic. Podophyllum, for example, was used to remove skin warts. Croton oil, which even in very small amounts is a true mucosal irritant, is now rarely if ever used.

Senna, like cascara, has an ancient history, and its use dates back to the pharoahs of Egypt. Previously it was consumed as the once-popular senna tea. Senna comprises a number of active glycosides, two of which have been isolated. They are called sennoside A and sennoside B. These glycosides have been standardized and their validity for human use has been established. These glycosides seem little absorbed in the small intestine in contrast to the free anthraquinone danthron, which is absorbed to an appreciable extent. It seems probable, too, that these glycosides require the presence of colonic bacteria for activity.

All of these laxatives, if taken regularly, can result in excessive loss of water and electrolytes and unabsorbed nutrients. Those acting in the small bowel, such as castor oil, can produce a degree of stearrhea and, over a long period of time and in excessive doses, could result in malabsorption of fat-soluble compounds.

Anthracene laxatives taken in excessive doses can result in the laxative or cathartic colon. The colon loses its motility and becomes a flaccid tube. Damage to nerve plexuses is irreversible. Another effect of overuse of anthracene laxatives is the occurrence of the pigmentation of the colonic mucosa known as melanosis coli. It is not clear if this pigmentation is of any pathological significance. It is, however, a useful marker to the physician that a patient is using large amounts of laxatives in cases of obscure, chronic diarrhea. Sigmoidoscopy should be performed in order to exclude this possibility.

III. SALINES

Saline laxatives include soluble sulphates, phosphates, or tartrates of sodium, potassium, or magnesium. The laxative effect of these materials depends on ionization of the solution, the osmotic action of their anions, and their low absorption. The salines most commonly used at present are magnesium salts, and their ingestion results in a retention in the gut lumen of large quantities of fluid, resulting in rapid intestinal transit and the discharge into the colon of extra quantities of fluid. A dose of 15 gm. of magnesium sulphate retains between 300 and 400 ml. of water in the intestinal lumen.

With excessive amounts of salines, there is loss of fluid, electrolyte imbalance, and potential disruption of absorptive mechanisms. In addition, magnesium compounds can be absorbed to a significant degree and result in hypermagnesemia and eventually magnesium poisoning, particularly in patients where there is defective renal function with poor excretion of magnesium ion by the kidney.

The magnesium ion stimulates the release of cholecystokinin and contraction of the gallbladder, the terminal ileum, and possibly the colon. Salines, therefore, can produce effects beyond those directly resulting from the osmotic effect of the saline load per se.

Sodium compounds are rarely used at the present time and are contraindicated in patients with hepatic, renal, or cardiac disease.

Lactulose is a specific disaccharide for which no corresponding enzyme exists in the small intestinal mucosa. Hydrolyzed by colonic bacteria to lactic acid, the compound regularly causes diarrhea and in some countries is used as a laxative. The laxative action is a combination of an osmotic effect in the small bowel with a pH change in the colon.

IV. STOOL SOFTENERS

Stool softener is not a specific term because practically all laxative materials result in stool softening. Under this heading are included those materials that cause a change in the consistency of the stool without any other marked effect. Dioctyl sodium sulfosuccinate has emulsifying, detergent, and weak bactericidal properties. Oral administration of dioctyl sodium sulfosuccinate may affect motor and secretory functions of the gut and may inhibit secretion of bile. For this reason nonionic poloxalkols may appear less objectionable than anionic dioctyl sodium sulfosuccinate. These materials are used in large quantity, and little evidence exists of a serious unwanted effect. However, the persistent use of detergents has, at least theoretically, the possibility of hazard.

V. BULKING AGENTS

Some natural fibers increase the bulk of the stool and the frequency of defecation and probably decrease transit time. Wheat bran and fibers derived from psyllium seed and other forms of cellulose, hemicellulose, and methylcelluloses result in increased bulk in the stool and relieve constipation.

These materials are safe, even when used in large quantities. The persistent use of very large amounts of fiber might cause zinc or calcium deficiency, especially in children or the elderly.

VI. LUBRICANTS

Mineral oil has been used for many years to soften feces. It has a sinister record of toxicity as a result of the absorption and deposition of oil, particularly in the lungs. This may be through seepage into the trachea during ingestion, but oil has also been noted in other body tissues and organs following absorption of part of the ingested dose. Parafinomas may occur in a variety of organ tissues, including the liver. Again, this is an irreversible situation resulting from a permanent deposition of the oil.

Mineral oils may also produce malabsorption of fats and vitamins A, D, E, and K. Anal seepage through the anal sphincter can result in troublesome pruritis, and where anal wounds or fistula in ano exist, delayed wound healing can result. Statistical evidence suggests that mineral oil may be a causative factor of gastrointestinal cancers. The deposition of mineral oil in the lungs as a foreign body may cause pneumonia to develop many years after the administration of the oil. Infants, the elderly, recumbent patients, and patients with gastroesophageal reflux or achalasia are particularly at risk and should not use mineral oil at night.

VII. CLINICAL FEATURES AND TREATMENT

The main unwanted effect of laxatives is excessive diarrhea with loss of water and electrolyte. Secretive laxative users may not admit to their habit, and the only telltale clues available to physicians are: (1) the testing of the urine for the presence of phenolphthalein—the addition of alkali turns the urine pink; (2) the inspection of the rectal mucosa with the proctoscope to detect melanosis coli.

The use of laxatives involving the small bowel, especially castor oil and mineral oils, may result in malabsorption with the increased fat content of the stool. Other indices of malabsorption may also exist. Treatment is to withdraw the laxative and to institute intravenous therapy with the use of appropriate volumes of water, sodium, and potassium. Potassium is particularly likely to be lost when there is excess loss of fluid from the colon.

The use of excessive amounts of bulk has occasionally been associated with the development of sigmoid volvulus in susceptible persons. This may resolve spontaneously, but if it persists, it is an acute surgical emergency.

Hypermagnesemia, such as might occur following inappropriate use of magnesium sulfate in a patient with chronic renal disease, can cause cerebral depression and respiratory arrest. Immediate treatment is intravenous calcium gluconate. Dialysis may have to be considered.

Excessive loss of magnesium can occur. Tetany may exist as a result of the associated hypercalcemia. Treatment is intramuscular or intravenous magnesium sulfate, 20 mEq. aliquots given slowly in 500 ml. of glucose in saline or water, usually along with potassium chloride. Calcium will return to normal, usually spontaneously.

Hypokalemia, or potassium depletion, may manifest as paralytic ileus, tendency toward cardiac arrhythmias, increased sensitivity to digitalis, and hyporeflexia. Many of these symptoms are potentially dangerous, and intravenous potassium replacement is necessary.

Protein-losing enteropathy can result from excessive use of phenolphthalein and bisacodyl.

Melanosis coli disappears between 4 months and 2 years after discontinuing an anthracene laxative, and in most cases disappears in less than 12 months.

BIBLIOGRAPHY

Boyd, J. T., and Doll, R.: Gastro-intestinal cancer and the use of liquid paraffin. Br. J. Cancer, *8:* 231–237, 1954.

Browne, J. C., McClure, E. V., Fairbairn, J. W., and Reid, D. D.: Clinical and laboratory assessments of senna preparations. Br. Med. J., *1:*436–439, 1957.

Conley, D. R., Coyne, M. J., Bonorris, G. G., Chung, A., and Schoenfield, L.: Bile acid stimulation of colonic adenylate cyclase and secretion of the rabbit. Am. J. Dig. Dis., *21:*453–458, 1976.

Ewe, K.: Effect of laxatives on intestinal water and electrolyte transport. Eur. J. Clin. Invest., *2:*283, 1972.

Ewe, K., and Holker, B.: Einflu eines diphenolischen laxans (Bisacodyl) augden Wasser-und Elektrolyt-transport im menschlichen colon. Klin. Woschenschr., *52:*827–833, 1974.

Findlay, J. M., Smith, A. N., Mitchell, W. D., Anderson, A. J. B., and Eastwood, M. A.: Effects of unprocessed bran on colon function in normal subjects and in diverticular disease. Lancet, *1:* 146–149, 1974.

Food and Drug Administration: Over-the-Counter Drugs: Proposal to establish monographs for OTC laxative, antidiarrheal, emetic and antiemetic products. Fed. Regist., *40:*12902–12944, 1975.

Hardcastle, J. D., and Mann, C. V.: Study of large bowel peristalsis. Gut, *9:*512–520, 1968.

Hofmann, A. F., and Poley, J. R.: Cholestyramine treatment of diarrhea associated with ileal resection. N. Engl. J. Med., *281:*397–402, 1969.

Lish, P. M.: Some pharmacologic effects of dioctyl sodium sulfosuccinate on the gastrointestinal tract of the rat. Gastroenterology, *41:*580–584, 1961.

Mekhjian, H. S., and Phillips, S. F.: Perfusion of the canine colon with unconjugated bile acids: effect on water and electrolyte transport, morphology and bile acid absorption. Gastroenterology, *59:*120–129, 1970.

Mertens, R. B., Mayer, S. E., and Wheeler, H. O.: Effect of cholera toxin on mucosal adenylate cyclase activity and in vivo fluid transport in rabbit gallbladder. Gastroenterology, *70:*919, 1976.

Smith, B.: Effect of irritant purgatives on the myenteric plexus in man and the mouse. Gut, *9:*139–143, 1968.

Teem, M. V., and Phillips, S. F.: Perfusion of the hamster jejunum with conjugated and unconjugated bile acids: inhibition of water absorption and effects on morphology. Gastroenterology, *62:* 261–267, 1972.

Williams, R. D., and Olmsted, W. H.: The effect of cellulose, hemicellulose and lignin on the weight of the stool: A contribution to the study of laxation in man. J. Nutr., *11:*433–449, 1936.

Zurrow, H. B., and Sergay, H.: Lipoid pneumonia in a geriatric patient. J. Am. Ger. Soc., *14:*240–243, 1966.

11. ANTIBIOTICS

Peter Frame, M.D.

Anti-infective drugs include the *antibiotics*, which are synthesized by microorganisms, the *semi-synthetic antibiotics*, which are chemically modified antibiotic compounds, and the *synthetic anti-infective agents*, which are synthetic compounds with inhibitory or killing activity against microbial pathogens. The antimicrobial mechanisms of action of these agents are quite varied, as are their toxic effects.

In addition to the specific toxic effects of the antibiotic agents, all of them cause some changes in the normal bacterial flora of the skin and mucosal surfaces. Most often, this effect is not clinically significant, but at times colonization by a pathogen can occur, or an organism which is not pathogenic in low numbers can overgrow to excessive numbers of organisms which can cause disease. Antibiotic-induced pseudomembranous colitis (discussed under clindamycin) and mucosal candidiasis are examples of disease caused by changes in normal bacterial flora. In general, the broad-spectrum antibiotics such as tetracyclines, chloramphenicol, cephalosporins, and broad-spectrum penicillins are more likely to cause clinically significant shifts in normal flora.

I. PENICILLINS

Penicillin G and its many analogs are the most widely used group of antibiotics. They inhibit bacterial cell wall synthesis and are relatively nontoxic to mammalian cells.

Penicillins are available in many oral and parenteral dosage forms. They are generally well distributed in the body, but cerebrospinal fluid levels are low in the absence of meningeal inflammation. The penicillins are excreted mainly by the kidney, but the liver is an important site of conjugation and excretion for some of them. Important pharmacological data for penicillins is outlined in Table 11-1.

Overdosage of penicillin G or its analogs in the presence of normal renal function should cause no serious side effects except for the risk of anaphylaxis. Patients tolerate short-term serum concentrations of greater than 500 μg./ml. with no complications. In the presence of massive overdose combined with severely reduced excretion of penicillin, such as with anuria and liver failure, reactions related to sustained high levels of penicillin such as encephalopathy or coagulopathy could theoretically occur. However, even in the face of anuria, the penicillin levels should fall into the nontoxic range within 6–24 hours, so there should be no need for specific therapy in penicillin overdose.

A. ACUTE TOXIC REACTIONS

1. Hypersensitivity

Immune-mediated reactions to penicillin G and its analogs can be divided into three groups:

"Immediate" allergic reactions, including anaphylaxis and accelerated urticaria.

"Late" allergic reactions, which include a number of skin reactions and "serum-sickness-like" reactions.

Possible "immune-mediated" reactions, which include hemolytic anemia, granulocytopenia, thrombocytopenia, nephritis, and hepatitis.

Fever can accompany any of these reactions or can occur as the only manifestation of penicillin allergy.

Table 11-1. **Pharmacology of the Penicillins**

Antibiotic	Dosage Forms	Cation Content per gram	Metabolism and Excretion*	Serum Half-Life (hrs.) Normal	Serum Half-Life (hrs.) Anuria	Dialysis[†]
Amoxicillin	P.O.		75% K; 25% L	1.0	7	H+/P ?
Ampicillin	P.O.		75% K; 25% L	1.0	8.5	H+/P−
	I.M., I.V.	3.12 mEq. Na+				
Carbenicillin	P.O.		85% K; 15% L	1.0	16	H+/P−
	I.V.	4.7 mEq. Na+				
Cloxacillin	P.O.		47% K; 53% L	0.5	0.8–2.2	H−/P ?
Dicloxacillin	P.O.			0.75	1.0	H−/P ?
Methicillin	I.V.	3.0 mEq. Na+	80% K; 20% L	0.5	4.0	H−/P−
Nafcillin	P.O.					
	I.M., I.V.	2.9 mEq. Na+	38% K; 62% L	0.5	1.2	H−/P ?
Oxacillin	P.O.					
	I.M., I.V.	3.2 mEq. Na+	47% K; 53% L	0.4	1.0	H−/P−
Penicillin G,	P.O.		80% K; 20% L	0.75	3–20	H+/P−
Crystalline	I.M., I.V.	1.5 mEq. K+/‡ 1.7 mEq. Na+‡				
Benzathine	I.M.					
Procaine (aqueous)	I.M.					
Penicillin V	P.O.		80% K; 20% L	0.5	?	?
Ticarcillin	I.V.	4.7 mEq. Na+	90% K; 10% L	1.2	11–15	H+/P+

*K = kidney; L = liver.
[†]Dialysis: H = hemodialysis, P = peritoneal dialysis, + = effective removal of the drug, − = not effective, ? = unknown.
[‡]Per million units.

a. "Immediate" Allergic Reactions

(1) Anaphylaxis

(a) Anaphylaxis occurs most commonly in patients known to be allergic to penicillin but can occur in patients without a penicillin allergy history who have received the drug before. Anaphylaxis has also been reported in patients with no previous exposure to any penicillin. Anaphylaxis is more likely to occur in atopic patients than in nonatopic patients.

(b) The incidence of anaphylaxis is about 15 to 40 patients per 100,000 receiving the drug, with a fatality rate of about 10% of those suffering anaphylaxis. Even though this incidence is low, penicillin use is so common that anaphylactic reactions are not unusual (estimated 300 deaths per year).

(c) Anaphylaxis can occur after any penicillin analog, any dose, any route of administration, or after any of the dosage forms, including oral penicillins and benzathine penicillin G.

(d) Anaphylaxis occurs within seconds to one hour after the dose. The severity of symptoms is variable and may be transient or progress to severe vasomotor collapse. They include palpitation, vertigo, dizziness, light-headedness, perspiration, tingling of the tongue, or just a "sick" feeling. Signs of laryngeal edema, hypotension, pallor, weak and thready pulse, clammy skin, and disorders of consciousness may be present.

(e) Treatment

i. Differentiate from procaine reaction (Table 11-2).

ii. Reverse Trendelenburg position.

iii. Epinephrine is the only drug of choice:

1) If no shock: 0.3–0.5 ml. 1:1,000 solution subcutaneously.

Table 11-2. **Differentiation of Anaphylaxis from Procaine Reaction**

	Anaphylaxis	*Procaine Reaction*
Type of penicillin	Any type	Aqueous procaine penicillin G only
Dose	Not dose related	More common with larger doses
Route of administration	Any route	I.M. (or inadvertent I.V.)
Onset after administration	1–60 min (parenteral) 15–120 min (oral)	1–15 min
Dizziness	Occasional	Common
Changes in mentation (confusion, hallucination, bizarre behavior)	No	Yes
Syncope	Common	Common
Unconsciousness	Occasional	Occasional
Seizures	No	Yes
Pulse rate	Increased	Increased
Blood pressure	Normal or decreased	Normal or increased
Sweating	Common	Uncommon
Allergic manifestations	Common	None
Duration of reaction	1–24 hours	10–15 min
Sequelae	Penicillin allergy	None

2) Shock: 0.5–1.0 ml. 1:1,000 solution slowly I.V.

3) Repeat if necessary, carefully monitoring for hypertension and cardiac arrhythmias.

iv. Establish and maintain airway. Emergency tracheostomy may be necessary.

v. If hypotension persists, I.V. volume expansion with saline, Ringer's solution, or plasma expanders.

vi. Hydrocortisone 100–200 mg. I.V. This drug does not reach maximum effect for several hours, and does not substitute for epinephrine.

vii. If wheezing is persistent after epinephrine, add I.V. aminophylline, 250 mg. I.V.

viii. Metaraminol as a continuous infusion should be used to maintain blood pressure if excessive epinephrine is required.

ix. Antihistamines have no place in the acute treatment of anaphylaxis, although they may be given after the patient is stable, for the management of other allergic phenomena.

x. Penicillinase is not indicated and is no longer commercially available.

xi. Patients should be hospitalized.

(2) Accelerated Urticaria

(a) Urticaria can appear early in the course of therapy from minutes to 48 hours after the dose. Patients with this reaction are in danger of progressing to anaphylaxis, particularly those occurring within the first hour after the dose.

(b) Treatment

i. Epinephrine, as above, for anaphylaxis without shock.

ii. Hydrocortisone, as above, for anaphylaxis.

iii. Antihistamines, orally or parenterally, e.g., diphenhydramine hydrochloride (Benadryl) 50 mg. I.M. or P.O.

iv. Patients with early onset urticaria should be observed in the hospital for 24 hours.

2. Procaine Reactions ("Pseudoanaphylaxis")

a. Patients may occasionally receive intravenous procaine penicillin G during an intramuscular injection or by erroneous intravenous infusion. The incidence of acute reactions to intravenous procaine penicillin is estimated at 1 in 100 to 1 in 400 injections, even when careful injections are given.

b. The symptoms occur within minutes of the injection and are characterized by extreme anxiety, a feeling of impending doom, hallucinations, seizures, tachycardia, and raised blood pressure. Cardiorespiratory arrests and death have been reported. Allergic manifestations are absent.

c. The mechanism of this reaction is most likely the toxic CNS effect of I.V. procaine, of which about 6% is unconjugated to penicillin.

d. The reaction rapidly subsides, usually within 15–30 minutes, and is without sequellae, unless a cardiorespiratory arrest has occurred.

e. Treatment

(1) Differentiate from true anaphylaxis (Table 11-2).

(2) There is no specific therapy indicated for any of the manifestations of procaine reaction, except for cardiorespiratory resuscitation when necessary.

(3) Seizures do not need antiseizure therapy.

3. Penicillin Encephalopathy

a. Encephalopathy is perhaps the only true toxic effect of penicillin G. It occurs when the level of penicillin in the CNS becomes excessive. There are three basic mechanisms by which penicillin can reach excessive levels in the CNS and thus cause toxic encephalopathy:

(1) By direct application of penicillin to the surfaces of the brain, such as in intrathecal or intraventricular instillation.

(2) When high serum levels are maintained because of massive doses of penicillin or impaired renal excretion.

(3) When the diffusion of penicillin into the CSF is enhanced, as in meningi-

tis, or diffusion out of the CSF is impaired, as in uremia and possibly with probenicid therapy.

b. The mechanism of toxicity appears to be a direct irritative effect on the cerebral cortex. There are no consistent pathologic changes described. Toxicity is most often associated with CSF penicillin G levels greater than 10 μg./ml. and with serum levels greater than 100 μg./ml.

c. Penicillin neurotoxicity is most often manifested by myoclonus, which may range from oculomotor twitching to generalized muscle jerking. Grand mal seizures and coma are common later findings, while asterixis and hyperreflexia are less often described.

d. Penicillin neurotoxicity occurs most often within 12 to 72 hours after starting therapy. Recovery also occurs within 12 to 72 hours after stopping the drug. Mortality in reported patients with penicillin neurotoxicity has been 25%, but it is difficult to assess the contribution of the severe underlying illnesses of these patients.

e. Treatment

(1) Differentiate from intracranial pathology causing seizures.

(a) History compatible with penicillin toxicity

(b) Normal neurological examination

(c) EEG-diffuse nonfocal dysrhythmia, with return to normal 24–48 hours after stopping penicillin

(d) High serum or CSF penicillin level

(2) Stop the penicillin.

(3) Standard supportive care for seizure patients should be used.

(4) Paraldehyde appears to suppress myoclonic jerking but should not be given to patients in coma.

(5) Anticonvulsants (phenytoin, phenobarbital, diazepam) are not effective against the seizure activity.

(6) Penicillin encephalopathy is not a contraindication for future penicillin therapy.

4. Penicillin-induced Coagulopathy

a. Clotting defects have been described with high blood concentrations of carbenicillin, ampicillin, penicillin G, ticarcillin, and methicillin.

b. Deficient platelet function is seen in vitro in all patients receiving the recommended doses of 30–40 gm. of carbenicillin per day. Serum carbenicillin concentrations at this dosage generally range from 100 to 500 μg./ml. With normal renal function, doses of penicillin G in excess of 50 million units per day are required to achieve these concentrations.

c. When carbenicillin concentrations exceed 500 μg./ml., an additional defect in plasma coagulation (fibrinogen-fibrin conversion) occurs with prolongation of prothrombin time and clotting time.

d. Bleeding from surgical sites, mucous membranes, and the gastrointestinal tract have occurred in patients with these coagulation defects, although this is a fairly unusual occurrence.

e. The platelet defect is reversed only after affected platelets are replaced by the marrow. The fibrinogen conversion defect is reversed after the carbenicillin concentration falls below 500 μg./ml.

f. Treatment

(1) In the absence of clinical hemorrhage, the drug may be continued.

(2) If bleeding occurs, stop the drug.

(3) Transfuse as necessary, using fresh whole blood if possible.

(4) Transfused platelets would be affected by the carbenicillin in the patient's serum, so that platelet transfusion is not indicated until carbenicillin levels have fallen to less than 50 μg./ml. and the patient continues to bleed.

B. OTHER REACTIONS

1. Late Allergic Reactions to Penicillins

Patients manifesting late allergic reactions do not develop anaphylaxis during the same course of penicillin administration, but have an increased risk of anaphylaxis during subsequent administration.

a. Late Cutaneous Manifestations

(1) Skin reactions to penicillins usually appear two or more days after the first administration of the drug. These may have any of the following characteristics:

Common	Rare
Morbilliform exanthems	Erythema nodosum
Generalized urticaria	Purpura
Vesicular eruptions	Erythema multiforme
	Acute toxic epidermal necrolysis
	Exfoliative dermatitis

(2) Treatment

(a) Stop the penicillin if possible.

(b) Administer antihistamine orally for symptomatic relief.

(c) In severe or recurrent cases, systemic steroid therapy is indicated.

2. Nonallergic Ampicillin Skin Rashes

In addition to allergic skin rashes as described above, ampicillin causes a nonallergic maculopapular rash. The incidence of all ampicillin rashes is 7–8% of patients receiving the drug, of which 2–3% are allergic, and the remainder are nonallergic. The incidence of this type of ampicillin rash is increased to 90% in patients with infectious mononucleosis or lymphatic leukemia who are given the drug. The concurrent administration of allopurinol increases the incidence of ampicillin rash to 22% of patients receiving both drugs.

3. Penicillin-induced Hemolytic Anemia

With prolonged high serum concentrations of penicillin G, a Coomb's positive hemolytic anemia rarely occurs. It has also been described with ampicillin, carbenicillin, and methicillin. The need for transfusions is uncommon. Coomb's positivity commonly occurs without hemolysis.

4. Penicillin-induced Granulocytopenia

On rare occasions low neutrophil counts, including agranulocytosis, have been described with penicillin G, methicillin, nafcillin, carbenicillin, and ampicillin. This complication seems to be most common when the drugs are given in high doses and has been described most often with methicillin. In all reported cases, the marrow was able to produce normal neutrophils within a few days of stopping the drug.

5. Penicillin-induced Nephritis

Most of the penicillins have been associated with the development of an allergic interstitial nephritis, but the incidence is the highest with methicillin administration, ranging from 4–16% in patients receiving prolonged high dosage. The incidence is probably much lower in patients receiving low doses and short duration therapy.

6. Penicillin Hepatotoxicity

Both symptomatic hepatitis and asymptomatic enzyme abnormalities have been occasionally described with ampicillin, carbenicillin, oxacillin, and cloxacillin therapy. Asymptomatic enzyme elevations are probably the more common, but their true incidence is unknown.

7. Cation Intoxication

a. All penicillins are administered as sodium or potassium salts. Patients receiving large doses of penicillins or patients with impaired renal function can develop congestive heart failure, hyperosmolar coma, hypokalemic metabolic alkalosis (sodium), or cardiac arrhythmias (potassium).

b. Table 11-1 indicates the cation content of the parenteral penicillins.

II. CEPHALOSPORINS

The cephalosporins are a rapidly expanding group of antibiotics that inhibit bacterial cell wall synthesis and, like penicillins, are relatively nontoxic to mammalian cells.

Cephalosporins are available in parenteral and oral dosage forms. The available oral forms are well absorbed except for cephaloglycine. The parenteral forms may be given either intravenously or intramuscularly, with some differences in their phlebitogenic and pain-producing tendencies. Cephalosporins are generally well distributed throughout the body except into the cerebrospinal fluid, where they penetrate very poorly. They all cross the placenta readily. Excretion of cephalosporins is mainly through renal tubular secretion of the unaltered drug. There is relatively minor liver conjugation of a few cephalosporins. In renal failure, hepatic metabolism becomes a significant factor, similar to the penicillins (Table 11-3).

Like the penicillins, overdosage of cephalosporins in the absence of renal dysfunction should cause no serious side effects other than the risk of anaphylaxis. Patients tolerate short-term serum concentrations up to 200 µg./ml. with no complications. In the presence of massive overdose in combination with severe renal failure, sustained high levels of cephalosporins could occur and theoretically could be associated with encephalopathy. It is unlikely that any special measures to remove cephalosporins would be necessary in this situation.

A. ACUTE TOXIC REACTIONS

1. Hypersensitivity

The cephalosporins induce the same types of allergic reactions as the penicil-

Table 11-3. **Pharmacology of the Cephalosporins**

Antibiotic	Dosage Forms	Cation Content per gram	Metabolism and Excretion*	Serum Half-Life (hrs.) Normal	Anuria	Dialysis†
Cefaclor	P.O.		71% K; 29% L	0.7	2.3	H−/P ?
Cefamandole	I.M., I.V.	3.3 mEq. Na+	80% K; 20% L	0.5	9	H−/P−
Cefazolin	I.M., I.V.	2.04 mEq. Na+	96% K; 4% L	1.8–2.0	40–50	H+/P−
Cefoxitin	I.M., I.V.	2.3 mEq. Na+	98% K; 2% L	0.8	21	H+/P ?
Cephalexin	P.O.		96% K; 4% L	0.9	15–22	H+/P ?
Cephaloridine	I.M.		85% K; 15% L	1.1–1.5	20–24	H+/P ?
Cephalothin	I.M., I.V.	2.8 mEq. Na+	55–65% K; 35–45% L	0.5	3–15	H+/P−
Cephapirin	I.M., I.V.	2.36 mEq. Na+	60% K; 40% L	0.5	1.8	H+/P ?
Cephradine	P.O.		96% K; 4% L	0.8	?	? / ?

*K = kidney; L = liver.
†Dialysis: H = hemodialysis; P = peritoneal dialysis; + = effective removal of the drug; − = not effective; ? = unknown.

lins, including anaphylaxis, skin rashes, and a "serum-sickness-like" syndrome; all with or without fever.

2. Cross-sensitivity with Penicillins

There are widely divergent opinions about the significance of cross-reactivity between the penicillins and cephalosporins, but a stance taken by many is that patients who have manifested penicillin allergy as anaphylaxis or immediate urticaria are at a higher risk for a similar reaction to cephalosporins. Conversely, patients who have had delayed skin rashes as a penicillin reaction can be given cephalosporins carefully if highly indicated.

3. Encephalopathy

The cephalosporins cause the same type of neurological disturbances as penicillins at very high serum or CSF concentrations.

B. OTHER REACTIONS

1. Late Allergic Reactions

These are similar to penicillin reactions.

2. Nephrotoxicity

a. Cephaloridine Nephrotoxicity

(1) Unlike the other cephalosporins, cephaloridine at high serum concentra-

tions causes proximal tubular dysfunction which can progress to tubular necrosis.

(2) In adult patients with normal renal function, this toxic effect can occur when the daily dose exceeds 4 gm. per day. When there is preexisting renal insufficiency, smaller doses are nephrotoxic.

(3) There are no longer any indications for the use of this drug, since less toxic intramuscular cephalosporins are now available.

b. Potentiation of Aminoglycoside Nephrotoxicity

When given to patients also receiving gentamicin or other aminoglycosides, the cephalosporins appear to increase the toxic potential of the aminoglycoside.

c. Allergic Interstitial Nephritis

A nephritis similar to that produced by the penicillins has been described.

3. Coombs'-positive Hemolytic Anemia and Neutropenia

See penicillins.

III. TETRACYCLINES

Tetracyclines are a large family of antibiotics that act by inhibiting bacterial protein synthesis. They are available for both oral and parenteral routes. The major distinguishing features between the tetracyclines are their pharmacology and, to some extent, their toxicology. Most tetracycline is administered orally, and all of the tetracyclines are well absorbed in the gastrointestinal tract. The absorption of all the tetracyclines is greatly impaired by food, particularly milk products, antacids and ferrous sulphate. For parenteral administration, certain tetracyclines are available for both intramuscular and intravenous use and some are recommended for intravenous use only. After administration, tetracyclines are widely distributed in body fluids and tissues. Tetracyclines penetrate into the cerebrospinal fluid in concentrations about one-tenth of the simultaneous serum concentration. They also cross the placenta. Tetracyclines are generally excreted unchanged by the kidney and to a lesser extent by the liver. High concentrations of active tetracycline is found in both the urine and the bile. Most tetracyclines are not metabolized, with the exception of chlortetracycline and doxycycline. These two compounds are metabolized in the liver, and the inactive metabolites are excreted in the urine. The biliary excretion of tetracyclines contributes to an enterohepatic circulation of the drugs.

In the presence of renal failure, all of the tetracyclines except chlortetracycline and doxycycline accumulate in the body because of the failure of renal excretion. None of the tetracyclines are significantly removed by peritoneal dialysis. Some tetracyclines are effectively removed by hemodialysis and some are not.

Overdosage of tetracyclines would most likely produce toxicity to the liver and azotemia. Most cases of hepatotoxicity or nephrotoxicity are functions of both the dosage level and the duration of the dosage. Management of oral overdoses of tetracycline should include removal of the unabsorbed tetracycline from the stomach with the induction of emesis or lavage, and the administration of antacids such as aluminum hydroxide gels or calcium salts and magnesium salts to chelate the remaining tetracycline and prevent its absorption. Further management of tetracycline overdoses would consist of observation for the development of liver or renal dysfunction. Hemodialysis would have little place in the management of tetracycline intoxication because most of the tetracyclines are poorly dialyzed. However, dialysis would be appropriate to manage azotemia associated with renal dysfunction.

A. ACUTE TOXIC EFFECTS

1. Liver Toxicity

a. Liver toxicity of tetracycline is uncommon but carries a high mortality rate. The toxicity is histologically manifested by fine fatty vacuolizatons without hepatocellular necrosis. It results in elevations of SGOT, SGPT, alkaline phosphatase, and bilirubin.

b. The overall incidence is unknown, but hepatotoxicity is more common in women than in men and most common in pregnant women. It occurs most often in patients receiving intravenous tetracycline, but it has been reported in patients receiving intramuscular or oral tetracycline. Patients developing hepatotoxicity have most often received high doses (usually more than 1–2 gm. per day) or have renal function impairment. This suggests that hepatotoxicity is directly related to serum levels of the drug, an observation supported by animal toxicity studies.

c. The clinical manifestations of tetracycline hepatotoxicity include nausea, vomiting, and fever followed by jaundice. The syndrome may then progress to hematemesis, renal failure, acidosis, hypoglycemia, hypotension, and death.

d. No patient should receive more than 1 gm. total dose per day intravenously or more than 2 gm. total daily dose orally. Tetracycline should not be given to pregnant women and to patients with renal failure.

e. Treatment

(1) Stop the drug.

(2) Maintain fluid and electrolyte balance and correct acidosis with bicarbonate.

(3) Monitor for and treat hypoglycemia with intravenous glucose.

(4) If renal function is normal, dialysis should not be necessary. However, if renal failure is present and measured tetracycline concentrations are excessive (greater than 5 μg./ml. of serum), hemodialysis may very slowly remove tetracycline and oxytetracycline.

2. Uremia and Nephrotoxicity

a. Uremia

(1) Tetracycline causes a modest rise in the blood urea nitrogen (BUN) in nearly all patients who receive it. In patients with borderline or preexisting renal failure, a terminal uremic syndrome can be precipitated by the tetracyclines.

(2) The mechanism of azotemia in patients receiving tetracycline is mainly from its antianabolic effect on human cells, which increases the nitrogen load to be excreted by the kidneys. In patients with limited renal capacity for nitrogen excretion, BUN elevation can be marked.

(3) The clinical features of renal failure induced by tetracycline are nonspecific and include anorexia, nausea, vomiting, weakness and lethargy, as well as heart failure or dehydration, progressive anemia, and metabolic acidosis. Pericardial effusions and bleeding disorders are common in advanced uremia.

(4) Patients with previously unrecognized mild renal dysfunction may develop the uremic syndrome only after a delay of several days after receiving tetracycline. This fact, coupled with the nonspecific character of the syndrome, may lead to nonrecognition of the relationship to tetracycline administration.

(5) The antianabolic effect of tetracycline is often synergistically affected by other catabolic events such as infection, neoplasia, malnutrition, and steroid administration.

(6) Concomitant deterioration of renal function as a result of salt and water depletion is a common feature of tetracycline-induced uremia. This is caused by poor intake or loss of salt from anorexia and vomiting and by concomitant use of diuretics. Tetracycline may also cause a sodium diuresis. The falling cardiac output of uremia further potentiates reduction in glomerular filtration rate.

(7) Tetracycline-induced azotemia may be reversible on stopping the drug if the patient does not succumb to the uremia syndrome.

(8) Treatment

(a) Stop the drug.

(b) In the absence of uremic symptoms, close observation is all that is required.

(c) In uremia, hemodialysis is required to clear the urea nitrogen, and this may clear some of the tetracycline. Prolonged dialysis may be required. Peritoneal dialysis can partially correct the uremia but will not remove the tetracycline.

b. Renal Failure

(1) In addition to the prerenal effect of tetracyclines on nitrogen metabolism, they also appear to have a direct effect on renal function.

(a) Tetracycline may cause increased sodium and water excretion which reduces the glomerular filtration rate through hypovolemia.

(b) Nephrogenetic diabetes insipidis (excess water loss) has been described with demethylchlortetracycline. This is reversed when the drug is discontinued.

(c) In the past, outdated tetracycline was associated with a reversible Fanconi syndrome (proteinuria, glucosuria, phosphaturia, and hypokalemia). With new drug formulations, this has not occurred and should no longer be a problem.

(d) In patients given tetracycline in association with methoxyflurane anesthesia, fatal renal failure has occurred with calcium oxylate crystals in the kidneys at autopsy.

2. Treatment

Mild renal impairment caused by these mechanisms is generally reversible when the drug is discontinued.

3. Vestibular Toxicity

A large number of patients receiving minocycline in the usual recommended doses experience reversible vertigo associated with nausea, vomiting, and ataxia within 24 hours of the first dose. Patients receiving minocycline should be cautioned about this possibility. This vertigo disappears when the drug is discontinued. Other tetracyclines do not cause this effect.

4. Intracranial Hypertension

a. This toxic effect is an uncommon complication of tetracycline therapy usually described in infants, but it has been rarely described in children or adults.

b. The symptoms of this toxic effect are severe headache, blurring of vision and papilledema, which rapidly resolve when the drug is withdrawn.

B. OTHER TOXIC EFFECTS

1. Cutaneous Reactions

a. Phototoxicity

1. All the tetracyclines, but particularly demeclocycline, can produce a mild or severe reaction of skin exposed to sunlight.

2. The reaction is characterized by a bright red rash similar to sunburn, which affects only the skin exposed to light and does not spread to other nonexposed skin. It may also be associated with eosinophilia and high fever.

b. Hypersensitivity Skin Reaction

Allergic cutaneous reaction such as maculopapular rashes, urticaria, fixed drug eruptions, and exfoliative dermatitis occur after tetracycline administration.

2. Teeth and Bones

a. All the tetracyclines have high affinity for bones and teeth and are concentrated in these structures at high levels.

b. The major effect of administering tetracycline to an infant or child during the time of tooth formation is a yellowish discoloration of the teeth. There is some controversy whether the teeth are functionally inferior and more prone to dental caries.

c. Tetracycline deposition in bones of the fetus, infant, or child is known to occur during tetracycline administration. Temporary arrest of bone growth is also known to occur, but the ultimate significance of this finding is not known.

IV. CHLORAMPHENICOL

Chloramphenicol is an antibiotic that inhibits bacterial protein synthesis, acting at the 50s subunit of the ribosome (the same site as erythromycin, lincomycin, and clindamycin). The drug is available for oral, I.V., and topical use. The oral forms are: chloramphenicol capsules at 125 and 250 mg., and chloramphenicol palmitate suspension. Chloramphenicol is well absorbed from the gastrointestinal tract, but because the palmitate must be hydrolyzed first, lower serum levels are achieved with the suspension. Intravenous chloramphenicol is only available as the succinate ester. This compound is bacteriologically inactive and must be hydrolyzed to free chloramphenicol by the tissue. Thus, serum concentrations achieved with intravenous chloramphenicol succinate are very similar to those concentrations achieved with a similar oral dose of chloramphenicol.

After absorption or hydrolysis, chloramphenicol is widely distributed in the body, including the cerebrospinal fluid, brain, and eye; and it readily crosses the placenta. Chloramphenicol is conjugated in the liver, and the inactive conjugate and some free chloramphenicol are excreted in the urine. Conjugated chloramphenicol appears to be nontoxic. In liver immaturity (newborn) and liver failure, active chloramphenicol can accumulate to toxic levels. In renal failure, the nontoxic conjugate accumulates. Chloramphenicol is not significantly dialyzed through the peritoneum but is readily removed from the blood by hemodialysis.

Overdosage of chloramphenicol may cause encephalopathy or circulatory collapse. The other toxic effects of chloramphenicol are idiosyncratic or related to more extended drug administration.

A. ACUTE TOXIC EFFECTS

1. Circulatory Collapse (Gray Syndrome)

a. First described in infants, particularly premature infants receiving large doses of chloramphenicol, this syndrome has also been described in older children receiving high doses of chloramphenicol, and in adults and children following overdoses of chloramphenicol.

b. The clinical picture is one of shock, with hypotension, pallor, cyanosis, and coma. The hypotension appears to be on the basis of peripheral vascular collapse. Abdominal distension and vomiting are seen in infants and children. Hypothermia and metabolic acidosis are also described.

c. Active drug levels are high, in the range of 75 μg./ml. or greater. These levels are achieved by an inability of the liver to conjugate the drug or by excessive doses of the drug.

d. Treatment

(1) Discontinue the drug.

(2) Establish and maintain airway and respiration.

(3) Intravenous fluids should be given to expand blood volume.

(4) In adults unresponsive to fluids, intravenous dopamine therapy for shock may be indicated.

(5) In overdose cases, prevent absorption with gastric emptying and activated charcoal.

(6) Hemodialysis may be useful in patients with severe liver failure. In the absence of liver immaturity or liver failure, drug levels should decline rapidly.

(7) Exchange transfusions have been used in infants to lower blood levels.

2. Chloramphenicol-associated Encephalopathy

a. A few patients who have received excessive doses of chloramphenicol (8 gm. or more per day) or who have received large doses in the presence of liver disease have developed a reversible encephalopathy. The reactions usually begin with nausea and a bitter taste in the mouth after a few days of therapy, followed by lethargy, disorientation, hallucination, and asterixis.

b. Treatment

(1) The symptoms are reversible on stopping the drug or reducing the dose.

(2) No data are available relating serum chloramphenicol levels to this toxic effect.

B. OTHER TOXIC EFFECTS

1. Anemia

There is a commonly occurring, dose-related suppression of red cell formation which may occur to some extent in all patients receiving chloramphenicol. Detectable suppression occurs when 6-hour serum concentrations exceed 15 μg./ml. Neutropenia and thrombocytopenia appear in more advanced cases. This is a separate effect from marrow aplasia.

2. Bone Marrow Aplasia

Aplasia is a rare idiosyncratic reaction that is unrelated to dose or duration of therapy. It may be a genetically determined sensitivity of DNA synthetic pathways. The risk is approximately 1 in 40,000 chloramphenicol-treated patients.

The onset of pancytopenia is often delayed weeks or months after the drug is stopped. The most common clinical presentations are the bleeding complications of thrombocytopenia. Symptoms of anemia or infections from neutropenia may also be present. The peripheral blood picture is one of pancytopenia, and the marrow is hypocellular or aplastic.

3. Optic Neuritis

Some patients who receive prolonged courses (more than six weeks) of chloramphenicol develop optic neuritis which may lead to blindness.

4. Hemolytic Anemia in Glucose-6-Phosphate Dehydrogenase Deficiency

Cloramphenicol may produce hemolytic anemia in some patients with glucose-6-phosphate dehydrogenase deficiency.

V. ERYTHROMYCIN

Erythromycin is a commonly used antibiotic that acts by inhibiting bacterial protein synthesis by attachment to the ribosomes at the same location as chloramphenicol, lincomycin, and clindomycin. It is generally effective against gram-positive organisms and ineffective against gram-negative enteric organisms. Erythromycin is available in a number of parenteral and oral forms. The oral forms are erythromycin base in tablets; erythromycin sterate in tablets, capsules, and oral suspension; erythromycin estolate in tablets, capsules, chewable tablets, and oral suspension; erythromycin ethyl succinate as chewable tablets and oral suspension. Erythromycin for intramuscular administration is available as erythromycin lactobionate and erythromycin gluceptate. As described below, the toxicities of erythromycin appear to be more related to the dosage form than to erythromycin itself.

When administered orally, erythromycin base is destroyed by gastric acid and absorption is interfered with by food. The various esters are designed to increase the acid resistance of the compound and improve gastrointestinal absorption. Peak serum levels achieved with erythromycin base taken on an empty stomach, erythromycin sterate, and erythromycin ethyl succinate are approximately the same, and occur two to four hours after the administration of the drug. Erythromycin estolate is absorbed as the ester as well as after dissociation in the intestine, so that serum concentrations of total drug are higher than with the other preparations. However, the circulating estolate is not an active antibacterial compound.

Erythromycin is widely distributed in the body tissues and fluids. It does not achieve significant concentrations in spinal fluid, however, and penetration across the placenta is low. About 85–95% of erythromycin is excreted through the liver in both an active and inactive form. The remainder of erythromycin is excreted in the active form in the urine. Erythromycin excretion is little affected by the presence of renal failure, but erythromycin may accumulate in patients with severe liver disease. There is no data currently available on the effect of dialysis on erythromycin.

Erythromycin overdosage has not been described.

A. ACUTE TOXIC EFFECTS

1. Hypersensitivity

Erythromycin is a rare cause of skin rashes and fever. Anaphylaxis has not been described.

2. Gastrointestinal Irritation

Erythromycin causes nausea, vomiting, diarrhea, and sometimes abdominal pain more often than most other antibiotics when given orally. These side effects are occasionally severe enough to cause the drug to be discontinued.

B. Other Toxic Effects

1. Liver Toxicity

a. Hepatotoxicity occurs in some patients after administration of erythromycin estolate, but not after other dosage forms of erythromycin, oral or parenteral.

b. The clinical syndrome usually occurs after one to two weeks of therapy and is manifested by nausea, vomiting, and abdominal pain similar to that of acute cholecystitis. Fever, jaundice, and pruritis may occur. Hepatomegaly may be present. Laboratory tests reveal elevated liver enzymes and bilirubin, and peripheral blood eosinophilia and leukocytosis. Liver biopsy has revealed interhepatic cholestasis without liver cell necrosis.

c. The mechanism of erythromycin estolate toxicity appears to be a hypersensitivity reaction and is not dose-related. Patients previously exposed to the drug may manifest the syndrome within a day or two after receiving the drug.

d. The hepatotoxicity of erythromycin estolate is reversible when the drug is stopped. There have been no deaths reported from this toxicity, but the jaundice has persisted on occasion for several weeks. Patients who have manifested toxicity to erythromycin estolate should not receive the drug again, although they may receive other forms of erythromycin without apparent ill effects.

2. Sensorineural Hearing Loss

a. Eight cases of reversible sensorineural hearing loss have been described in patients receiving intravenous erythromycin lactobionate. The doses given were large. The effect has appeared early in the course of therapy as well as after several weeks. Patients have a high-tone hearing loss that progresses to mid-range hearing loss if the drug is continued.

b. This form of eighth nerve toxicity is apparently completely reversible when the drug is discontinued.

3. Pyloric Stenosis

A relationship between the administration of erythromycin estolate to newborns and the development of hypertrophic pyloric stenosis has been described.

VI. CLINDAMYCIN AND LINCOMYCIN

Lincomycin and clindamycin are closely related antibiotics that act by inhibiting bacterial protein synthesis at the same ribosomal site as erythromycin.

Lincomycin and clindamycin are both available in oral and parenteral preparations. Oral lincomycin is absorbed much more poorly than clindamycin. Absorption is also impaired by food, whereas for clindamycin it is not. The serum levels after oral administration of clindamycin are approximately twice as high as a similar dose of lincomycin. Intramuscular clindamycin and lincomycin achieve serum levels roughly the same as oral clindamycin in the same dosage. Intravenous administration of the drugs results in peak levels that are about twice as high as a similar dose given intramuscularly. Both drugs are widely distributed in body tissues and fluids, including sputum. However, neither drug crosses the normal blood brain barrier. Both drugs cross the placenta, achieving levels in the cord blood of about one-quarter that in the maternal serum.

The majority of the administered dosage of both drugs is inactivated by the liver, with metabolic products being excreted in both urine and bile. The serum half-life of clindamycin in normal patients is about 2.5 hours, and the serum half-life of lincomycin is about twice as long. In the presence of renal failure, clindamycin half-life is increased by about 1 hour and lincomycin half-life is increased to 10 hours. Because of the long lincomycin half-life in the presence of renal failure, recommended doses of lincomycin are reduced in renal failure, whereas those of clindamycin are not. In the presence of liver failure, either drug can accumulate, and significant dosage reduction is indicated. Neither drug is significantly affected by peritoneal dialysis or hemodialysis.

Clindamycin or lincomycin overdosage is probably not particularly dangerous aside from the unlikely possibility of a severe hypersensitivity reaction. The cardiac arrest syndrome described with intravenous linocomycin (see below) would be unlikely with oral administration of either drug. Thus, the treatment of clindamycin or lincomycin overdosage would consist only of observation.

A. ACUTE TOXIC EFFECTS

1. Cardiac Arrest

When large doses of lincomycin have been given intravenously very rapidly, such as with bolus injection or with rapid infusion, a number of patients have been described with either hypotension or cardiac arrest. At least one patient has experienced concomitant nausea, vomiting, and shortness of breath and had electrocardiographic changes lasting 20 minutes. These effects have not occurred when infusions were given over a 30-minute period or longer.

2. Hypersensitivity

a. Anaphylactoid reactions have rarely been described with lincomycin and clindamycin.

b. Skin rashes including urticaria and a rare report of Stevens-Johnson syndrome have been reported. The incidence of maculopapular rashes was as high as 10% in one study.

B. OTHER TOXIC EFFECTS

1. Diarrhea and Pseudomembranous Colitis

a. Both diarrhea and pseudomembranous colitis have been described after

lincomycin administration as well as after several other antibiotics, including ampicillin, tetracycline, and chloramphenicol. However, the clinical syndromes appear to be the same and occur at approximately the same incidence.

b. The incidence of diarrhea associated with clindamycin therapy ranges from 4% to 33% with the two largest studies reporting 6.6% and 18%.

c. Pseudomembranous colitis may be present in as many as half the patients who develop diarrhea or up to 10% of the patients receiving the drug.

d. Variations in the incidence of colitis among different regions of the country and at different times in the same location have suggested a cofactor in the etiology of this disease. Recent research has implicated a toxin producing *Clostridium* as the cause of pseudomembranous colitis. This organism is resistant to clindamycin and produces an enterotoxin that causes colitis.

e. Both diarrhea and colitis have the same incidence whether they occur after oral or parenteral therapy. There seems to be no relationship between the daily dose or the total dose and the development of diarrhea.

f. Treatment

(1) In patients receiving clindamycin or lincomycin, the drug should be discontinued if diarrhea develops.

(2) Treat hypokalemia and electrolyte disturbances with electrolyte-containing fluids.

(3) Observe for colonic perforation and toxic megacolon by physical examination and x-rays.

(4) Sigmoidoscopy should be done to differentiate between diarrhea alone and pseudomembranous colitis. Colonic biopsy can be done if there is a question about the presence of pseudomembranes.

(5) The offending *Clostridium* species is sensitive to vancomycin. In patients with pseudomembranous colitis, give 500 mg.

vancomycin (10 ml. intravenous solution) in 30 ml. water orally, or by nasogastric tube, every eight hours until symptoms abate.

(6) Diphenoxylate and atropine (Lomotil) is contraindicated. In experimental animals, the colitis is potentiated by this medication.

(7) Steroids are of no benefit in the treatment of this disease.

g. Hepatotoxicity

Mild to moderate elevations of SGOT and SGPT and alkaline phosphatase have been seen in up to 50% of patients receiving clindamycin. This effect has been reported most often when the drug is given parenterally. When the drug has been discontinued, there has generally been no progression of a liver disease in these cases. Jaundice and hepatocellular damage are rare, but they have been reported in a few isolated cases.

VII. SULFONAMIDES

The sulfonamides are synthetic antibacterial agents that interfere with folic acid synthesis in bacterial cells. Because mammalian cells do not synthesize their own folic acid, sulfonamides do not interfere with DNA synthesis in humans.

There are a large number of sulfonamides, all of which are administered by mouth. The sulfonamides are divided into three groups, depending on their pharmacology:

1. Short-acting sulfonamides, which include sulfadiazine, sulfisoxazole, and triple sulfa.
2. Medium-acting sulfonamides, which include sulfamethoxazole.
3. Long-acting sulfonamides; none of these drugs are currently available in the United States.

The short- and medium-acting sulfonamides are rapidly absorbed from the gastrointestinal tract after oral administration. Peak serum concentrations are usually achieved after two to three hours. The sulfonamides are widely distributed throughout the body including the spinal fluid, the aqueous humor of the eye, the placenta, and the fetal circulation. There is some acetylation of the sulfonamides in the liver. The amount of acetylation varies among drugs and also varies with genetically determined rates of acetylation.

Both free and acetylated sulfonamides are excreted in the urine by glomerular filtration and tubular excretion. The short-acting sulfonamides have half-lives of approximately 2 to 5 hours, and the medium-acting sulfamethoxazole has a half-life of 10 to 11 hours in adults. The excretion of sulfamethoxazole is more rapid in children over the age of 1 year with a half-life of 4 to 5 hours. In infancy, the half-life is even longer than that for adults. Sulfisoxazole and sulfamethoxazole are both rapidly removed by hemodialysis and peritoneal dialysis.

The toxic effects of sulfonamides which are of special concern in overdosage are central nervous system toxicity, renal toxicity, and hypoglycemia. Additionally, hypersensitivity reactions and hemolytic anemia caused by glucose-6-phosphate dehydrogenase deficiency, which are unrelated to dosage, also occur. In addition to the specific therapy described below for these toxic effects, hemodialysis or peritoneal dialysis may play an important part in the removal of sulfonamides.

A. ACUTE TOXIC EFFECTS

1. Kidney Toxicity

a. Sulfonamides and their acetylated metabolites form crystals in the urine because of their high concentration and low solubility. Crystallurea can be present without obstruction or can cause anuric renal failure when the tubules, renal pelvis, or ureters become obstructed.

b. Crystallization and obstruction are potentiated by low urine volume and low urine pH (acid urine).

c. Crystallurea is now less common than it was with the older sulfonamides. However, the potential for crystallization is still present, especially with sulfadiazine —the currently available sulfa which is most likely to cause crystallurea. Sulfamethoxazole is the next most likely because of its relatively insoluble acetylated form. Crystallurea is least likely with sulfisoxazole.

d. Patients with crystallurea may have flank pain, ureteral colic, and hematuria; however, there may be no symptoms even in the presence of significant azotemia.

e. Treatment

(1) Stop the drug.

(2) Establish a high urine flow by oral or parenteral administration of fluids.

(3) If the patient is anuric, cytoscopy should be performed to remove obstructing crystal deposits from the bladder outlet and the utero vesical junction.

(4) Bicarbonate should be administered orally or parenterally to achieve a urine pH of greater than 7.15.

2. Central Nervous System Toxicity

a. Sulfonamides occasionally cause minor disturbances of central nervous system function, such as anorexia, nausea, and vomiting of central origin.

b. Higher sulfonamide levels may cause tremor, ataxia, confusion, and mental depression.

c. Acute toxic psychosis has been described with the sulfonamides. These are characterized by an acute delirium with disorientation, overactivity, and hallucinations. These reactions were much more common with the older sulfonamide compounds that are no longer available.

d. The central nervous system manifestations of sulfonamide toxicity are rapidly reversible when the drug is discontinued and tissue levels decrease.

3. Hypoglycemia

a. There have been a few case reports of severe hypoglycemia associated with excessive levels of sulfonamide.

b. In addition to hypoglycemia caused by excessive levels of sulfonamide, a drug interaction with tolbutamide has also been described. In these instances, diabetics had greatly increased serum tolbutamide levels and significant hypoglycemia.

c. Patients receiving sulfonamides who have renal failure or are undergoing tolbutamide therapy or who receive excessive doses of sulfonamides may develop this complication. Monitoring of serum glucose should be performed. If hypoglycemia occurs, sulfonamides should be discontinued and intravenous glucose should be administered. As with tolbutamide-induced hypoglycemia, the effect of the drug may be prolonged, and close observation is necessary for recurrence of hypoglycemia after glucose therapy has been stopped.

4. Acute Hemolytic Anemia

a. Most hemolytic episodes occurring with sulfonamide administration are the result of hemolysis of glucose-6-phosphate-dehydrogenase–deficient red cells. See section IX, "Nitrofuration," for a discussion of this deficiency.

b. Sulfonamides also may produce a hemolytic anemia on the basis of a hypersensitivity reaction. This type of hemolysis usually does not appear until after the patient has been on the drug for several days.

B. OTHER TOXIC EFFECTS

1. Bone Marrow Suppression

a. Any of the marrow elements can be suppressed by sulfonamides, most commonly the neutrophil, resulting in neutropenia or agranulocytosis.

b. Neutropenia occurs in roughly 1% of patients receiving sulfadiazine, and the incidence of agranulocytosis about 0.1%. Thrombocytopenia and erythroid hypoplasia are much less common. Aplastic anemia, with complete suppression of all marrow activity, is very rare.

c. Most of the marrow suppression syndromes are reversible when the drug is stopped, although aplastic anemia may not be reversible.

2. Skin Rashes

a. A wide variety of allergic skin rashes have been described with the sulfonamides, occurring in about 3% of patients receiving these drugs.

b. Bullous erythema multiforme (Stevens-Johnson syndrome) is a serious skin and mucous membrane eruption that is associated most often with long-acting sulfonamides not currently available in the United States. However, this syndrome has rarely been described with other sulfonamides. The onset of the Stevens-Johnson syndrome is usually about the 10th day of therapy and may be accompanied by high fever and bullous ulcerating mucous membrane lesions. Management consists of stopping the drug and usually requires the administration of high-dose corticosteroids. Secondary infections of skin lesions sometimes occur.

3. Liver Toxicity

a. Hepatic injury and necrosis have been described rarely with sulfonamides. The mechanism appears to be a hypersensitivity reaction. This complication appears to be less common with the currently available sulfonamides.

b. Sulfonamides competitively displace unconjugated bilirubin from serum albumin. Thus, jaundice and kernicterus have been described in infants born of mothers who were receiving sulfonamide at delivery and in infants who received the drug.

VIII. TRIMETHOPRIM-SULFAMETHOXAZOLE

Trimethoprim is a synthetic compound that interrupts bacterial purine synthesis at a stage immediately following the step blocked by sulfonamides. Although this step (the reduction of dihydrofolic acid to tetrahydrofolic acid) is also present in mammalian cells, trimethoprim has an affinity 10,000 times greater for bacterial enzymes than human enzymes.

Trimethoprim is available in the United States only in combination with sulfamethoxazole in a fixed ratio of five parts sulfamethoxazole to one part trimethoprim. It is generally available for oral use only.

Trimethoprim is well absorbed after oral administration and reaches a peak blood level approximately two hours after administration. The drug is widely distributed throughout all body tissues and fluids including cerebrospinal fluid, prostatic tissue, bile, and sputum. Trimethoprim readily crosses the placenta and achieves tissue levels in the fetus approximately equal to that of the mother.

Approximately half of a dose of trimethoprim is excreted unchanged in the urine with a serum half-life of approximately 13–16 hours. The remaining portion of trimethoprim is metabolized in the body to antibacterially inactive compounds which are also excreted in the urine. In contrast to sulfamethoxazole, the excretion of trimethoprim is increased by acid loading. Trimethoprim and sulfamethoxazole are rapidly removed from the blood by hemodialysis.

In overdosage of trimethoprim-sulfamethoxazole, patients should be observed for the toxic effects of the sulfamethoxazole. There are no available data on the toxic effects of trimethoprim.

IX. NITROFURANTOIN

Nitrofurantoin is a synthetic antibacterial compound used specifically for urinary tract infections. It is available for oral use in a crystalline or a macrocrystalline form.

Nitrofurantoin is rapidly absorbed from the gastrointestinal tract. The drug is rapidly metabolized in tissues and excreted through the kidneys with a serum half-life of 20–60 minutes. Significant concentrations of the drug are not achieved in serum or in body tissues because of the rapid metabolism and excretion. Urine alkalinization depresses tubular reabsorption of the drug and thus enhances the renal excretion. Significant amounts of nitrofurantoin are also excreted in the bile, with concentrations 200 times higher than those in the serum. Nitrofurantoin is effectively removed from the serum by hemodialysis.

In the event of nitrofurantoin overdosage, the most likely toxicity would be that of nausea and vomiting. Acute hemolytic anemia related to glucose-6-phosphate dehydrogenase deficiency might also be seen. Polyneuropathy would be unlikely except if the overdosage was associated with renal failure. Treatment of nitrofurantoin overdosage consists of the administration of high volumes of intravenous fluids and alkalinization of the urine. In the presence of renal failure, hemodialysis might remove some of the nitrofurantoin from the blood; however, this maneuver would probably not be necessary because of rapid metabolism of the drug in the tissues.

A. ACUTE TOXIC EFFECTS

1. Nausea and Vomiting

a. Nausea and vomiting are the most common and troublesome side effects of nitrofurantoin therapy, occurring in about 9% of patients to a degree severe enough to stop the drug. Nausea and vomiting are probably a toxic effect of nitrofurantoin on the central nervous system, rather than directly on the gastrointestinal tract.

b. These effects are directly related to the serum concentration of the drug and thus are more common when higher doses are used (7 mg./kg. or more), or when the patient has impairment of renal function which increases serum concentrations of the drug. Nausea and vomiting are less common in men and are also somewhat

less common with the macrocrystalline form.

c. Treatment

(1) Stop the drug.

(2) Maintain fluid and electrolyte balance as needed.

(3) Do not give phenothiazine antiemetics because both drugs are causes of cholestatic jaundice.

2. Hemolytic Anemia (G-6-P-D Deficiency)

a. Patients of African or Mediterranean background have a high incidence of genetically determined deficiency of glucose-6-phosphate dehydrogenase in aged red cells. Additionally, young infants are deficient in this enzyme. When G-6-P-D-deficient red cells are exposed to nitrofurantoin (or a large number of other drugs), acute hemolysis of the deficient cells occurs.

b. The patient may experience an acute hemolytic episode within hours of exposure to the drug. The clinical manifestations may be quite mild or can be severe enough to cause hemoglobinuria and peripheral vascular collapse. Because hemolysis is limited to the older cells that are deficient in the enzyme, the hemolytic episode is generally self-limited. The extent of hemolysis may be more severe in patients of Mediterranean origin.

c. Laboratory features of an acute hemolytic episode include a rapid fall in hematocrit and plasma haptoglobin and a concomitant rise in serum hemoglobin and unconjugated bilirubin.

d. Treatment

(1) Stop the drug.

(2) Maintain a high volume of urine flow to prevent hemoglobin nephropathy.

(3) Blood transfusions should not be required since the younger red cells will not be hemolyzed.

(4) A G-6-P-D screening test is of no

value after an acute hemolytic episode because G-6-P-D-deficient cells are no longer present. However, this test should be performed as confirmation of the deficiency after several months.

B. OTHER TOXIC EFFECTS

1. Peripheral Neuropathy

a. Peripheral neuropathy, a fairly uncommon toxic effect of nitrofurantoin therapy, can be fatal. Neurotoxicity appears most often in patients with renal insufficiency, but can occur in patients with normal or near-normal creatinine clearances. More than half of the patients receiving the drug chronically have nerve conduction defects on electromyography.

b. The onset of neuropathy may be as early as 3 days or longer than 200 days after the beginning of therapy. Most cases begin within one to two months.

c. The neuropathy is partially or completely reversed when the drug is stopped, but the recovery period may require several months.

2. Hypersensitivity

Common hypersensitivity reactions of drug fever, skin rashes, and eosinophilia occur in about 4% of patients receiving nitrofurantoin.

3. Interstitial Pneumonitis

a. Patients receiving nitrofurantoin may develop acute or chronic interstitial pneumonitis, presumably on an allergic basis. The acute form may occur within hours if the patient has been previously exposed to nitrofurantoin. However, it most commonly occurs after a more prolonged period of therapy.

b. The clinical manifestations of acute interstitial pneumonitis include the sudden onset of cough, fever, and shortness of breath. The radiographic picture resembles pulmonary edema, but the heart size is usually normal.

c. Treatment

(1) Stop the drug. In most cases this is sufficient to reverse the clinical picture rapidly.

(2) In severe cases short-term therapy with corticosteroids may be necessary.

d. Chronic interstitial pneumonitis is associated with irreversible interstitial fibrosis and is a sequel of long-term nitrofurantoin therapy.

4. Liver Toxicity

Cholestatic jaundice or hepatocellular necrosis have been described rarely with nitrofurantoin administration. These may be associated with eosinophilia and other evidence of hypersensitivity.

X. NALIDIXIC ACID

Nalidixic acid is a synthetic chemotherapeutic agent that is chemically unrelated to any other antibacterial agent. Its mechanism of action is presumed to be interference with bacterial DNA function.

Nalidixic acid is available for oral use in both tablets and in a suspension of 50 mg./ml. It is variably absorbed from the gastrointestinal tract, resulting in serum levels in the range of $20-50$ μg./ml., two hours after an oral dose of 1 gm. The drug is poorly distributed in body fluids other than the blood and urine. It is rapidly conjugated in the liver to inactive monoglucuronides, which are rapidly excreted by the kidney. About 15% of the active drug is also excreted in the urine, accounting for its antibacterial effect in urinary tract infections. In patients with renal failure, there is no accumulation of the active drug, but there is accumulation of the glucuronide in patients with severe renal failure. The accumulated glucuronide may contribute to the toxic effects of the drug.

In cases of overdosage of nalidixic acid, the toxic effects most likely to be seen are central nervous system effects such as hallucinations, psychosis, seizures, and increased intracranial pressure. Other toxic effects described with overdosage are hyperglycemia and metabolic acidosis. The treatment of overdose of nalidixic acid is supportive. Dialysis to remove nalidixic acid should not be necessary.

A. ACUTE TOXIC EFFECTS

1. Central Nervous System Toxicity

a. Seizures

(1) Seizures due to nalidixic acid are rare and most likely to occur in patients with high serum levels of the drug. This may be seen in conjunction with hyperglycemia.

(2)Treatment

(a) Stop the drug.

(b) Unless status epilepticus is present, there is no need to treat with antiseizure medication, since the seizures will disappear as the serum concentration of nalidixic acid falls.

b. Psychosis

Acute toxic psychosis ranging from mild visual disturbances to paranoia is a rare complication of nalidixic acid in high doses. The psychosis is reversible within days after stopping the drug.

c. Intracranial Hypertension

Infants and children receiving nalidixic acid in a therapeutic dose range have rarely developed reversible signs of increasing intracranial pressure, with papilledema, ocular palsy, and bulging fontanelles. This complication is reversible when the drug is stopped.

2. Hyperglycemia

a. Overdosage of nalidixic acid causes mild transient elevation of blood glucose, usually in association with central nervous system toxicity. The level of blood glucose rarely exceeds 300 mg./100 ml. and does not require insulin therapy be-

cause the glucose rapidly falls to normal ranges when the drug is stopped.

b. Nalidixic acid causes a false positive glucosuria with Clinitest tablets. In conjunction with central nervous system toxicity and mild hyperglycemia, diabetic acidosis is simulated. However, the serum and urine ketones are generally negative. The venous CO_2 is usually normal, although it is mildly depressed in the presence of metabolic acidosis.

3. Metabolic Acidosis

a. Patients with excessive overdosage of nalidixic acid or with normal doses in the presence of severe renal failure can develop metabolic acidosis, presumably as a result of the acid metabolic products of nalidixic acid. Metabolic acidosis usually appears in conjunction with central nervous system symptoms such as seizures and with mild hyperglycemia. The venous CO_2 content may be depressed.

b. Treatment

(1) Stop the drug.

(2) Bicarbonate therapy is probably not necessary in this syndrome because the acidosis is generally mild and is reversed as the nalidixic acid is cleared. In patients with severe renal failure with significant acidosis, hemodialysis may be necessary to more rapidly correct the acidosis.

B. OTHER TOXIC EFFECTS

1. Skin Rashes

a. Allergic rashes, both maculopapular and urticarial, have been described but are relatively uncommon.

b. Photosensitivity Reactions

(1) Nalidixic acid is one of the most common causes of photosensitivity reactions. It is more common in women than in men and occurs with moderate to heavy exposure to sunlight, at varying times after beginning the drug. A latent

period of one to two weeks after onset of drug therapy is most common, but reactions can occur on exposure to sunlight after having been on the drug for up to one year, and it may appear upon exposure to sunlight up to six months after discontinuing the drug. Recurrent exposure to sunlight can cause a recurrence of the reaction whether or not the drug has been stopped. The reaction is a bullous photodermatitis which occurs on exposed skin other than the face.

(2) Treatment

(a) Avoidance of sunlight will result in disappearance of the skin lesion.

(b) The drug should be discontinued although some patients have had no further reaction, if sunlight is avoided.

3. Hemolytic Anemia

G-6-P-D-deficient patients may have hemolysis precipitated by nalidixic acid. See the discussion under nitrofurantoin for management of this problem.

XI. GENTAMICIN AND OTHER AMINOGLYCOSIDES

Aminoglycosides are broad-spectrum antibiotics that are minimally absorbed from the gastrointestinal tract and thus are prepared for parenteral and topical use only. The members of this class of drugs are: streptomycin, neomycin, kanamycin, gentamicin, tobramycin, and amikacin. Spectinomycin is a closely related antibiotic that is available only for the treatment of uncomplicated gonorrhea. Neomycin, because of its excessive toxicity, is only used for topical therapy and as a nonabsorbed antibiotic given by mouth for modification of bowel flora.

Streptomycin dosage is usually 15 mg./kg. body weight per 24 hours in one dose or divided into two doses. The recommended dosage of kanamycin and amikacin is 5–7.5 mg./kg. of lean body weight per 12 hours, and the recommended dosage for gentamicin and tobra-

mycin is 1–1.7 mg./kg. of lean body weight per 8 hours. All the drugs are rapidly absorbed from an intramuscular injection site and reach a peak serum concentration within 30 minutes following administration. Whether given intravenously or intramuscularly, there is some variability in the peak serum concentration of these drugs. The doses listed above are designed to give peak concentrations of kanamycin and amikacin between 16 and 32 μg./ml. of serum; gentamicin and tobramycin, between 5 and 12 μg./ml. of serum.

The distribution of each of these drugs is similar. They diffuse readily into interstitial, pleural, ascitic, and other body fluids. Penetration into secretions such as saliva and sputum approximate 30–40% of the serum concentrations. All of these drugs penetrate very poorly into the cerebrospinal fluid. These drugs are present in the bile in approximately the same concentrations as found in the serum, except in the presence of biliary obstruction where the concentrations are quite low.

Excretion of all of the aminoglycosides is through the kidney in an unchanged form. There is a high concentration of each of the drugs in the kidney parenchyma and in the urine. In patients with normal renal function, the serum half-life for kanamycin and amikacin is approximately four hours; and for gentamicin and tobramycin, approximately three hours. In newborn infants, the excretion of these drugs is somewhat prolonged, but within a few days of birth, the excretion approximates that in adults; in older infants and children the excretion is more rapid than in adults.

There is no significant inactivation of any of these drugs in the body. All of the drugs are easily removed from the serum by both hemodialysis and peritoneal dialysis.

The toxic effect of aminoglycosides most likely to be seen in a case of overdosage would be neuromuscular blockade. Eighth nerve and nephrotoxicity would be unlikely sequelae of transient overdosage. In the presence of neuromuscular blockade, excessive levels of aminoglycosides can be removed by dialysis if the patient is in renal failure. If no renal failure is present, the drugs should be rapidly cleared by the kidney, and dialysis would be unnecessary.

A. ACUTE TOXIC EFFECTS

1. Neuromuscular Blockade

a. All of the aminoglycosides can cause competitive inhibition of the neuromuscular junction. This complication was most often described when large doses of the drugs were given intraperitoneally for postoperative lavage. The doses given were in excess of the doses which would be used systemically, and presumably very high blood levels of the drug were achieved. However, neuromuscular blockade has also been described with systemic administration of these drugs and is more likely to occur in patients who have other impairment of the neuromuscular junction, such as concomitant surgical anesthesia with ether or muscle relaxants, myasthenia gravis, and hypocalcemia.

b. Neuromuscular blockade induced by aminoglycosides is usually manifested as respiratory insufficiency. Apnea may occur. Generalized muscular weakness also occurs.

c. Treatment

(1) Stop the drugs.

(2) Obtain serum for aminoglycoside levels and serum electrolyte concentrations including calcium and magnesium.

(3) Obtain atrial blood gases, and maintain respiration with intubation and mechanical ventilation if necessary.

(4) Monitor the blood pressure and support with infusions of sympathomimetic amines if necessary.

(5) Administer neostigmine methysulfate, 1 mg. intravenously, combined with 0.5–1 mg. of atropine sulfate.

(6) If significant renal failure is present, hemodialysis or peritoneal dialysis may be necessary to remove excess aminoglycosides.

B. OTHER TOXIC EFFECTS

1. Eighth Cranial Nerve Toxicity

a. All aminoglycosides damage the vestibular and auditory portions of the eighth nerve as their major toxicity. Some of them are more selective for the vestibular portion, such as gentamicin and streptomycin, and some are more toxic to the auditory portion, such as kanamycin. However, toxicity to both portions of the nerve are possible with any of the drugs.

b. The clinical manifestations of vestibular toxicity range from tinnitus to vertigo to acute Ménière's disease. Toxic effects on the auditory portion of the nerve are manifested first by high-tone hearing loss detectable only by audiograms and then progressive loss of hearing in the mid and lower ranges. Complete deafness is rare. Toxicity to both vestibular and auditory portions may be partially reversible, and patients are also able to partially compensate for the loss of eighth nerve function.

c. Eighth nerve toxicity has been associated with serum concentrations of gentamicin and tobramycin greater than 12 μg./ml. of serum. Similarly, eighth nerve toxicity from kanamycin and amikacin has been associated with peak serum concentrations of 32 μg./ml. Vestibular and auditory toxicity have also occurred in patients receiving prolonged courses of low doses of the drug without elevated serum concentrations.

d. Eighth cranial nerve toxicity appears more commonly in patients with renal dysfunction, patients in older age groups, patients who have received previous courses of aminoglycoside therapy, and patients receiving concomitant therapy with ethacrynic acid.

e. Prevention and Treatment

(1) Patients receiving aminoglycosides, particularly gentamicin, tobramycin, kanamycin, and amikacin should have frequent measurements of serum aminoglycoside concentrations. This is especially true for those receiving high doses and those with renal failure. The therapeutic ranges of the drugs are narrow (5–12 μg./ml. for gentamicin and tobramycin and 16–32 μg./ml. for kanamycin and amikacin). The pharmacology of the drugs varies widely within the same patient and among patients over the course of their illnesses.

(2) The single most important measure for preventing eighth nerve toxicity is to stop the drug when the indications for its use have passed. Often the drugs are started empirically in very ill patients. Also, all too commonly, the drugs are continued even when subsequent cultural and clinical data do not support their continued use.

(3) In the event that vestibular or auditory symptoms occur in patients receiving these drugs, they should be stopped. There is no other therapy for eighth nerve toxicity.

2. Renal Toxicity

a. All aminoglycosides have the potential to cause renal damage. This is less common than eighth nerve toxicity and is generally reversible. The toxicity is mainly tubular and is manifested by proteinuria, rising BUN, and rising creatinine. Occasionally hypokalemia due to excessive renal potassium loss has been reported.

b. Attempts to relate nephrotoxicity to peak or trough serum levels have been generally inconclusive. There has been some correlation with elevated trough levels and the development of subsequent renal failure, but since these drugs are cleared through the kidney, the elevated levels may merely reflect retention of the drug by the kidney rather than directly causing the kidney failure.

c. Prevention and Treatment

(1) Patients receiving these drugs should have serum concentrations monitored frequently, particularly those with renal failure and those receiving high doses of the drugs.

(2) Renal dysfunction is not a contraindication to the use of these drugs, but the dosage regimen must be changed to ensure that excessive levels do not accumulate. The most common method for empirical modification of dosage is to lengthen the time interval between doses while continuing to give the same dose of the drug. A less commonly used method is to continue to administer the drug at a fixed time interval such as 8 or 12 hours but to reduce the amounts of the drug given in each dosage interval. Neither of these methods is accurate enough to assure that patients will receive adequate or nontoxic dosage. Thus, whatever dosage modification regimen is decided, serum concentrations must be measured and dosage intervals adjusted to maintain the appropriate concentrations.

(a) Gentamicin and tobramycin are frequently given according to the "rule of eights." This method fixes the gentamicin or tobramycin dosage interval at eight times the patient's serum creatinine.

(b) Similarly, the "rule of nines" is used for modification of kanamycin and amikacin dosage. With this rule, nine times the serum creatinine is the dosage interval in hours between doses.

(3) In the face of deteriorating renal function from whatever cause, the need for these drugs should be reevaluated. If continued therapy with aminoglycosides is necessary, the drugs can generally be continued with meticulous monitoring of serum concentrations so that they are clinically effective and do not accumulate to excessive levels.

(4) Generally, when the drugs are stopped, renal function returns to near its baseline. Occasionally, patients receiving these drugs in the face of renal failure and without serum concentration monitoring have developed complete anuria.

XII. ISONIAZID

Isoniazid (INH) is a drug available for oral use for both the treatment and prophylaxis of tuberculosis. It acts by interfering with nucleic acid metabolism as well as interfering with an enzyme system unique to the mycobacteria.

Isoniazid is rapidly absorbed from the intestine and reaches a peak serum level within the first one to two hours after administration. It is widely distributed in body fluids and tissues, including cerebrospinal fluid, pleural fluid, and caseous tissue. The drug crosses the placenta and is also excreted in human milk. The majority of isoniazid is metabolized in the liver by acetylation. The acetylated inactive metabolites are excreted along with active drug through the kidney. The speed of actylation is genetically determined, and humans can be classified as "slow inactivators" and "rapid inactivators." Slow acetylators excrete a higher proportion of active isoniazid in the urine and have a longer serum half-life of the active drug. The rate of acetylation of the drug is probably not important in routine use of the drug, but in patients with severe renal failure, slow acetylators may require a reduction in dosage. Isoniazid is effectively dialyzed by both hemodialysis and peritoneal dialysis.

Overdosage of isoniazid has been reported repeatedly in the literature. The manifestations of isoniazid overdosage are nervous system toxicity, with dizziness and stupor associated with repeated seizures. Metabolic acidosis, shock, and death can occur. Treatment of isoniazid overdosage is described below under central nervous system toxicity. Peritoneal dialysis and hemodialysis have been used in severe cases.

A. ACUTE TOXIC EFFECTS

1. Hypersensitivity

a. Skin rashes and fever are rare but can occur with isoniazid therapy.

b. There have been some case reports of systemic vasculitis with positive antinuclear antibodies.

c. Allergic bone marrow suppression, including neutropenia, thrombocytopenia, anemia, and eosinophilia, has been rarely described.

2. Central Nervous System Toxicity

a. Convulsions

(1) Patients receiving an overdose of isoniazid frequently develop multiple generalized seizures. However, patients with preexisting seizure disorders, slow acetylators of isoniazid, and patients with renal failure have rarely developed seizures while taking relatively normal doses of the drug.

(2) Treatment

(a) Standard anticonvulsants have little effect on isoniazid-induced seizures.

(b) Pyridoxine (vitamin B_6) should be given intravenously as a slow bolus. The amount that has been given varies, but an estimated dose is 1 gm. pyridoxine hydrochloride for each estimated gram of isoniazid ingested. If the amount is unknown, 5 gm. should be given over 5 minutes. The dose should be repeated every 5–20 minutes until the seizures are controlled. Intravenous pyridoxine should also be given to known isoniazid overdose patients even if seizures have not occurred.

(c) Correction of metabolic acidosis may be required to make pyridoxine therapy effective.

(d) In patients whose seizures are controlled with pyridoxine, dialysis should not be necessary. However, in patients who have renal failure and uncontrollable seizures, hemodialysis or peritoneal dialysis may be useful adjunctive therapy.

(e) Pyridoxine therapy should be considered in other patients with controllable seizures of unknown etiology, particularly when isoniazid has been available to the patient.

(3) Most patients with seizures have responded within 24 hours to pyridoxine and supportive therapy.

b. Coma

(1) Disorders of consciousness ranging from mild drowsiness to deep coma can occur with isoniazid overdosage. Coma may be present with or without seizures, and seizures may be present without coma.

(2) The treatment of unconsciousness related to isoniazid overdose is supportive with appropriate management of convulsions and metabolic acidosis.

c. Psychological Effects

(1) Isoniazid therapy has not infrequently been associated with changes in memory, mood, and affect. These changes may range from minor losses in memory to severe psychosis. Most cases of psychosis are described in patients who have a previous history of this type of illness.

(2) Mentation changes associated with isoniazid are not related to dose and are generally reversible when the drug is discontinued.

3. Metabolic Acidosis

a. Massive ingestions of isoniazid may lead to severe metabolic acidosis, usually in conjunction with seizures and coma. The acidosis appears to be lactic and has been associated with a blood pH as low as 6.88. Occasionally, high blood glucose is reported, and acetonuria has been reported.

b. Treat the metabolic acidosis with intravenous sodium bicarbonate. Correction of the acidosis may be necessary before seizures can be terminated by pyri-

doxine. Pyridoxine is incompatible with sodium bicarbonate and must be given separately.

B. OTHER TOXIC EFFECTS

1. Peripheral Neuropathy

a. Isoniazid therapy is associated with the development of peripheral neuropathy on the basis of pyridoxine deficiency. All patients receiving isoniazid excrete excessive amounts of pyridoxine in their urine.

b. The incidence of neuropathy ranges from 2% of adult patients receiving the usual dose of 300 mg. per day (approximately 3–5 mg./kg.) to as high as 20% in patients receiving 10 mg./kg. per day. The incidence of neuropathy is also more common in patients who have other predisposing causes to peripheral nerve disease such as alcoholism and diabetes. Peripheral neuropathy is also more common in patients who are "slow acetylators" of isoniazid.

c. The onset of neuropathy usually appears within five to six weeks in the higher dose patients and up to six months after starting the drug in the lower dose patients. The initial symptoms are tingling or numbness of the hands and feet which progresses to loss of pain and temperature sensation in a typical stocking-glove distribution. Motor symptoms are relatively uncommon unless the neuropathy is allowed to progress.

d. The symptoms are reversible with withdrawal of the drug, usually within several weeks unless the neuropathy was severe. In patients who require isoniazid therapy, the drug can be restarted in patients who develop neuropathy, usually at a lower dose and with pyridoxine supplementation in a dose of 50 mg. daily.

e. Patients who are receiving high doses of isoniazid should receive pyridoxine supplementation routinely from the onset of therapy, but this is unnecessary in patients receiving 5 mg./kg. per day.

2. Liver Toxicity

a. Isoniazid therapy is associated with a wide clinical range of hepatic toxicity, which can be separated into two clinical types.

b. Subclinical hepatic toxicity can occur in up to one-fourth of patients receiving the drug, and is manifested by mild elevations of liver enzymes (SGOT or SGPT two to five times the normal value). Occasionally mild elevations of bilirubin occur, but clinical jaundice is rare. This type of hepatotoxicity may subside even though the drug is continued, or the elevated enzymes may remain constant throughout the course. There is no apparent relationship between the acetylation rate and the development of subclinical hepatitis.

c. Clinically apparent isoniazid hepatitis is manifested by signs and symptoms indistinguishable from viral hepatitis. The histology of the hepatitis is also indistinguishable from viral hepatitis. There is some controversy about whether the hepatitis is caused by a direct toxic effect of the drug or its metabolites, a hypersensitivity reaction, or a concomitant viral infection. Symptomatic hepatitis occurs most often during the first two months of therapy, but it occasionally may be as late as one year after the onset of therapy. The incidence of severe liver damage increases with age as follows: (1) age less than 20, rare; (2) age 20–34, 0.3% of isoniazid recipients; (3) age 35–49, 1.2% of isoniazid recipients; (4) age over 50, 2.3% of isoniazid recipients.

d. The mortality rate of clinical hepatitis induced by isoniazid is reported at 12%. The mortality is higher in black women, in patients developing hepatitis after two months of therapy, and in patients with bilirubin over 20 mg./100 ml.

e. Treatment

Patients who have mild elevations of serum enzymes and are not symptomatic can be continued on the drug with close observation and frequent monitoring of enzymes. Patients with more severe forms of hepatic injury should not take the drug. In most cases, the hepatitis resolves quickly when the drug is stopped. Supportive therapy such as for viral hepatitis should be used.

3. Optic Neuritis

Optic neuritis has been reported very rarely with isoniazid therapy and appears to be unrelated to dose. When the drug is stopped early there are no sequelae, but if the drug is continued, optic atrophy can occur.

XIII. RIFAMPIN

Rifampin is an antibiotic with a wide spectrum of activity, but it is currently approved in the United States only for the treatment of tuberculosis and the meningococcal carrier state. It acts by interfering with bacterial RNA synthesis but does not interfere with RNA synthesis in mammalian cells. Rifampin is available for oral use. It is rapidly absorbed from the gastrointestinal tract and reaches its peak serum concentration in about two to four hours. Absorption is somewhat inhibited by food and by PAS. After absorption, rifampin is widely distributed in all body tissues including spinal fluid, sputum, tears, and saliva. Rifampin also has the capacity to penetrate mammalian cells and is thus effective against intracellular organisms.

Approximately 30% of an orally administered dose of rifampin is excreted unchanged in the urine. Most of the remainder is excreted through the biliary tract. Some active drug is excreted by the liver, but most is deacetylated in the liver and undergoes enterohepatic recirculation. The serum half-life of rifampin is one and a half to five hours. Rifampin is an inducer of hepatic enzymes, and its half-life decreases considerably after a few weeks of therapy. The presence of hepatic insufficiency can result in elevated serum concentrations of rifampin; the presence of renal insufficiency does not significantly affect excretion of rifampin. Both peritoneal and hemodialysis partially remove rifampin from the blood.

Rifampin overdose has been reported twice by Newton and Forrest (1975). They described a patient with a massive overdose who had red discoloration of the skin, urine, serum, and sweat. Recovery was complete without other toxic effects. Patients with an overdose of rifampin should be observed for renal toxicity, thrombocytopenia, liver disease, and those syndromes associated with intermittent therapy.

A. ACUTE TOXIC EFFECTS

1. Intermittent Therapy

A number of clinical syndromes have been described in patients who were on antituberculus regimens that called for intermittent doses of a few days to a week. In addition, the same syndromes have been described in patients who have discontinued and restarted their rifampin. Some of these syndromes have been described after intervals of more than one year off the drug.

a. Flu syndrome, characterized by the onset of fever, headache, malaise, and generalized myalgia, can occur within a few hours of taking a dose of rifampin after an intermittent period without the drug. This clinical picture may occur alone or may be associated with other toxic syndromes.

b. Like the flu syndrome, the abdominal syndrome occurs within a few hours after an intermittent dose of rifampin and is characterized by abdominal pain, nausea, vomiting, and diarrhea.

c. The respiratory syndrome is characterized by shortness of breath usually accompanied by wheezing.

d. There are apparently two types of acute renal failure which can develop with intermittent rifampin therapy.

(1) Within a few hours of receiving a reinstituted dose of rifampin, the patient may develop the acute onset of fever and lumbar pain followed by oliguria and anuria. This may be associated with the symptomatology of one of the syndromes mentioned above and may or may not be associated with other manifestations of rifampin toxicity.

Both clinically and histologically, the disease appears to be acute tubular necrosis with complete recovery. Patients may require maintenance dialysis until renal function returns to normal.

(2) A few patients have been reported in which renal failure did not have a symptomatic onset, but occurred gradually after reinstitution of rifampin therapy. Unlike the patients with acute oliguric renal failure, these patients had recovery of some but not all baseline renal functions. Renal biopsy demonstrated glomerular disease as well as tubulointerstitial disease. The glomeruli in some cases contained deposits of immunoglobulins and complement.

e. Acute hemolytic anemia is usually seen in association with one of the other syndromes associated with intermittent rifampin therapy. Acute hemolysis can occur within two or three hours after a dose of rifampin. Occasionally, hemolysis is severe enough to cause acute renal failure (acute hemolysis does not account for all of the reported episodes of renal failure).

f. Treatment

(1) Available evidence suggests that most or all of the intermittent therapy syndromes have an immunological etiology. However, many patients have rifampin antibodies and do not have these syndromes.

(2) Patients who have the less serious syndromes have been maintained on daily doses of rifampin without untoward effects. They have been satisfactorily main-

tained on intermittent therapy with a shortened drug-free interval or with a lower dose of the drug. Thus, patients who experience flu syndrome, abdominal syndrome, or respiratory syndrome can probably be continued on rifampin on a daily basis if the drug is necessary.

(3) Patients who have one of the more serious complications of intermittent rifampin therapy should never be given the drug again.

(4) Management of acute hemolytic anemia is primarily the prevention of renal failure by maintaining a high urine volume. Alkalinazation of the urine has been suggested as a means of preventing renal failure from hemolysis, but cautious administration of sodium salts to patients who already have renal insufficiency is essential to prevent fluid overload.

(5) Acute oliguric renal failure is managed similarly to acute tubular necrosis of other etiologies. Dialysis may be necessary.

2. Thrombocytopenia

a. Thrombocytopenia can occur as a manifestation of intermittent rifampin therapy, either alone or in association with one of the other intermittent rifampin syndromes. However, thrombocytopenia may also occur in patients who are on well-supervised daily therapy.

b. As with the intermittent syndromes, the onset of thrombocytopenia may occur within a few hours of receiving a dose of rifampin, and if the drug is discontinued, the platelets return to normal.

c. Most patients have not had significant bleeding problems with thrombocytopenia, but bleeding diseases ranging from cutaneous purpura to fatal intracerebral hemorrhage have been described.

d. Treatment

(1) In patients with bleeding from rifampin, the drug should be discontinued and never given again.

(2) The mechanism appears to be anti-body-dependent which requires the presence of rifampin. Thus, discontinuing the drug allows the platelet count to rapidly return to normal. There does not seem to be any interference with platelet production.

(3) Platelet transfusion should not be necessary since rifampin is excreted from the blood within a few hours. Also, the patient's platelet production is not impaired; the platelets are being destroyed peripherally.

(4) In the event of massive hemorrhage, blood transfusion may be necessary.

3. Hypersensitivity

a. As with virtually any other drug, allergic reactions have been described with rifampin. The most common reaction is skin rash or flushing. These reactions appear to be more common in patients receiving large doses of the drug. Many patients who have had mild cutaneous reactions have been continued on rifampin without consequences.

b. Very rare anaphalactoid reactions have been described.

c. There is no cross-reaction with any other antibiotic.

B. OTHER TOXIC EFFECTS

1. Liver Toxicity

a. Rifampin, like many other antituberculous drugs, has been found to cause mild transient elevation of liver enzymes early in the course of therapy. When the drug is continued in the asymptomatic patients, the enzymes generally return to normal levels.

b. In addition to enzyme elevation, rifampin may have several interactions with bilirubin. Rifampin may compete with bilirubin for serum carrier sites and for bilirubin excretion so that after a single dose of rifampin, there is a transient and reversible increase in serum bilirubin level. Thus, after the first dose of rifampin in a normal patient, the serum bilirubin level may rise from less than 0.5 to 1.5 within 4–5 hours. By the end of the 24-hour period, serum bilirubin has returned to normal. In addition, rifampin imparts a reddish color to body fluids and may interfere with colorimetric determination of bilirubin concentrations. Thus, serum bilirubin measurement should be performed before the daily administration of rifampin or 24 hours after the last dose to avoid a falsely elevated bilirubin value.

c. Rarely, patients on rifampin either intermittently or continuously develop serious symptomatic hepatitis. The risk of hepatitis appears to be increased with large doses and also appears to be higher in patients who have preexisting liver disease. In patients with minimal hepatic reserves, this toxic hepatitis may be fatal.

d. Treatment

(1) Although rifampin is not contraindicated in patients with preexisting liver disease, these patients should be monitored closely for the development of symptomatic hepatitis. Since most of these patients are also receiving isoniazid or other antituberculous drugs, the presence of elevated liver enzymes or symptomatic liver disease may be related to the rifampin or to one of the other drugs. Synergistic toxicity of rifampin and isoniazid probably does not occur.

(2) Stop the drug.

(3) Patients who have manifested symptomatic liver disease induced by rifampin should not be given the drug again. Patients who have a symptomatic enzyme elevation can probably be continued on the drug if necessary, although careful monitoring of the patient is necessary.

2. Drug Interaction

Rifampin is an inducer of hepatic enzymes and thus affects the metabolism of a number of other drugs. In addition to

accelerating its own metabolism, rifampin accelerates the metabolism of oral anticoagulants, oral hypoglycemic agents, oral contraceptive agents, corticosteroids, digitoxin, and methadone. These interactions may necessitate the modification of dosage of these drugs or alternative therapy.

XIV. FLUCYTOSINE

Flucytosine (5-fluorocytosine) is an oral compound used for the treatment of yeast infections, such as candidiasis and cryptococcosis. The drug is rapidly converted to 5-fluorouracil inside the fungal cell that interferes with RNA metabolism. There is no enzyme in mammalian cells capable of making this conversion.

Flucytosine is absorbed rapidly from the gastrointestinal tract and reaches a peak serum level approximately two to four hours after administration. The drug is widely distributed in body fluids and tissues and penetrates well into the spinal fluid, bronchial secretions, saliva, and eye. Flucytosine is excreted unchanged by the kidney through glomerular filtration. Very little of the drug is excreted by the liver or in the feces. Flucytosine is removed by hemodialysis and peritoneal dialysis.

Intentional overdosage of flucytosine has not been reported. In a case of flucytosine overdose, the likely toxic effects would be on the bone marrow and liver. If excessive overdosage of flucytosine is documented in the presence of renal failure, dialysis may be necessary to remove the drug.

A. ACUTE TOXIC EFFECTS

1. Bone Marrow Suppression

a. Flucytosine is capable of suppressing all of the elements of bone marrow. Neutropenia and thrombocytopenia are the most common toxic manifestations. Bone marrow toxicity, particularly neutropenia, seems to be related to concentrations greater than 125 μg./ml. of serum.

b. Since the drug is excreted entirely by the kidney, the presence of impaired renal function predisposes to elevated serum levels of flucytosine. This is particularly a problem in patients who are receiving both flucytosine and amphotericin B, which causes renal dysfunction. The marrow toxicity appears to be readily reversible if the drug is stopped or the drug dosage lowered before the onset of marrow aplasia.

c. Fatal marrow aplasia has been described in at least four cases. All of these patients were receiving large doses of flucytosine and had concomitant renal failure. At least one patient had markedly elevated flucytosine levels for two weeks.

d. Treatment

(1) Flucytosine given in conjunction with amphotericin B or in any patient who has even mild renal dysfunction should be monitored by frequent measurements of serum concentrations, and the dose adjusted accordingly.

(2) If neutropenia or thrombocytopenia occur, the drug should be stopped until the serum concentration falls below 100 μg./ml.

(3) If the drug is absolutely necessary, it may be reinstituted at a lower dosage, again monitoring serum flucytosine concentrations.

(4) In the presence of marrow aplasia, the drug should not be restarted. If the patient's renal function is significantly impaired, dialysis should be undertaken to reduce the serum concentrations of flucytosine to well under 100 μg./ml.

2. Gastrointestinal Toxicity

a. Approximately 6% of patients receiving flucytosine have gastrointestinal intolerance, which may be manifested by copious diarrhea, nausea, and vomiting. Pseudomembranous colitis does not seem to be the mechanism of the diarrhea.

b. Rare cases of intestinal ulceration and perforation have been described.

B. OTHER TOXIC EFFECTS

1. Liver Toxicity

Approximately 5% of patients receiving flucytosine have asymptomatic elevation of liver enzymes, usually serum transaminase or alkaline phosphatase. Significant hepatic dysfunction has been rarely reported, with biopsy evidence of patchy necrosis of hepatic cells. Serum flucytosine concentrations have not been measured in these cases.

2. Hypersensitivity

Skin rashes and eosinophilia have been described with flucytosine therapy. Anaphylactic reactions have not been described.

XV. GRISEOFULVIN

Griseofulvin is an antibiotic produced by *penicillium* mold which is administered orally for the therapy of dermatophytosis.

After oral administration, griseofulvin is partially absorbed in the gastrointestinal tract and reaches peak serum levels about four hours after administration. Absorption is increased by the presence of fat in the intestine. The drug is widely distributed in body tissues and is concentrated in liver fat, skeletal muscle, and keratinized tissues. Griseofulvin is slowly inactivated by the liver, and the inactive metabolite is excreted in the urine. Barbiturates accelerate the metabolism of griseofulvin.

A. ACUTE TOXIC EFFECTS

1. Headache

a. In as many as 15% of patients receiving griseofulvin, mild to severe headaches have been described. The headaches frequently disappear even when the drug is continued.

b. The headaches are not associated with any other apparent CNS disorder.

2. Gastrointestinal Irritation

As with many other antibiotics, nausea, vomiting, and diarrhea are not uncommon with griseofulvin. Dry mouth and thirst have also been described.

B. OTHER TOXIC EFFECTS

1. Skin Rashes

A wide variety of lesions has been described with griseofulvin therapy including maculopapular, urticarial, photosensitive, and erythema multiformelike rashes.

2. Hepatotoxicity

a. Griseofulvin interferes with porphyrin metabolism, although this is not of clinical significance in normal patients. Patients with porphyria have had aggravation of their condition during griseofulvin administration.

b. There have been very rare case reports of liver enzyme abnormalities with griseofulvin therapy.

3. Drug Interaction

a. Griseofulvin reduces the anticoagulant effect of warfarin.

b. Phenobarbital accelerates the metabolism of griseofulvin.

BIBLIOGRAPHY

I. PENICILLINS

Baldwin, D. W., Levine, B. B., McCluskey, R. T., and Gallo, G. R.: Renal failure and interstitial nephritis due to Penicillin and methicillin. N. Engl. J. Med., *279*:1245–1252, 1968.

Beirman, C. W., Pierson, W. E., Zeitz, S. J., Hoffman, L. S., and Van Arsdel, P. P., Jr.: Reactions associated with ampicillin therapy. J.A.M.A., *220*:1098–1100, 1972.

Brown, C. H., Natelson, E. A., Bradshaw, M. W., Williams, T. W., Jr., and Alfrey, C. P.: The hemostatic defect produced by carbenicillin. N. Engl. J. Med., *291*:265–270, 1974.

Fossieck, B., Jr., and Parker, R. H.: Neurotoxicity during intravenous infusion of penicillin: a review. J. Clin. Pharm., *14*:504–512, 1974.

Green, R. L., Lewis, J. R., Kraus, S. J., and Frederickson, E. L.: Elevated plasma procaine concentrations after administration of procaine penicillin G. N. Engl. J. Med., *291*:223–226, 1974.

Kerr, R. O., Cardamone, J., Dalmasso, A. P., and Kaplan, M. E.: Two mechanisms of erythrocyte destruction in penicillin-induced hemolytic anemia. N. Engl. J. Med., *287*:1322–1325, 1972.

Klastersky, J., Vanderkelen, B., Danegu, D., and Mathieu, M.: Carbenicillin and hypokalemia. Ann. Intern. Med., *78*:774–775, 1973.

Luciano, J. R., and Tarpay, M.: Penicillin allergy. South. Med. J., *69*:118–120, 1976.

Olans, R. N., and Weiner, L. B.: Reversible oxacillin hepatotoxicity. J. Pediar., *89*:835–838, 1976.

Yow, M. D., Taber, L. H., Barrett, F. F., Mintz, A. A., Blankenship, G. R., Clark, G. E., and Clark, D. J.: A ten-year assessment of methicillin-associated side effects. Pediatrics *58*:329–334, 1976.

II. CEPHALOSPORINS

Gralnick, H. R., McGinniss, M., Elton, W., and McCurdy, P.: Hemolytic anemia associated with cephalothin. J.A.M.A., *217*:1193–1197, 1971.

Mandell, G. L.: Cephaloridine. Ann. Intern. Med., *79*:561–565, 1973.

Moellering, R. C., Jr., and Schwartz, M. N.: The newer cephalosporins. N. Engl. J. Med., *294*:24–28, 1976.

Sanders, W. E., Johnson, J. E., Taggart, J. G.: Adverse reactions to cephalothin and cepharpirin. N. Engl. J. Med., *290*:424–429, 1974.

Weinstein, L., and Kaplan, K.: The cephalosporins: microbiological, chemical, and pharmacological properties and use in chemotherapy for infection. Ann. Intern. Med., *72*:729–739, 1970.

III. TETRACYCLINES

Robinson, M. J., and Rywlin, A. M.: Tetracycline-associated fatty liver in the male. Dig. Dis., *15*:857–862, 1970.

Tetracycline and blood urea. Br. Med. J., *3*:370, 1972.

Williams, D. N., Laughlin, L. W., and Lee, Y. H.: Minocycline: possible vestibular side-affects. Lancet, *2*:744–746, 1974.

IV. CHLORAMPHENICOL

Cocke, J. G., Jr., Brown, R. E., and Geppert, L. J.: Optic neuritis with prolonged use of chloramphenicol. J. Pediar., *68:*27–31, 1966.

Craft, A. W., Brocklebank, J. T., Hey, E. N., and Jackson, R. H.: The 'grey toddler': chloramphenicol toxicity. Arch. Dis. Child, *49:*235–237, 1974.

Levine, P. H., Regelson, W., and Holland, J. F.: Chloramphenicol-associated encephalopathy. Clin. Pharmacol. Ther., *11:*194–199, 1970.

McCaffery, R. P., Halsted, C. H., Wahab, M. F. A., and Robertson, R. P.: Chloramphenicol-induced hemolysis in Causasian glucose-6-phosphate dehydrogenase deficiency. Ann. Intern. Med., *74:*722–726, 1971.

Thompson, W. L., Anderson, S. E., Jr., Lipsky, J. J., and Lietman, P. S.: Overdoses of chloramphenicol. J.A.M.A. *234:*149–150, 1975.

Yunis, A. A., and Bloomberg, G. R.: Chloramphenicol toxicity: clinical features and pathogenesis. Prog. Hematol., *4:*138–159, 1964.

V. ERYTHROMYCIN

Cacace, L. G., Schweigert, B. F., and Gildon, A. M.: Erythromycin estolate induced hepatotoxicity: report of a case and review of the literature. Drug Intell. Clin. Pharmacol., *11:*22–25, 1977.

Karmody, C. S., and Weinstein, L.: Reversible sensorineural hearing loss with intravenous erythromycin lactobionate. Ann. Otol., *86:*9–11, 1977.

San Fillipo, J. A.: Infantile hypertrophic pyloric stenosis related to ingestion of erythromycin estolate: a report of five cases. J. Pediatr. Surg., *11:*177–180, 1976.

VI. CLINDAMYCIN AND LINCOMYCIN

Elmore, M., Rissing, J. P., Rink, L., and Brooks, G. F.: Clindamycin associated hepatotoxicity. Am. J. Med., *57:*627–630, 1974.

George, W. L., Sutter, V. L., and Finegold, S. M.: Antimicrobial agent-induced diarrhea: a bacterial disease. J. Infect. Dis., *136:*822–828, 1977.

Gurwith, M. J., Rabin, H. R., Love, K., et al.: Diarrhea associated with clindamycin and ampicillin therapy: preliminary results of a cooperative study. J. Infect. Dis., *135:*S104–S110 (suppl.), 1977.

Tedesco, F. J., Barton, R. W., and Alpers, D. H.: Clindamycin associated colitis. Am. Intern. Med., *81:*429–433, 1974.

VII. SULFONAMIDES

Craft, A. W., Brocklebank, J. T., and Jackson, R. H.: Acute renal failure and hypoglycemia due to sulfadiazine poisoning. Postgrad. Med. J., *53:*103–104, 1977.

Dujovne, C. A., Chan, C. H., and Zimmerman, H. J.: Sulfonamide hepatic injury. N. Engl. J. Med., *277:*785–788, 1967.

Lehr, D.: Clinical toxicity of sulfonamides. Ann. N. Y. Acad. Sci., *69* (3):417–447, 1957.

Weinstein, L., Madoff, M. A., and Samet, C. M.: The sulfonamides. Part II. N. Engl. J. Med., *263:*952–957, 1960.

VIII. TRIMETHOPRIM-SULFAMETHOXAZOLE

Frisch, J. M.: Clinical experience with adverse reactions to trimethoprim-sulfamethoxazole. J. Infect. Dis., *128* (suppl.):S607–S611, 1973.

IX. NITROFURANTOIN

Hailey, F. J., Glascock, H. W., and Hewitt, W. F.: Pleuropneumonic reactions to nitrofurantoin. N. Engl. J. Med., *281:*1087–1090,1969.

Koch-Weser, J., Sidel, V. W., Dexter, M., et al.: Adverse reactions of sulfisoxazole, sulfamethoxazole, and nitrofurantoin. Arch. Intern. Med., *128:*399–404, 1971.

Toole, J. F., and Parrish, M. L.: Nitrofurantoin polyneuropathy. Neurology, *23:*554–559, 1973.

X. NALIDIXIC ACID

Anderson, E. E., Anderson, B., and Nashold, B. S.: Childhood complications of nalidixic acid. J.A.M.A., *216:*1023–1024, 1971.

Brauner, G. J.: Bullous photoreaction to nalidixic acid. Am. J. Med., *58:*576–580, 1975.

Dash, H., and Mills, J.: Severe metabolic acidosis associated with nalidixic acid overdose. Ann. Intern. Med., *84:*570–571, 1976

Islam, M. A., and Sreedharan, T.: Convulsions, hyperglycemia, and glycosuria from overdose of nalidixic acid. J.A.M.A., *192:*1100–1101, 1965.

XI. GENTAMICIN AND OTHER AMINOGLYCOSIDES

Appel, G. B., and Neu, H. C.: The nephrotoxicity of antimicrobial agents. N. Engl. J. Med., *296:*722–728, 1977.

Barza, M., and Scheife, R. T.: Antimicrobial spectrum, pharmacology, and therapeutic use of antibiotics. IV., Aminoglycosides. Am. J. Hosp. Pharm., *34:*723–737, 1977.

Pittinger, C., and Adamson, R.: Antibiotic blockade of neuromuscular function. Ann. Rev. Pharmacol., *12:*169–184, 1972.

XII. ISONIAZID

Brown, C. V.: Acute isoniazid poisoning. Am. Rev. Resp. Dis., *105:*206–216, 1972.

Byrd, R. B., Horn, B. R., Griggs, G. A., and Soloman, D. A.: Isoniazid chemoprophylaxis: association with detection and incidence of liver toxicity. Arch. Intern. Med., *137:*1130–1133, 1977.

Cameron, W.: Isoniazid overdose. Can. Med. Assoc. J., *118:*1413–1415, 1978.

Goldman, A. L., and Braman, S. S.: Isoniazid: a review with emphasis on adverse effects. Chest, *62:*71–77, 1972.

Mitchell, J. R., Zimmerman, H. J., Ishak, K. G., Thorgeirsson, U. P., Timbrell, J. A., Snodgrass, W. R., and Nelson, S. D.: Isoniazid liver injury: clinical spectrum, pathology, and probable pathogenesis. Ann. Intern. Med., *84:*181–192, 1976.

Neff, T. A.: Isoniazid toxicity: reports of lactic acidosis and keratitis. Chest, *59:*245–248, 1971.

XIII. RIFAMPIN

Girling, D. J.: Adverse reactions to rifampicin in antituberculosis regimens. J. Antimicrob. Chemother., *3:*115–132, 1977.

Newton, R. W., and Forrest, A. R. W.: Rifampicin overdosage: "the red man syndrome." Scot. Med. J., *2:*55, 1975.

XIV. FLUCYTOSINE

Bennett, J. E.: Flucytosine. Ann. Intern. Med., *86:*319–322, 1977.

Kauffman, C. A., and Frame, P. T.: Bone marrow toxicity associated with 5-fluorocytosine therapy. Antimicrob. Agents Chemother., *11:*244–247, 1977.

XV. GRISEOFULVIN

Anderson, D. W.: Griseofulvin: biology and clinical usefulness: A review. Ann. Allergy, *23:*103, 1965.

Blank, H., et al.: Griseofulvin for the systemic treatment of dermatomycoses. J.A.M.A., *171:*2168, 1959.

12. ANTIHISTAMINES

Edward C. Conradi, M.D., and T. Douglas Cowart, Pharm.D.

Histamine-1 receptor antagonists have been in use for about 30 years with more than 100 prescription or nonprescription compounds available. These drugs are substituted ethylamines and may be divided into five different classes (Table 12-1).

The antihistamines are readily absorbed following both oral and parenteral administration. Diphenhydramine and triplennamine rapidly leave the blood and achieve maximal effect and tissue concentrations within one to two hours after an oral dose. Tissues are free of these compounds within six hours. Little free drug is excreted in the urine.

Chlorpheniramine is rapidly and almost completely absorbed after oral administration and reaches peak plasma concentration in about two hours. The volume of distribution is much greater than body water, suggesting one or more deep pools for the drug. Metabolism is rapid, and enterohepatic recirculation of the drug has been suggested. Recovery of the drug or its metabolites as much as 48 hours after a single dose suggests slow release from tissue. In overdose, slow tissue release and rapid metabolism of the drug would probably decrease the effectiveness of dialysis procedures. The significance and therapeutic implication of enterohepatic recirculation in overdose remain to be determined.

With the use of timed-release antihistamine preparations, onset of action and peak effect are delayed, and excretion is prolonged. This becomes important in the management of toxicity with these preparations.

I. CLINICAL FEATURES

It is estimated that 20–50% of people taking antihistamines experience some side effects (Table 12-2). Many of these are mild and easily corrected by stopping or changing the drug being used. However, the most serious toxic effects are a result of central nervous system stimulation or depression. These adverse effects occasionally occur with therapeutic doses of antihistamines but are usually the result of overdose.

Antihistamine poisoning occurs in all age ranges. In children, the most likely cause of poisoning is accidental ingestion of either proprietary or prescription drugs, although iatrogenic overdose has occurred. In adults, acute poisoning is usually a result of a suicide attempt or intentional abuse specifically for hallucinatory effect. In some instances, the toxic dose has been absorbed through the skin. The lethal dose in humans is not known for most of the antihistamines; however, 20–30 tablets of most available antihistamines represent a lethal or near-lethal dose for children. Children are particularly susceptible to the central nervous system stimulatory effects of the antihistamines with seizure activity predominant. Most fatalities have occurred in children, and it appears that as age increases, death from acute antihistamine toxicity is less likely.

Concomitant use of other drugs may complicate toxicity, and the combination of antihistamines with other anticholinergic drugs may potentiate CNS depression. Alcohol and barbiturates may potentiate CNS depression, and phenothiazines may have an additive effect.

Therapeutic and toxic doses of antihistamines may either depress or stimulate the central nervous system. In the therapeutic dose range, depression of the central nervous system is most commonly seen and is manifested as drowsiness, dizziness, or weakness. Central nervous system stimulation results in insomnia, nervousness, restlessness, and headache. In an antihistamine overdose, the CNS effects of the drug are predominant, and any of the toxic manifestations listed in Table 12-2 may be seen; however, the clinical picture tends to differ between children and adults. In children there is CNS stimulation with excitement, tremors, hyperactivity, hallucinations, hyperreflexia, and tonic-clonic convulsions. Children are more likely to have signs and symptoms of anticholinergic poisoning with flushed skin, fever, tachycardia, and fixed dilated pupils. Children that die usually have uncontrolled seizures progressing to coma and cardiorespiratory arrest. Acute poisoning in adults usually results in CNS depression with somnolence and coma. Anticholinergic effects are not as apparent, but several instances of seizures have been reported in younger adults.

II. TREATMENT

A. HISTORY

The following points should be emphasized since they bear directly upon the subsequent observation and management of the intoxicated patient:

1. Time of ingestion: Unless gastric emptying has been delayed (i.e., food, other drugs), the antihistamines are rapidly absorbed and gastric lavage may not return any ingested drug.

2. Type and quantity of drug: Combinations of drugs may potentiate one another and require specific therapeutic interventions not necessarily required for antihistamines alone. Especially important is the ingestion of a timed-release preparation. In this case, the observation period should be prolonged, and an attempt should be made to remove any portion of the drug not absorbed.

B. PHYSICAL EXAM

1. Vital signs.
2. Check for evidence of anticholinergic

Table 12-1. **Classes of H-1 Receptor Antagonists**

Class	Example	Major Secondary Effect
Ethanolamines	Diphenhydramine	Sedation
	Dimenhydrinate	Motion sickness
Alkylamines	Chlorpheniramine	Sedation
	Tripolidine	Sedation
Ethylenediamines	Triplennamine	Sedation
	Methapyrilene	Sedation
	Pyrilamine	Sedation
Piperazines	Cyclizine	Antinauseant
	Meclizine	Antinauseant
Phenothiazines	Promethazine	Sedation Antinauseant

effects (elevated temperature, arrhythmia, mydriasis, etc.).

C. EMERGENCY TREATMENT

1. Maintain adequate airway.
2. Control seizures.
   a. Diazepam: Children, 0.04–0.3 mg./kg. I.V. Adults, up to 10 mg. total dose I.V. Diazepam may produce respiratory arrest; however, it does not have the prolonged respiratory depression associated with the barbiturates.
   b. Physostigmine: Children, 0.5 mg. slowly I.V., 5 minutes between doses. If not effective, administer no more than 2 mg. If effective, the lowest effective dose should be repeated as indicated. Adults, 1 mg. slowly I.V., 20 minutes between doses. If no effect, the 1-mg. dose may be repeated once more to determine efficacy. If effective, a 1–2-mg. dose is repeated as indicated. If physostigmine is given too rapidly or in too large a dose, seizures may result.

   Indications include seizures which are difficult to control; extreme hyperpyrexia, severe hallucinations, hypertension, and arrhythmias.

Table 12-2. **CNS Side Effects and Acute Toxicity of Antihistamines**

Common CNS Side Effects	Acute Poisoning
Sedation	Hallucinations
Dizziness	Ataxia
Tinnitus	Athetosis
Incoordination	Excitement
Nervousness	Hyperactivity
Euphoria	Toxic psychosis
Insomnia	Incoordination
Tremors	Tremors
Blurred vision	Convulsions
	Restlessness
	Disorientation
	Drowsiness
	Somnolence
	Coma
	Hypotension
	Hypertension

Anticholinergic Effects	Other Effects
Flushing	Asthma
Mydriasis	Hematopoietic
Tachycardia	Agranulocytosis
Fever	Neutropenia
Dry mouth	Gastrointestinal
	Nausea
	Diarrhea
	Constipation
	Peripheral neuro-
	pathy
	Dermatitis
	Abnormal hepatic
	enzymes

Relative contraindications include asthma, gangrene, mechanical obstruction of the genitourinary or gastrointestinal tract, and cardiac disease.

D. DRUG REMOVAL

1. Emesis

a. Give syrup of ipecac 30 ml. orally. This should not be used in a situation where aspiration may occur. The dose may be repeated in 20 minutes. If there is no vomiting, the ipecac and any ingested drug should be recovered by gastric lavage.

b. Apomorphine 0.1 mg./kg. This drug should be restricted to adults with no evidence of cardiovascular disease. It may or may not be effective in overdoses of antinausea antihistamines. Apomorphine may produce respiratory depression.

2. Gastric Lavage

a. Use large bore tube #30.

b. Use lukewarm water or saline in aliquots not greater than 100 ml. Larger amounts may force the ingested drug into the small intestine.

c. If comatose, insert cuffed endotracheal tube prior to gastric lavage to prevent aspiration.

3. Activated Charcoal

Administer 30 to 60 gm. as a water slurry.

4. Catharsis

Sodium sulfate: Children, 250 mg./kg. Adults, 20–30 gm. This in combination with activated charcoal placed in the intestine may be very important in the management of overdose of delayed-release preparations.

5. Forced Diuresis, Peritoneal Dialysis, Hemodialysis

No data is available for these methods of treatment. One would not expect them to be beneficial because the antihistamines are rapidly taken up by tissues and rapidly metabolized with very little free drug present in plasma.

E. HYPERTHERMIA

1. Sponge with tepid water.
2. Cover the patient with a thermal blanket.
3. See above for physostigmine.
4. No alcohol. This produces shivering and helps increase temperature.

F. LABORATORY WORK

1. Blood gases—monitor severity of respiratory depression.
2. ECG—monitor for arrhythmias.
3. Chest x-ray to assess for aspiration

and check the position of the endotracheal tube if patient is intubated.

4. Gastric, urine, and blood samples for drug identification (gastric and urine samples are the most helpful in antihistamine overdose).

III. USES: TYPES OF PREPARATIONS THAT CONTAIN ANTIHISTAMINES

Antihistamines are used in the treatment of various allergic diseases and are most efficacious in acute allergies. They are also used as sedatives, antinauseants, and to prevent motion sickness. There are several oral and topical preparations for pruritus and various dermatoses. Antihistamines are present in many cough syrups, and multiple proprietary and prescription preparations contain different combinations of one or more antihistamines, caffeine, analgesics, and sympathomimetic amines for symptomatic relief of the common cold. Methapyrilene and pyrilamine are present in several nonprescription hypnotic preparations in combination with salicylamide and different amounts of the anticholinergic drug, scopolamine (e.g., Sominex, Nytol, Compoz). The reader is referred to the American Drug Index for a comprehensive list of prescription and nonprescription preparations containing antihistamines.

BIBLIOGRAPHY

Bayley, M., Walsh, F. M., and Valaske, M. J.: Fatal overdose from bendectin. Clin. Pediatr. *14:*507, 1975.

Bayley, M., Walsh, F. M., and Valaske, M. J.: Report of a fatal acute triplennamine intoxication. J. Forensic Sci. *20:*539, 1975.

Douglas, W. W.: Histamines and antihistamines: 5-hydroxytryptamine and antagonists. *In:* Goodman, L. S., and Gilman, A. (eds.): The Pharmacological Basis of Therapeutics. pp. 590-629, New York, Macmillan, 1975.

Jones, I. H., Stevenson, J., Jordan, A., Connell, H. M., Heterington, H. D. G., and Gibney, G. N.: Pheniramine as an hallucinogen. Med. J. Aust. *1:* 382, 1973.

Lee, J., Turndorf, H., and Poppers, P. J.: Physostigmine reversal of antihistamine-induced excitement and depression. Anesthesiology, *43:*683, 1975.

Meadow, S. R.: Poisoning from delayed release tablets. Br. Med. J., *1:*512, 1972.

Reyes-Jacang, A., and Wenzl, J. E.: Antihistamine toxicity in children. Clin. Pediatr. *8:*297, 1969.

Soleymanikashi, Y., and Weiss, N. S.: Antihistamine reactions: A review and presentation of two unusual examples. Ann. Allergy, *28:*486, 1970.

Wyngaarden, J. B., and Seevers, M. H.: The toxic effects of antihistaminic drugs. J.A.M.A. *145:*277, 1951.

Zepp, E. A., Thomas, J. A., and Knotts, G. R.: Some pharmacologic aspects of the antihistamines. Clin. Pediatr., *14:*119, 1975.

13. ALCOHOLS AND GLYCOLS

Charles L. Mendenhall, M.D., Ph.D., and Robert E. Weesner, M.D.

I. ALCOHOLS

A. ETHANOL

Ethanol (ethyl alcohol) is the most commonly encountered organic solvent and is used as a topical antiseptic, chemical intermediate, and beverage. For many commercial uses ethanol is denatured with other solvents, methanol, acetone, methyl isobutyl ketone, tertiary butanol, and diethyl phthalate, which may contribute to its toxicity. When consumed in small to moderate amounts, toxicity is low. However, larger amounts produce significant pathophysiological changes and even death.

1. Clinical Features

Excess alcohol results in central nervous system (CNS) depression beginning with the primitive reticular activating system, which is responsible for much of the integration of activity in various parts of the nervous system. This results in disruption of motor and thought processes and produces the clinical picture of intoxication.

Blood alcohol levels are used to diagnose intoxication. The American Medical Association House of Delegates, in 1960, recommended that persons with alcohol levels of 100 mg./100 ml. or more be considered intoxicated. However, many persons with levels of 50 mg./100 ml. or less may be intoxicated. In most legal jurisdictions in the United States, a person is judged legally intoxicated with blood alcohol of 100 to 150 mg./100 ml.

a. Central Nervous System

Acute toxic effects include CNS depression, beginning with mood changes and progressing to psychomotor retardation, reflex slowing, lethargy, sleep, and ultimately coma and death.

Alcoholic coma occurs at blood levels exceeding 300 mg./100 ml., with death occurring at levels above 400 mg./100 ml. However, survival has been reported at 700 mg./100 ml. Death results from respiratory center paralysis with apnea.

Death usually occurs after 5 to 10 hours of coma. Findings are similar to those seen with surgical anesthesia passing from stage 3 to deep stage 4, in which lid and gag reflexes are progressively decreased, with flaccidity of the limbs, dilatation of pupils, and diminished thoracic respiration. Abdominal respiration first increases and then fails. If respiration is supported, cardiovascular collapse ensues with irreversible shock.

The LD_{50} consumption in humans is 5 gm. alcohol/kg. of body weight. See Table 13-1 for contents of common alcoholic beverages.

2. Differential Diagnosis

The odor of alcohol on breath is not pathognomonic for alcoholic coma. The presence of a high blood alcohol (more than 300 mg./100 ml.) does not exclude the concomitant existence of other equally serious and life-threatening processes. To be considered are:

Head trauma
Drug overdose
Hypoglycemia
Diabetes mellitus with coma
Hepatic coma
Heat or cold exposure
Overwhelming infection
Cardiac arrhythmia
Postconvulsive state

Head trauma must be ruled out by the history and physical findings of trauma, skull x-rays, and spinal tap.

Table 13-1. **Ethanol Content of Alcoholic Beverages***

Alcoholic Beverage	Ethanol Content (gm./oz.)
Beers	
Lager: 3% to 6% (vol) ethanol; mean 4.5% 12 oz. can contains 12.8 gm.	1.07
Ale: 3% to 8% (vol) ethanol; mean 5.5% 12 oz. can contains 15.6 gm.	1.30
Wines (24.0–25.6 oz. bottle)	
Table wines (red, rosé, white, champagne) 10% to 14% (vol) ethanol; mean 12%	2.84
Dessert or cocktail wines (muscatel, port, sherry, vermouth) 16% to 22% (vol) ethanol	4.74
Liqueurs 22% to 50% (vol) ethanol; mean 32%	7.58
Distilled Spirits	
80 proof: 40% (vol) ethanol	9.47
100 proof: 50% (vol) ethanol	11.84

*Leake, C. D., and Silverman, M.: Chemistry of alcoholic beverages. *In* Kissin, B., and Begleiter, H. (eds.): The Biology of Alcoholism. vol. 1, pp. 575–610. New York, Plenum Press, 1971.

Drug overdose in the alcoholic patient is frequent. Synergistic reaction between ethanol and other CNS depressants is of special significance in the differential diagnosis of coma. Competitive inhibition of hepatic drug metabolizing enzymes, as well as the synergestic CNS depression, has resulted in death when the individual levels were far below those considered dangerous.

Hypoglycemia is frequently associated with excess ethanol consumption. The occurrence may be as long as 36 to 48 hours after the last drink and does not correlate with the blood alcohol level. Usually but not necessarily, it is associated with malnutrition or vomiting and food deprivation. Blood sugar is diagnostic.

Diabetic coma may be confused with alcoholic coma. The two are unrelated and can be differentiated by blood sugar.

Hepatic coma is associated with severe liver disease and, hence, may be seen in alcoholics with alcoholic liver disease. Liver function tests (SGOT, bilirubin, alkaline phosphatase, prothrombin time), if severely abnormal, are consistent with hepatic coma but not pathognomonic. Arterial blood ammonia (NH_3) and EEG findings may be helpful.

Overwhelming infection with secondary shock must be considered. Presence or absence of leukocytosis and fever are suggestive. Chest x-rays, urinalyses, and blood cultures may be diagnostic.

Convulsions in the alcoholic, so called run fits or alcoholic epilepsy, are frequent. They occur during the withdrawal phase but may be associated with drinking as recent as six hours previously. Duration of drinking episodes range from five days to many months (mean, three weeks). Seizure is grand mal. The EEG is usually normal, and diagnosis is one of exclusion.

3. Treatment

1. Remove unabsorbed alcohol by gastric lavage.
2. Maintain adequate airway and respiration.
3. Maintain body temperature—hypothermia is a frequent complication.
4. Avoid all CNS depressant drugs.
5. Maintain blood sugar with I.V. glucose (10 –50% solutions)—hypoglycemia is a frequent complication.
6. Correct lactic acid acidosis, a frequent complication, with sodium bicarbonate.
7. Hemodialysis is indicated if blood alcohol levels exceed 400 mg./100 ml.

Acute alcohol excess not infrequently

produces a moderate to severe hemorrhagic erosive gastritis or duodenitis. This is especially true when combined with salicylates.

Clinical features include nausea, vomiting, hematemesis, melena, and epigastric pain. Endoscopy is diagnosic.

Remove remaining ethanol by gastric lavage and suction. Antacids or Cimetadine reduce and inhibit gastric acidity. Surgical intervention may be necessary if bleeding persists.

B. METHANOL

Methanol (methyl alcohol, wood alcohol, Columbian Spirits) is the simplest of the alcohols used as a solvent to denature or contaminate ethyl alcohol, to make it unfit for human consumption but acceptable for industrial use. The toxic dose varies with individual susceptibility, ranging from 15 to 250 ml., 0.2 to 2.8 gm./kg., and usually requiring more than 70 ml. for death.

1. Clinical Features

Toxic effects are usually superimposed or mixed with signs of ethyl alcohol excess. CNS depression is of minor significance. As a result of metabolic conversion of methanol to formic acid, acidosis is severe. Optic neuropathy that produces blindness may result from formaldehyde formation.

Symptoms include headache, vertigo, nausea, vomiting, diarrhea, blurring of vision, and tenderness of eyes. Abdominal pain associated with acute pancreatitis is frequent. Lethargy and restlessness may progress rapidly to confusion, convulsions, coma, and death.

Symptoms of toxicity lag 8–36 hours behind the ingestion. Visual disturbances may be the first sign and occur as early as 6 hours. Visual recovery occurs within six days with treatment; permanent impairment is usually present when severe retinal edema is present.

2. Treatment

a. Gastric lavage with 1 teaspoon sodium bicarbonate added to 2–4 liters of tap water, (20 gm./liter).

b. Ethyl alcohol will competitively inhibit methanol oxidation and can be given 0.4–0.6 gm./kg. orally in a 5–10% solution every two hours for four days. Blood ethanol levels should be maintained in the range of 100–200 mg./ml.

c. Combat acidosis with sodium bicarbonate.

d. Hemodialysis is indicated if blood methanol exceeds 50 mg./100 ml. or if symptoms progress rapidly and do not respond to administration of ethyl alcohol or alkalinating agents.

C. ISOPROPYL ALCOHOL

Isopropyl alcohol (Isopropanol, 2-propanol and N-propanol, 1-propanol) is an important industrial solvent and disinfectant. Most frequent home uses are in rubbing alcohol, skin lotions, hair tonic, and deicing and antifreeze preparations. Isopropanol is intermediate in toxicity—less toxic than methanol but more toxic than ethanol.

1. Clinical Features

a. Central Nervous System

As a CNS depressant it is about twice that of ethanol. The LD_{50} dose is 5.8 gm./kg. with a lethal dose of 2.7 gm./kg. or 240 ml. in a 70 kg. adult. Blood levels of 150 mg./100 ml. are associated with deep coma.

Symptoms include dizziness, incoordination, headache, and confusion, progressing to stupor and coma. Hypothermia, hypotension, and circulatory collapse are not infrequent. Death is usually due to respiratory failure.

b. Digestive System

Gastritis and duodenitis are usually more prominent than with ethanol; symptoms include nausea, vomiting, and hemorrhage.

2. Laboratory Findings

Because isopropanol is metabolized to acetone, severe acetonuria without acidosis is present. Tests of liver and kidney function are usually abnormal, but severe changes are rare.

3. Treatment

Treatment is similar to that for ethanol.
a. Gastric lavage with water.
b. Maintain adequate airway, respiration, body temperature.
c. Hemodialysis reduces blood and tissue levels.
d. Gastritis is managed in a manner identical to ethanol.

N-propanol is used as a solvent resin but is not commonly available for home use. It is reportedly slightly more toxic than isopropanol but produces essentially the same biological effects and clinical symptoms. The LD_{50} is 1.87 gm./kg. Treatment is identical to that for isopropanol.

II. GLYCOLS

The glycols are heavy, colorless, odorless, water-soluble liquids with a sweet, acrid taste which may contribute to their popularity as suicide agents and as a poor person's substitute for alcohol. They are represented by ethylene glycol, diethylene glycol, hexylene glycol, and propylene glycol. Diethylene glycol has an ether linkage not present in ethylene glycol, which produces more intense renal damage. Unlike ethylene glycol, diethylene glycol is not metabolized to oxalate and is not associated with hypocalcemia. Propylene glycol is essentially nontoxic and is an unusual example of a foreign compound entirely catabolized by normal metabolic pathways.

Because most clinical experience with glycols comes from ethylene glycol, the discussion will be limited to this agent. Ethylene glycol was discovered as a substitute for glycerine and is found in detergents, paints, lacquers, pharmaceuticals, polishes, cosmetics, and most often in deicers and antifreezes. The metabolites of ethylene glycol are much more toxic than the parent compounds. Since alcohol dehydrogenase is the first enzyme involved in the degradation of ethylene glycol, ethanol is used as a blocking agent. The estimated lethal dose of ethylene glycol is 100 ml.

A. CLINICAL FEATURES

1. Inhalation is rare because of low vapor pressure (BP 198°C). Nystagmus, lymphocytosis, and recurrent attacks of unconsciousness have been reported in workers chronically exposed to ethylene glycol heated above 100°C.

2. Irritation and penetration of skin is minor. Acute iridocyclitis has followed accidental eye contact.

3. Acute ingestion has the following CNS effects 30 minutes to 12 hours after ingestion.
   a. Intoxication without alcoholic odor on breath.
   b. Nausea, vomiting, headache, coma, convulsions, nystagmus, ophthalmoplegia, papilledema (with subsequent optic atrophy), depressed reflexes, generalized or focal seizures, myoclonic jerks, and tetanic contractions.
   c. Cerebrospinal fluid findings compatible with meningoencephalitis.

4. Metabolic effects include leukocytosis (10,000–40,000/cu. mm.), acidosis (bicarbonate often < 10 mEg./liter), anion gap > 20, hyperkalemia, hypocalcemia.

5. Cardiopulmonary effects occur 24 to 72 hours following ingestion and include tachypnea, tachycardia, mild hypertension, cyanosis, pulmonary edema, bronchopneumonia, cardiac enlargement, and congestive failure.

6. Renal effects include oliguria, which

can occur within 12 hours of ingestion and can last as long as 50 days.

    a. Urine: calcium oxalate crystals, hippurate crystals, low specific gravity, proteinuria, microscopic hematuria, pyruria, and cylinduria.

    b. Costovertebral angle tenderness and acute tubular necrosis.

B. TREATMENT

1. Gastric lavage with water.

2. Provide oxygen and artificial respiration as needed for CNS depression.

3. Intravenous mannitol to produce an osmotic diuresis, thus promoting excretion of ethylene glycol and its metabolites. Continue until crystalurea ceases (contraindicated if oliguria has already occurred).

4. Correct acidosis with sodium bicarbonate.

5. Correct hypocalcemia with calcium gluconate.

6. Ethanol, 0.1mg./kg. per hour of 100% ethanol intravenously as a 5% solution in D_5W (only beneficial if given within the first four to eight hours of ingestion).

7. Hemodialysis or peritoneal dialysis to reduce blood and tissue levels of ethylene glycol and metabolites, as well as to correct uremia and acidosis. Perform if above treatment is ineffective.

8. Give large doses of thiamine and pyridoxine, precursors to cofactors needed to degrade ethylene glycol to less toxic products than oxalic acid.

9. Treat convulsions if intense or persistent with a short-acting barbiturate drug.

10. Treat shock if present.

BIBLIOGRAPHY

Gonda, A., Gault, H., Churchill, D., et al.: Hemodialysis for methanol intoxication. Am. J. Med., *64:* 749, 1978.

Keyvan-Larijarni, H., and Tannenberg, A. M.: Methanol intoxication. Arch. Intern. Med., *134:* 293, 1974.

Parry, M. F., and Wallach, R.: Ethylene glycol poisoning. Am. J. Med., *57:*143, 1974.

Sellers, E. M., and Kalant, H.: Alcohol intoxication and withdrawal. N. Engl. J. Med., *294:*757, 1976.

14. CORROSIVES

Irwin B. Hanenson, M.D., and Amadeo J. Pesce, Ph.D.

Corrosives, including acids and bases, are chemicals which destroy tissue on exposure by inhalation, ingestion, or contact with skin or eyes. These agents destroy tissue by dissolution and precipitation of cellular protein. The lesion produced is analogous to a burn.

The concentration of the corrosive agent is the single most important property related to its toxicity. Lethality is related not only to quantity of a chemical but also to the physical effect of the corrosive action (e.g., esophageal penetration, pulmonary edema). Therefore, when possible, dilution of these agents is an important factor in reducing toxicity.

This chapter will include acids, alkali, gases, and oxidizing agents which are responsible for the majority of medically significant corrosive poisonings.

I. ACIDS

The corrosive acids include acetic, hydrochloric, hydrofluoric, nitric, oxalic, phosphoric, and sulfuric acids. Oxalic and hydrofluoric acids are also metabolic poisons. Oxalic acid reduces the plasma ionized calcium and forms calcium oxalate stones in the kidney. The fluoride ion also combines with calcium and, in addition, interferes with enzyme activity. Acids readily dissolve in the fluids of mucous membranes and lung tissue to produce inflammation.

A. CLINICAL FEATURES

1. Inhalation

a. Acute chemical pneumonitis and/or pulmonary edema manifested by cough, chest pain, cyanosis, dyspnea, hemoptysis, and diffuse rales. Blood pressure may be high or low.

b. Chronic cough with bronchial pneumonia.

2. Ingestion

a. Corrosive burns of the oropharynx, esophagus, and stomach accompanied by burning pain; vomiting with or without blood; melena. Associated physical findings include hypotension, fever, rigid abdomen, perforation of the esophagus or stomach, with mediastinitis or peritonitis. Stricture of the pyloris and esophagus may subsequently develop.

b. Oxalate ingestion may also produce respiratory collapse and renal stones with or without anuria.

3. Contact

a. Skin: burns, pain, and brownish or yellowish stains.

b. Eyes: pain, tearing, sensitivity to light, conjunctival edema, and corneal destruction.

B. TREATMENT

1. Inhalation

a. Respiratory support: artificial respiration, patent airway by endotracheal intubation or tracheostomy, respirator.

b. Shock: I.V. fluids and transfusion if necessary.

c. Pulmonary edema: sedation, oxygen, bronchodilators and rapidly acting diuretics.

d. Pneumonia: provide appropriate chemotherapy.

e. Pulmonary fibrosis: prevent by prednisone, 2 mg./kg. per day for 7–14 days.

2. Ingestion

a. Avoid gastric lavage or emesis.

b. Dilute acid by having patient drink large quantities of water or milk.

c. Intravenous fluid replacement.

d. Relieve pain with morphine sulfate, 5–10 mg. every four hours as necessary.

e. Neutralize with milk of magnesia, 100–200 ml.

f. Maintain airway to prevent asphyxia secondary to glottal edema.

g. For suspected perforation, give nothing by mouth until endoscopic examination.

h. Esophageal stricture formation may be suppressed by prednisone, 2 mg./kg. per day for 7–14 days.

i. Oxalate: measure calcium; if low, give milk, limewater, or intravenous calcium gluconate to replenish the ionized calcium.

3. Contact

a. Skin: flush with water; burns, same manner as for thermal burns.

b. Eyes: flush with water; burns, consult ophthalmologist; pain, systemic analgesics.

II. BASES

The most commonly encountered corrosive bases contain ammonium, sodium, or potassium hydroxide. In contrast to acids, bases are not volatile with the exception of ammonium hydroxide, which upon neutralization produces the gas ammonia. Inhalation of ammonia produces inflammation of the respiratory passages and pneumonitis.

A. Clinical features and treatment are the same as for acids with the following exceptions:

1. Neutralization is often not necessary since this will be accomplished by the stomach acids.

2. The ammonium ion, in contrast to sodium and potassium, is a systemic poison producing convulsions and coma.

III. CORROSIVE GASES

The corrosive gases include chlorine, the nitrogen oxides, the sulfur oxides, and ammonia. With the exception of ammonia, they are oxidizing agents that form strong acids when dissolved in mucous fluids and produce an inflammatory reaction of the respiratory tract when inhaled.

A. CLINICAL FEATURES

Upon inhalation or on contact with eyes, clinical features are as described for acids. The nitrous oxides are inhaled for their psychodelic effects. Observe for this possibility.

B. TREATMENT

Treat as for acid.

IV. OXIDIZING AGENTS

These include iodine, hydrogen peroxide, silver nitrate, and potassium permanganate. As corrosives, they cause severe burns. Iodine and silver nitrate are both oxidizing agents and precipitate cellular protein; hydrogen peroxide destroys cells by oxidation alone.

There are no toxic metabolic products of either hydrogen peroxide, which is quickly broken down by enzymes, or silver nitrate, which precipitates with chloride ion.

A. CLINICAL FEATURES

1. Inhalation

Hydrogen peroxide forms a gas that acts as an irritant to the respiratory passages.

2. Ingestion

a. Signs and symptoms are the same as those for acids.

b. Hydrogen peroxide breaks down rapidly and releases oxygen gas, which distends the stomach.

c. Iodine and potassium permanganate may cause anuria.

3. Skin

a. Clinical features of burns are the same as those for acids.

b. Hydrogen peroxide penetrates the skin, yielding subcutaneous bubbles.

4. Eyes

a. Clinical features are the same as those for acids.

b. Hydrogen peroxide produces punctate lesions of the cornea that appear immediately or several days later.

B. TREATMENT

1. Inhalation

Treat as for acids.

2. Ingestion

a. Treat as for acids.

b. For hydrogen peroxide, dilute and insert nasogastric tube to relieve distention.

c. For iodine, neutralize with starch, 30 gm. corn starch per liter of water given orally, or by a 1% solution of sodium thiosulfate.

d. Treat acute renal shutdown by conventional techniques.

3. Skin

Treat as for acids.

4. Eyes

Treat as for acids.

BIBLIOGRAPHY

Arena, J. M.: Poisoning Toxicology Symptoms, Treatments. 3rd ed. Springfield, Ill., Charles C Thomas, 1974.

Christian, M. S.: Principles of emergency treatment for swallowed poisons. Proc. R. Soc. Med., *70:* 764–778, 1977.

Rumack, B. H.: Poisindex. Denver, Micromedex, 1978.

15. HYDROCARBONS AND HOUSEHOLD CHEMICALS

HYDROCARBONS

Amadeo J. Pesce, Ph.D., and Edward J. Otten, M.D.

I. PETROLEUM DISTILLATES

This classification refers to carbon compounds that are liquid at room temperature and usually found as solvents, fuels, and additives in household cleaners, polishes, and cements. They may contain a mixture of straight- and branched-chain aliphatic hydrocarbons. Substances such as kerosene, naphtha, gasoline, and mineral spirits, because of their low surface tension and vapor pressure, tend to spread over a large surface area such as the lungs. This accounts for the major toxicity of these compounds. It was originally thought that the presence of these substances in the lungs was secondary to the vomiting that usually accompanies their ingestion. However, it has been shown that even without vomiting and subsequent aspiration, the mere presence of the substance in the hypopharynx can cause chemical pneumonitis. Pathologically, the lesions show alveoli filled with proteinaceous material, interstitial edema, and occasionally frank hemorrhage. Weakened alveolar wall may lead to emphysema and pneumothorax. There usually are associated central nervous system symptoms secondary to systemic absorption and rarely liver, kidney, myocardial, and bone marrow injury.

A. CLINICAL FEATURES

1. Inhalation

a. Acute chemical pneumonitis is manifested by cough, rales, hemoptysis, dyspnea, and respiratory failure. This may develop immediately or up to 12 hours after ingestion. Classically the chest x-ray shows basilar infiltrates. Acute pulmonary edema, emphysema, and pneumothorax may also occur.

b. CNS depression develops with absorption of large amounts (see Ingestion).

2. Ingestion

a. Acute chemical pneumonitis can occur (see Inhalation).

b. Gastrointestinal irritation is manifested by severe abdominal pain, nausea, and vomiting. Often there is the odor of hydrocarbons on the patient's breath.

c. CNS depression initially presents as euphoria, mania, and excitement, and later progresses to headache, irritability, depression, confusion, coma, and convulsions. The degree of CNS involvement is related to the individual constituents of the ingested substance and the dose.

d. Rarely, there is kidney, liver, and bone marrow involvement.

e. Myocardial sensitization with potentially fatal cardiac arrhythmias have been reported.

3. Contact

a. With prolonged contact, there is often a first-degree burn exhibiting red, painful areas.

b. The substance may be absorbed through the skin and produce systemic manifestations, especially when large surface areas are involved.

B. TREATMENT

1. Inhalation

a. Provide respiratory support: oxygen, endotracheal intubation, and mechanical ventilation as indicated. Follow with serial arterial blood gases and chest x-rays.

b. Steroids have not been shown to be useful.

c. Antibiotics are indicated in the treatment of specific bacterial infections but are probably not useful prophylactically.

2. Ingestion

a. A great deal of controversy has arisen over whether the stomach should be emptied. In general, the stomach should probably be emptied if:

(1) The amount of hydrocarbon ingested is more than 1 ml./kg. of body weight.

(2) If the hydrocarbon is particularly toxic, i.e., trichloroethane.

(3) If the hydrocarbon contains an organophosphate insecticide, heavy metal, or other toxic substance. Each case should be judged individually, and the risk of aspiration should be weighed against the benefit of removing the toxin. Vomiting should be induced only in an awake patient with an intact gag reflex. The patient should be placed in the left lateral recumbent, head down position to minimize the chance of aspiration. In patients without a gag reflex, a cuffed endotracheal tube should be inserted before gastric lavage is performed. In children under 6 years of age, a cuffed endotracheal tube is not used; the cricoid ring provides the necessary seal at this age.

b. The use of vegetable oil to increase the viscosity of the ingested hydrocarbon is probably not beneficial, and some studies have shown an increased incidence of pneumonitis with this procedure.

c. General supportive care should include cardiac monitoring, baseline laboratory studies, chest x-ray, and ECG.

d. Intravenous diazepam may be used to control convulsions.

e. Because of the possibility of myocardial sensitization by the hydrocarbon, epinephrine should be avoided if possible. There have been reports of fatal arrhythmias secondary to the use of myocardial stimulants.

3. Contact

a. Flush the area involved with water.

b. Watch for signs of systemic toxicity.

II. AROMATIC HYDROCARBONS
(Benzene, Xylene, Toluene)

These substances are solvents which evaporate readily at room temperature and are commonly found in paint and varnish removers, lacquers, and rubber and plastic cements. The volatility and aromatic smell of these compounds, coupled with the CNS effects that they produce, make them popular with "glue sniffers." The compound, in cases of solvent abuse, is placed in a plastic bag and inhaled until the desired effect is reached. The acute inhalation or ingestion is very similar to the petroleum distillates with one exception: most of the deaths related to solvent abuse are probably due to suffocation by the plastic bags or some activity of the person while under the influence of the inhaled substance. Tolerance and dependence rapidly develop with chronic abuse, but serious withdrawal symptoms have not been noted. Patients with a history of long exposure or chronic abuse may develop bone marrow suppression, liver failure, kidney failure, and irreversible CNS changes.

A. CLINICAL FEATURES

1. Inhalation

a. The patient may present with a number of CNS manifestations including euphoria, staggering gait, dizziness, violent behavior, hallucinations, blurred vision, tremors, confusion, coma, and convulsions. The presentation may resemble acute alcohol intoxication.

b. Gastrointestinal symptoms of nausea, vomiting, abdominal pain, or burning of nose and mouth are common.

c. Tracheobronchitis and signs of chemical pneumonitis occur (see petroleum distillates for description).

d. There is myocardial sensitization with various arrhythmias.

e. Chronic exposure may cause liver or kidney failure, bone marrow suppression, and focal or generalized CNS changes.

2. Ingestion

Clinical features are the same as those for inhalation.

3. Contact

a. Depending on the compound and length of exposure, there may be anything from dry, peeling, scaly skin to burning, red, blistering skin.

b. Although uncommon, systemic signs may be present if a large amount of the substance was absorbed through the skin.

c. Superficial burns of the eyes are common, as is inflammation of the mucous membranes with contact of the solvent or its fumes.

B. TREATMENT

Treatment is the same as for petroleum distillates. Baseline studies such as CBC, prothrombin time, platelet count, liver and renal profiles, urinalysis, ECG, and chest x-ray should be done in severe cases or with a history of prolonged exposure.

III. ALDEHYDES AND KETONES

A. ALDEHYDES

This group of compounds is very reactive and combines with many cellular constituents such as proteins, sugars, and nucleic acids. Unlike strong bases or acids, which actually may be considered to "burn" through tissue, aldehydes destroy tissue by "fixing" it in place. These compounds are usually strong irritants and if ingested can have metabolic effects. The most commonly encountered aldehyde is formaldehyde.

1. Formaldehyde

a. Clinical Features

(1) Inhalation
This causes irritation of the pharynx and trachea.

(2) Ingestion
(a) This produces burning abdominal pain with gastritis, collapse, coma, and possible anuria. There is CNS depression.

(b) Hemolysis of red cells and liver injury may be present.

(3) Eyes
Irritation conjunctivitis may be present.

(4) Skin
Brown discoloration and dermatitis are common.

b. Treatment

(1) Ingestion
(a) Treatment is the same as that for corrosives. Dilute with milk, water, or activated charcoal. Most protein-containing material will react to neutralize formaldehyde.

(b) Removal by gastric lavage or emesis is controversial because of the risk of esophageal damage and aspiration. However, if a large volume of formaldehyde has been taken, there may be less risk with emesis or with gastric lavage than allowing the toxin to remain in the stomach.

(c) If patient has severe hemolysis, alkalinize and replace blood as necessary.

(d) Maintain urine flow.

2. Ketones

The most commonly encountered ketone is acetone, which is found in many household products. It is a natural metabolic product, and its major effects are from drying of mucous membranes and possible CNS depression. Large amounts ingested can result in hypoglycemia.

If large quantities are ingested, emesis should be induced or gastric lavage performed.

Other ketones vary in their toxicity. Since many are volatile, the patient may present with the effects of inhalation. The clinical features are upper respiratory irritation and pulmonary edema. The pulmonary effects are less severe than other hydrocarbons such as lower boiling point petroleum distillates.

HOUSEHOLD CHEMICALS

Irwin B. Hanenson, M.D., and Amadeo J. Pesce, Ph.D.

The toxic agents present in household chemicals are quite varied. For a variety of technological and legal reasons, formulations change rapidly or differ by region. Thus, the date of manufacture and place of production are of importance in establishing the toxic substance. Several toxic agents may be present in a particular product. Drug and Poison Information Centers have the most accurate information on formulations and toxic chemicals and should be called if the contents are not known.

For many products, the toxicity is quite low. The order of frequency of lethal ingestion by toxic agent is petroleum distillates, insecticides and herbicides, soaps, shampoos, detergents, cleaners and cleansers. (Table 15-1).

I. BORATES

Various forms of borate compounds (alkaline in strong laundry soaps to acid for eyewash) are used in household products. All borates in high concentration are cellular poisons. Because they are concentrated and excreted by the kidney, renal failure is a possible lethal effect.

A. ALKALINE BORATES

These are often corrosive.

1. Clinical Features

a. Corrosive effect of bases is evident.

b. Vomiting and diarrhea, convulsions, cyanosis, hypotension, coma, and possible renal failure are common.

2. Treatment

a. See corrosive bases (Chap. 14).

b. If on skin or eyes, wash thoroughly and treat as corrosive base.

c. If ingested, emesis or gastric lavage, depending upon mental status of patient.

d. Give I.V. fluids to maintain urine output.

e. Treat convulsions with diazepam.

f. For extreme toxicity, perform dialysis or exchange transfusion.

B. ACID BORATES

1. Clinical Features

Vomiting, diarrhea, shock, coma, and renal failure are common.

2. Treatment

Follow (b) to (f) above.

Table 15-1. **Classes of Household Products and Most Likely Toxic Agents**

Products	Examples of Products	Toxic Agents
Adhesives	Duro Plastic Rubber, Duco, Testors	Trichloroethane Epoxy resins Cyanoacrylate Toluene, acetone nitrocellulose, hexane
Bleaches	Clorox, Purex	Sodium hypochlorite Alkaline borates Anionic detergents
Cleaners	Vanish, Windex, Spic & Span, Mr. Clean	Soaps Alkaline, borates Anionic detergents Nonionic detergents Polyphosphates, glycols
Cleansers	Comet, Ajax	Sodium hypochlorite Anionic detergents
Detergents	Cascade, Tide	Anionic detergents Alkaline borates Alkaline polyphosphates
Disinfectants	Lysol, Lestoil	Anionic detergents Nonanionic detergents Cationic detergents Phenol Isopropyl alcohol Hydrocarbons Petroleum distillates Nitrites Nitrates
Deodorants	Secret, Ban	Anionic detergents Nonionic detergents Ethanol Soaps
Deodorizers	Pinesol, Airwick	Chlorinated hydrocarbon Insecticides Detergents, anionic, nonionic Hydrocarbons Petroleum distillates
Drain cleaners	Drano, Liquid Plummer	Sodium hydroxide Trichloroethane Sodium hypochlorite Surfactants
Fertilizers	Scotts	Nitrogen Phosphorus Potassium Insecticides, if present, major toxic chemicals
Glues	Elmer's, Super Glue	Cyanoacrylate

Table 15-1. **Classes of Household Products and Most Likely Toxic Agents—Continued**

Products	Examples of Products	Toxic Agents
Glues (cont.)		Glycols Toluene/xylene
Glycols	Prestone	Ethylene glycol Diethylene glycol
Herbicides	Orthotriox, Weed Killer	Chlorophenylalkyl ureas Chlorophenylalkoxy ureas
Insecticides	Raid, Terminex	Carbamates Chlorinated hydrocarbons Hydrocarbons Organophosphates Petroleum distillates Pyrethrin
Liquid polishers and wax	Pledge, Johnson, Aero	Hydrocarbons Petroleum distillates Isopropyl alcohol Borates Xylene/toluene
Moth balls		Naphthalene Chlorinated hydrocarbons Insecticides
Paint	Rustoleum, Sears	Alkaline corrosives (white wash) Linseed oil Hydrocarbons Petroleum distillates Toluene diisocyanates (urethanes)
Perfumes and colognes	Avon, Revlon, etc.	Ethanol Essential oils
Shampoo (hair)	Head & Shoulders, Johnson's	Detergents Soaps Anionic detergent Nonanionic detergent Cationic detergent
Shampoo (carpet)	Glory, Blue Luster	All above hydrocarbons Petroleum distillates

II. ANIONIC DETERGENTS

These usually have minimal toxicity.

A. CLINICAL FEATURES

These include vomiting, diarrhea, and intestinal distention.

B. TREATMENT

1. Administer intravenous fluids to the patient.

2. Control excessive vomiting by administering antiemetics.

III. CATIONIC DETERGENTS

Some forms of these detergents are cellular poisons (zephirin, benzaconium chloride, quaternary ammonium forms, nalteyl dimethyl ethyl benzyl ammonium chloride). If ingested, they are readily absorbed. Often they are formulated with a strong acid; this may be the toxic agent.

A. CLINICAL FEATURES

Vomiting, collapse, and coma are common.

B. TREATMENT

1. Emesis if patient is awake and alert.
2. Lavage if patient obtunded.
3. Milk or activated charcoal.

IV. SODIUM HYPOCHLORITE

This is occasionally found in bleaching agents and cleaners. On contact with body fluids present on mucous membranes, there is a release of hypochlorous acid which acts as a corrosive.

A. CLINICAL FEATURES

These are similar to, but less severe than corrosive acids.

B. TREATMENT

Treatment is the same as for acid corrosives.

V. NONIONIC DETERGENTS

These are usually forms of alkylaryl polyethersulfates and are included in various household formulations. Symptoms and treatment are identical to the anionic detergents.

VI. POLYPHOSPHATES

Polyphosphates may be considered to belong to the class of corrosive alkalis because they are usually present as the sodium form. These compounds are readily absorbed and have a strong affinity for calcium.

A. CLINICAL FEATURES

1. Skin and eye: similar to corrosive alkali.
2. Ingestion: corrosive effect is most marked. Hypocalcemic convulsions may occur.

B. TREATMENT

1. Treat as for corrosive alkali.
2. If ingested, a solution of 5 milliliters of 10 per cent calcium gluconate slowly infused intravenously may be used to treat the hypocalcemic convulsions.

BIBLIOGRAPHY

Beamon, R. F., et al.: Hydrocarbon ingestion in children: a six year retrospective study. J.A.C.E.P., 5:771, 1976.

Gosselin, R. E., Hodge, H. C., Smith, R. P., and Gleason, M. N.: Clinical toxicology of commercial products. *In* Acute Poisoning. 4th ed. Baltimore, Williams & Wilkens, 1976.

Grant, W. M.: Toxicology of the Eye. 2nd ed. Springfield, Ill. Charles C Thomas, 1974.

Hayden, J. W., Comstock, E. G., and Comstock, B. S.: The clinical toxicology of solvent abuse. Clin. Toxicol., 9:169, 1976.

Ng, R. C., Darwish, H., and Stewart, D. A.: Emergency treatment of petroleum distillate and turpentine ingestion. Canadian Medical Association Journal, 111:537, 1974.

Porter, J. A. H.: Acute respiratory distress following formalin ingestion. Lancet, 2:603, 1975.

Steele, R. W., et al.: Corticosteriods and antibiotics for the treatment of fulminant hydrocarbon ingestion. J.A.M.A., 219:1434, 1972.

U.S. Department of Health, Education and Welfare: Handbook of Common Poisonings in Children. Washington, D.C., Superintendent of Documents, U.S. Government Printing Office, Stock No. 017-012-00240-4, 1976.

Wyse, D. G.: Deliberate inhalation of volatile hydrocarbons: a review. Can. Med. Assoc. J., 108: 71, 1973.

16. METALS

Paul Hammond, D.V.M., Ph.D.

There are approximately forty elements that are classified as metals. They vary considerably as to toxicity. In many cases little is known about toxicity for humans, simply because human contact in the toxic range has been either nonexistent or very infrequent. For most of the remaining metals, poisoning results mainly from occupational exposure. There are notable exceptions of course, as in the case of alkyl mercurials and cadmium, which have caused episodes of poisoning by introduction into the food chain.

Toxicity from overdoses taken with suicidal intent is rare and is limited mainly to occasional cases involving arsenic and thallium. Similarly, toxicity in young children is largely limited to three metals—lead, iron, and thallium.

It must be emphasized that a good medical history is essential in unveiling metal poisoning. The presenting signs and symptoms seldom constitute an adequate basis for diagnosis. They are too variable and nonspecific to lead to any firm conclusions. An awareness about occupational or other activities resulting in exposure to toxic metals is almost essential for a proper diagnosis. For this reason, sources of exposure to the metals may well be the single most important element in discovery of exposure.

I. LEAD

The most common source of lead poisoning is probably occupational. The major occupational hazards exist among workers employed in primary or secondary lead smelters and in the manufacture of storage batteries. Workers engaged in cutting structural steel with acetylene torches also are at risk if the metal has been previously painted with red lead paint. The dust emitted during cutting may contain high concentrations of lead. Other trades in which potentially toxic lead exposure may occur are plastics manufacture and typesetting.

Illicitly distilled whiskey often contains toxic concentrations of lead and, among heavy consumers, has been the cause of lead poisoning. Acidic foods and beverages stored in improperly glazed earthenware may also cause poisoning if the container is used consistently for storage of food or beverage.

Children 1 to 5 years of age are prone to pica. If they chew on chips of lead-base paint or plaster, lead poisoning may result. It is also suspected, though not proved, that street and house dust may similarly be a source of poisoning if consumed in sufficient quantities. The source is fallout of lead from the exhaust of motor vehicles that burn leaded gasoline.

A. CLINICAL FEATURES

Rarely, cases of poisoning are reported in which massive single oral doses of lead have been taken as an abortifacient or, perhaps, with suicidal intent. Presenting signs and symptoms are drowsiness, abdominal pain, and nausea. Jaundice and petechial hemorrhages are usually noted. Extensive degeneration of the kidneys leads to albuminuria or anuria.

Most cases of poisoning occur as a result of repeated exposure over a period of weeks or months. Signs and symptoms progress in approximately the following sequence, depending on severity and duration of exposure.

1. Anemia (nonhemolytic)
2. Gastrointestinal disturbances, mainly nausea, abdominal colic, diffuse abdominal pain, constipation

3. Weakness and lethargy
4. Tubular nephritis manifested mainly as aminoaciduria and glycosuria, but also including hyperphosphaturia in the presence of hypophosphatemia
5. Interstitial nephritis and renal insufficiency
6. Encephalopathy progressing from lethargy, drowsiness, and irritability to clumsiness, ataxia, stupor, and finally to tremor, coma, and convulsions

B. LABORATORY FINDINGS

Excessive lead exposure is readily established on the basis of concentration of lead in whole blood. None of the signs and symptoms described above are encountered when the blood lead concentration remains in the normal range of 10–40 μg./dl. There is, however, no clear proportionality between degree of blood lead elevation and severity of poisoning. Elevation of free erythrocyte porphyrin concentration is also a good index of lead exposure, although it is nonspecific and is also associated with iron deficiency anemia. Elevation of δ-aminolevulinic acid coproporphyrin in the urine are also useful indices of excessive lead exposure which correlate reasonably well with the degree of blood lead elevation. Elevations of indices of excessive exposure are particularly valuable in the case of lead because they persist for many weeks after cessation of exposure.

C. TREATMENT

Regardless of the severity of poisoning, measures must first be taken to remove the patient from the source of exposure. This of itself will usually not effect a prompt termination of elevated circulating lead or of signs and symptoms. The rate of disappearance of lead from even the more readily exchangable body stores is slow. The biological half-life for lead in blood, for example, ranges from several weeks to several years, depending on the duration of exposure.

The need to take additional measures will depend on the severity of illness. Even when signs and symptoms are only very moderate, it is usually justified to institute chelation therapy. For this purpose three drugs have received fairly extensive evaluation in humans, calcium disodium ethylenediamine tetracetate (CaEDTA), dimercaptopropanol (BAL), and D-penicillamine (PCA). PCA is available only for investigational purposes. All three drugs act by markedly and promptly enhancing the urinary excretion of lead. CaEDTA and BAL are effective only by parenteral administration, whereas PCA is effective parenterally and orally. CaEDTA may be administered either intravenously or intramuscularly. The intravenous route is preferred. Ideally, the dose should be given by intravenous drip over six hours. A slow infusion has been found to mobilize appreciably more lead than infusion over one hour. The adult dosage of CaEDTA is 1–2gm. per day given on four or five successive days. Courses of therapy may be repeated after several days of rest. BAL is not commonly used in adults for the treatment of lead poisoning.

The treatment of lead poisoning in children also entails courses of CaEDTA therapy, either alone or in combination with BAL. Combined therapy is initiated with BAL, 4 mg./kg., intramuscularly. Four hours later and every four hours for the next five to seven days, CaEDTA (12.5 mg./kg.) and BAL (4 mg./kg.) are given concurrently at separate intramuscular sites.

D. PROGNOSIS

The prognosis depends entirely on the severity of poisoning. Mild anemia is readily reversible. This usually is also the case for gastrointestinal and renal tubular effects. If exposure is sufficiently severe; permanent renal and central nervous system effects can occur.

II. MERCURY

There are three general forms of mercury: (1) elemental mercury and inorganic salts of mercury, (2) alkyl mercury compounds, and (3) aryl organic mercurial compounds. Perhaps the most frequently encountered type of mercury poisoning results from inhalation of vapors of elemental mercury. Occupationally, exposure to mercury vapors occurs in the chloralkali industry. Large pools of mercury are used as cathodes in the electrolytic conversion of sodium chloride to sodium hydroxide and chlorine gas. Hazardous exposures also occur in the manufacture or repair of instruments such as barometers, thermometers, switches, and ultraviolet lamps. Dangerous accumulations can also occur in laboratories as a result of repeated spillage. Salts of mercury are used in the manufacture of fungicides and bactericides. Here the danger is mainly from accidental oral intake.

Whereas inhalation of elemental mercury vapor is quite hazardous, oral intake such as swallowing mercury from broken thermometer bulbs is relatively harmless. When injected intravenously, as in suicide attempts, elemental mercury is moderately toxic. Slow release of mercuric mercury from resultant emboli of mercury can cause chronic systemic poisoning.

Inorganic salts of mercury are not commonly a problem. At one time mercuric chloride was used as a disinfectant. Accidental and suicidal ingestion of tablets or concentrated liquid occurred. Mercurous chloride (calomel) was used as a laxative, and excessive doses has caused fatal mercury intoxication. Its toxicity is considerably lower, however, than is the toxicity of mercuric chloride.

Alkyl mercurial compounds, notably methyl and ethyl mercury salts, have been used extensively as fungicides. A major application has been to protect seed grain from mold infestation. On occasion, mercury-treated seed grain has found its way into the market for human consumption as flour. As a result, hundreds of people have been poisoned, often fatally. Notable episodes occurred in Iraq, Guatemala, Pakistan, and Ghana, the most recent being in Iraq, 1971–1972. Methyl mercury has also been found to contaminate fish under certain circumstances. Contamination is due to synthesis of methyl mercury by aquatic microorganisms with subsequent transfer and biomagnification up the food chain to carnivorous fish. In many instances the original source of mercury has been traced to contamination of streams with inorganic mercury from industrial processes, e.g., chloralkali plants. Heavy fish consumers are suspected of approaching dangerous levels of methyl mercury intake, but clear-cut intoxication is not demonstrable.

A. CLINICAL FEATURES

1. Inorganic Mercury

Salts of mercury are locally corrosive, causing necrotic, vesicular, and inflammatory effects at the point of contact, particularly mucous membranes. After ingestion of large doses, diarrhea occurs. Blood and shreds of intestinal mucosa may be passed. Nausea, vomiting, and abdominal pain occur, along with salivation.

The major target organs for inorganic mercury after systemic absorption are the kidneys. Extensive renal tubular damage occurs fairly promptly. An initial phase of diuresis occurs, followed by oliguria or anuria within a few days.

In chronic oral intake, excessive salivation occurs, along with inflammatory changes of the gums and mouth (stomatitis and gingivitis). Teeth also may become loose. If the route of intake is inhalation, as is more commonly the case, these effects are usually not seen.

The systemic effects of chronic mercury absorption are primarily neurological and behavioral, but at low levels of exposure certain nonspecific effects occur. These are mainly, loss of weight and appetite. Insomnia and nervousness also occur at low levels of exposure. Objective signs most commonly seen are tremors of fingers, eyes, and tongue. Sudden attacks of anger, loss of memory, and drowsiness also occur, but probably at higher levels of exposure.

2. Organic Mercury

The effects of alkyl mercury compounds are primarily neurological. The neurological effects are primarily sensorimotor. This is in contrast to the effects of chronic inhalation of elemental mercury in which the effects are more of a psychic character. Major effects are paresthesia, ataxia, constriction of the visual field, slurred speech, motor weakness, slowed cerebration, and impaired hearing. More severe cases exhibit stupor, inability to speak, incontinence and choreo-athetotic movements. In ethyl mercury poisoning, renal disorders are common, whereas in methyl mercury poisoning, these are rare. Gastrointestinal symptoms also are more common in ethyl mercury poisoning than in methyl mercury poisoning. Although salts of phenyl mercury are also used as fungicides, the toxic effects are more like those of inorganic salts of mercury. This is because of the rapid breakdown of phenyl mercury in the body to inorganic mercury.

B. LABORATORY FINDINGS

1. Inorganic Mercury

As with lead, the most helpful laboratory aid to diagnosis is determination of the concentration of metal in biological fluids. Urine and whole blood are equally valuable as indices of exposure. The normal range for mercury in urine is approximately < 0.1–0.1 mg./liter (corrected to specific gravity = 1.018), and for whole blood it is approximately < 1–5 μg./dl. The correlation between urinary and blood mercury is fairly good, at least among people with elevated exposure. In interpreting blood mercury values, it must be borne in mind that the mercury is concentrated mainly in the erythrocytes. Even in mild cases of poisoning, urinary mercury may exceed 10 mg./liter, and

blood mercury may exceed 25 μg./dl., but any value outside the normal range must be viewed as supportive of a diagnosis of mercury intoxication.

2. Organic Mercury

Again, as with inorganic mercury poisoning, the most helpful laboratory aid is analysis for mercury in the patient. The concentration of mercury in the whole blood and hair are the most useful indices of exposure. The lowest concentration of mercury in whole blood that has been observed in association with alkyl mercury toxicity is 20 μg./dl. Severely intoxicated people often have whole blood values of several hundred micrograms per deciliter. Extensive studies of mercury in hair indicate a concentration ratio, hair to whole blood, of roughly 100 to 1.

C. TREATMENT

In acute cases of inorganic mercury intoxication by oral intake, certain measures are recommended to neutralize mercury in the gastrointestinal tract. Milk combined with several egg whites should be taken. A generous dose of activated charcoal is also recommended. This should be followed by gastric lavage.

In the case of both acute and chronic inorganic mercury poisoning, chelating agents are useful for accelerating removal of the metal from the body. The choice of agents is limited to CaEDTA and BAL. PCA and its *N*-acetyl derivative (*N*-acetyl DL-penicillamine; NAP) both show more promise than CaEDTA or BAL but are available for investigational use only. BAL is probably more efficacious in mobilizing mercury than CaEDTA, based on experimental animal studies. Because it enhances mercury excretion through the bile as well as the urine, it is the obvious choice in cases of severe oliguria or anuria. It should be administered at 3–5 mg./kg. intramuscularly every four hours for up to one week.

In the treatment of alkyl mercury intoxication, the efficacy of chelating agents has been highly equivocal. Neither PCA nor NAP, two drugs which are probably more efficacious than BAL, effected any notable improvement in the clinical status, although their use was accompanied by a modest reduction of blood mercury levels.

D. PROGNOSIS

In acute inorganic mercury poisoning, the greatest danger is renal shutdown, particularly if it occurs early in the course of illness. In such circumstances, the outlook is grave. Generally, however, recovery is complete if therapy is instituted promptly. Even the more insidious effects seen in chronic inorganic mercury poisoning are slowly reversed after termination of exposure.

The outlook for patients with poisoning from methyl or ethyl mercury is not good. Severe cases of poisoning are often fatal despite therapeutic efforts, but some mildly and moderately severe cases make a full recovery. Even some severe cases show considerable improvement one or two years after exposure.

III. ARSENIC

Toxicity from excessive exposure falls into two general categories, occupational and nonoccupational. The most serious occupational exposures occur as a result of arsenic-bearing dusts and fumes generated in connection with the smelting of copper, lead, zinc, and other ores. Less frequent and severe exposure occurs in the manufacture of arsenical chemicals, e.g., arsenical rodenticides, herbicides, and insecticides. Cleaning of arsenic-containing storage tanks with acids sometimes leads to the generation of toxic amounts of arsine gas (AsH_3). At one time, agricultural uses of arsenates as orchard sprays and herbicides constituted a widespread occupational hazard. These applications have largely been replaced by use of organic compounds with greater degrees of selective toxicity. Needless to say, these occupational exposures are of a chronic nature, with the exception of exposure to arsine.

Nonoccupational exposures, by contrast, are almost invariably of an acute nature. Historically, arsenic has been a major poison used in suicide and homicide. These uses have diminished considerably over the years. Its use as a rodenticide and for the control of roaches and ants has also diminished. Similarly, its use as a herbicide is no longer extensive in agriculture, but it is still a common ingredient in weed control formulations sold to the home gardener.

A. CLINICAL FEATURES

1. Acute

Massive single doses of arsenic cause death within a few hours with few if any clinical signs. The cause of death in such cases is heart failure. Cardiomyopathy is also frequently a feature of arsenic poisoning when it runs a more protracted course.

Acute arsenic poisoning may not be rapidly fatal. If the subject survives more than a few hours, a profuse diarrhea usually develops. This is accompanied by vomiting and abdominal pain, inflammation of the conjunctivae and respiratory mucous membranes, cardiomyopathy, erythematous or vesicular rash, and renal and hematological dysfunction. Facial and ankle edema commonly develop.

Neuropathy commonly develops 7–14 days following severe acute arsenic poisoning. A numbing and tingling paresthesia progresses from the distal portions of the lower extremities upward. Subjects often complain of a burning sensation on the soles of their feet. Upper extremities are less commonly and less severely involved. Foot drop, wrist drop, distal wasting, abnormal gait, and loss of limb reflexes follow. The neuropathy is generally symmetrical. Central neuropathy is much less common than peripheral neuropathy.

2. Chronic

Chronic exposure to arsenic results in such nonspecific effects as malaise, loss of weight, loss of appetite, and irritability. The most characteristic effects of chronic poisoning are skin changes. These are a fine, mottled brown pigmentation and hyperkeratosis, especially of the palms and soles. The nails become irregularly thickened. A characteristic white line develops above the lunulae. This is also seen four to six weeks after acute poisoning.

There is a strong body of epidemiological evidence indicating that arsenic is a low-grade carcinogen. Several studies show that occupational exposure to arsenic results in an increased incidence of lung cancer.

3. Arsine Toxicity

Arsine gas has unique toxicological effects in comparison to other forms of arsenic. Within as little as one hour of toxic exposure, vertigo, headaches, nausea, and vomiting occur. Pricking sensations may be felt. Hematuria occurs very early. Within a day, a bronze jaundice develops. Severely affected subjects also develop somnolence or psychomotor disturbances. The main problem at this point is severe kidney damage, often with anuria, which persists for as long as several weeks in spite of vigorous dialysis.

B. LABORATORY FINDINGS

As with most other metallic poisons, the most valuable laboratory diagnostic aid is determination of the concentration of the metal in the patient. In the case of arsenic, the concentration of arsenic in the urine and hair is most useful. The concentration of arsenic in the urine normally does not exceed 0.1 mg./liter, except after ingestion of seafood, in which case arsenic excretion may rise transiently to as much as 0.4 mg./liter. Return back to baseline occurs with a half-time of less than 24 hours. In acute arsenic poisoning the concentration exceeds 1 mg./liter for a few days and most often is of the order of 5–10 mg./liter. The urinary concentration of arsenic in chronic poisoning has not been clearly specified in the literature.

The concentration of arsenic in hair is more useful as a diagnostic aid for chronic poisoning than arsenic in urine. Elevated concentrations persist for many weeks following acute exposure. The normal range is < 0.3–1 μg./gm. of hair. In a series of cases of acute poisoning the range was 10 –220 μg./gm. Hair should first be washed in detergent and ethanol if there is any suspicion of external contamination.

C. TREATMENT

In acute poisoning, appropriate supportive measures are important for the initial signs and symptoms. If there is adequate basis for suspecting that oral intake occurred within the previous several hours, gastric lavage is indicated. Special attention should then be directed toward potential heart failure and fluid and electrolyte imbalance. Chelation therapy should be instituted as soon as possible in order to avert subsequent neuropathy. The drug of choice is BAL, 3–5 mg./kg. every four hours by intramuscular injection for up to one week.

In the special case of arsine poisoning, the major problem is management of threatening anuria. The role of chelation therapy is uncertain.

Chronic arsenic poisoning is largely a matter of removing the patient from the source of exposure. Chelation therapy is probably not justified in view of the fact that circulating arsenic is cleared from the body spontaneously with a relatively short half-life—about two to three days.

D. PROGNOSIS

The prognosis for complete recovery from acute poisoning depends on early diagnosis. Modern symptomatic measures are usually adequate to carry the patient through the initial phase of dehydration, shock, and cardiomyopathy. The real problem is averting the subsequent development of neuropathy. If removal of arsenic from the body is not instituted early, by chelation therapy, neuropathy will develop. The neuropathic effects are often irreversible and are not much influenced by chelation therapy. The prognosis for recovery from chronic poisoning is good. The prognosis for recovery from arsine poisoning must be very guarded. Many patients die in spite of prompt institution of hemodialysis and other supportive measures.

IV. IRON

Iron poisoning is the result of the ingestion of iron preparations intended for therapeutic use. These consist principally of ferrous sulfate, ferrous fumarate, and ferrous gluconate in tablet form. The vast majority of cases of poisoning occur in children less than 6 years of age. Occasional cases of poisoning occur in adults due to the ingestion of these same therapeutic preparations with suicidal intent. As with most toxic substances, the acute lethal dose in humans is not clearly defined. The average lethal dose expressed in terms of elemental iron has been estimated to be 200–900 mg./kg. As little as 600 mg. may be fatal to infants, however.

A. CLINICAL FEATURES

Evidence of iron ingestion should be obtained as quickly as possible. Check for bottles containing an iron preparation and attempt to estimate the amount that might have been consumed. Staining of the hands and mouth may also be useful evidence of iron ingestion.

The onset of toxicity usually occurs within a few hours but may not be manifest for about six hours. Four successive stages of illness are generally recognized.

The first is a manifestation of the corrosive effects of iron on the gastrointestinal mucosa. Vomiting and diarrhea (sometimes bloody) may occur. Stool and emesis should be examined for iron tablets. Lethargy is a common early sign. It may progress to coma and be accompanied by shock.

The second stage is one of apparent improvement. It may begin within 6 hours of the onset of illness and last 20–48 hours.

This phase is then followed by a period of deterioration in which the patient may exhibit profound shock with circulatory collapse, hepatic damage, coma, convulsions, coagulation defects, and hyperpyrexia.

The fourth stage consists of sequelae due to corrosive effects on the gastrointestinal mucosa. This is mainly scarring and consequent stricture of the esophagus, stomach, and intestines. Patients who survive the initial three phases should be examined in five to six weeks for evidence of these possible complications.

B. LABORATORY FINDINGS

The most meaningful laboratory finding is evidence of excessive absorption as determined by serum iron. It is of diagnostic value if the analysis is performed from one to six hours after ingestion occurs. If the concentration exceeds 300 μg./dl., chelation therapy is indicated. Therapy should not be delayed, however, pending serum iron determination if the history and clinical evidence are strongly suggestive of iron poisoning.

C. TREATMENT

1. In the absence of substantial vomiting, induce emesis with syrup of ipecac. When the amount of ingested iron is large (greater than 200 mg. in children), gastric lavage should be instituted using 5% sodium bicarbonate or 5% sodium dihydrogen phosphate, which may be prepared by diluting Fleet brand enema 1:1 with water.

The purpose is to convert soluble ferrous salts to the less soluble carbonate and phosphate as well as to evacuate the stomach. A saline cathartic and an enema also frequently result in the removal of many iron tablets.

In severe cases, chelation therapy should be instituted along with appropriate supportive measures. As an aid to deciding whether to institute chelation therapy, a serum iron determination is very helpful. It should be determined within six hours of ingestion. Chelation therapy with deferoxamine is recommended when serum iron exceeds 300 μg./dl., regardless of whether or not clinical signs of poisoning are evident. However, opinion varies as to what level of serum iron calls for chelation therapy.

Deferoxamine should be administered intravenously. In young children, the dose is 80 mg./kg. up to 1 gm. The rate of infusion should be limited to 50 mg./kg. per hour to minimize the hazard of drug-induced hypotension. No dosage schedule can be recommended for adults. Experience is too limited. The treatment may be repeated at 4–12-hour intervals, depending on the clinical status. It is generally recommended that the dosage of repeat treatments be reduced to one-half the original level. Intramuscular administration is indicated in mild cases or in cases where hypotension is judged to pose a serious problem. Therapy should be continued until the serum iron level falls below the serum iron binding capacity or the urine returns to a normal color. The iron-deferoxamine complex imparts a reddish, salmon color to the urine. Disappearance of the color signals termination of iron mobilization.

2. Treat shock (see Chap. 1).

3. Treat convulsions (see Chap. 1).

D. Prognosis

The prognosis is very much dependent on the status of the patient at the time therapeutic measures are instituted. If shock or coma develops, the prognosis must be guarded, even with the use of definitive therapy as deferoxamine. In the absence of shock or coma, the prognosis for survival is good.

V. THALLIUM

Thallium was previously used rather extensively for control of rodents and ants. In 1972, the use of thallium as a pesticide was banned in the United States. In other countries its use is still fairly common. Occasional cases of poisoning are still reported, mainly in northern Europe. Thallous sulfate, the most commonly used form, is said to be tasteless and is readily soluble in water. The average oral toxic, nonfatal dose in humans is approximately 4–8 mg./kg., and the minimal fatal dose probably is somewhat less than 10 mg./kg. The toxic dose in children and adults is approximately the same.

A. Clinical Features

Initially, the signs and symptoms are gastrointestinal pain, diarrhea, and vomiting; paresthesia and pain in the upper and lower limbs. Dizziness, and facial weakness follow, usually in two to five days. Somnolence, delirium, or coma may occur. Electrocardiographic and electroencephalographic abnormalities have been reported frequently. Alopecia is a common sign. It occurs at least one week following the initial signs and symptoms.

B. Laboratory Findings

The only useful laboratory finding is the presence of thallium in the urine. Only traces of thallium occur normally, < 1.5 μg./liter. In cases of poisoning, the concentration is of the order of 0.1–10 mg./liter depending on the toxic dose and the time after ingestion. The half-life for urinary excretion is approximately 30 days. Therefore, abnormal concentrations of thallium in the urine persist for several months.

C. TREATMENT

If ingestion is suspected to have occurred within a few hours, gastric lavage is indicated to remove unabsorbed thallium. Several specific therapeutic agents have been found useful for the purpose of accelerating the removal of thallium. The agent of choice appears to be prussian blue. When given orally, it increases fecal excretion of thallium severalfold. It acts by binding thallium as it is excreted into the intestine, thereby short-circuiting enterohepatic recirculation. The recommended dose is 250 mg./kg. per day divided in four equally spaced doses. These doses are administered orally in 50 ml., 15% aqueous mannitol. If prussian blue is not available, activated charcoal (5 gm./kg. twice daily) and potassium chloride (3–5 gm. daily as a solution) can be given orally. Charcoal adsorbs thallium in the gastrointestinal tract, thereby enhancing fecal excretion, and potassium chloride enhances the urinary excretion of thallium. The latter should be used only if renal function is normal. Its use may be accompanied by transient aggravation of clinical signs of toxicity. If renal function is impaired, hemodialysis may be attempted to remove thallium.

D. PROGNOSIS

Recovery from thallium poisoning is slow, but the prognosis for complete recovery is good in adults. The prognosis for complete recovery in children must be more guarded. In one follow-up study it was found that neurological abnormalities could persist for at least four years.

VI. COPPER

The most frequently reported cause of copper poisoning is drinking from copper-containing beverages. Contamination is from containers either lined with copper or from copper components, such as tubing and spigots. Copper components of hemodialysis machines may leach sufficient copper to cause poisoning. Poisoning from accidental or suicidal ingestion of copper sulfate solutions has also been reported. Acidic liquids leach more copper than neutral or alkaline solutions.

A. CLINICAL FEATURES

In mild cases, nausea, vomiting, and occasionally, diarrhea occur. These effects probably are not entirely caused by local irritation because they are reported in cases involving contaminated hemodialysis units. In more severe cases copper causes hemolysis of erythrocytes with consequent hemoglobinuria and icterus. In the severest cases, death may occur within 24 hours, preceded by coma. It can occur later from hepatic or renal complications.

B. LABORATORY FINDINGS

Serum and whole blood copper concentrations are elevated, more or less in proportion to the severity of the case. Normal values in serum are approximately 80–140 μg./dl. The concentration in packed blood cells is similar, 63–107 μg./dl. In mild cases serum or whole blood copper may be only marginally elevated.

C. TREATMENT

Very little is known concerning the most effective means of managing severe cases of copper poisoning. In the few cases reported in the recent medical literature, little is noted about therapeutic measures. The most effective chelating agent for the mobilization of excessive copper in the body is D-penicillamine (Cuprimine), available from Merck Sharp & Dohme. The major application of D-penicillamine is in the treatment of hepatolenticular degeneration (Wilson's disease) resulting from an inherited abnormality of copper metabolism. D-penicillamine also may be of some benefit in acute copper poisoning. Use of this drug should be limited to serious cases of poisoning. For information on its use, it is recommended that expert advice be sought.*

D. PROGNOSIS

The prognosis for acute copper poisoning is highly variable. In mild cases characterized only by nausea, vomiting, and diarrhea, recovery usually is rapid and complete. When poisoning is accompanied by severe systemic effects such as hemolysis, the prognosis must be guarded.

VII. CADMIUM

Cadmium has long been recognized as a significant occupational poison from inhalation of cadmium oxide fumes and dust. Nonoccupational poisoning occurs infrequently. There is one report of suicidal poisoning. In Japan there has been one well-documented episode of chronic poisoning among residents of a limited area where the locally grown rice was extensively polluted with irrigation water that drained a mine located upstream. The minimal acute toxic dose is probably 1–3 mg./cu. m. by inhalation. The product of air concentration (milligrams per cubic meter) times minutes of exposure known to be acutely fatal is 2,600, e.g., 26 mg./cu. m. inhaled for 100 minutes. The minimal toxic dose for an 8-hour period is probably 1–3 mg./cu. m. Estimated oral lethal doses are not clearly known. The minimal dose may be as low as 350 mg. for an adult.

A. CLINICAL FEATURES

Acute poisoning by inhalation is characterized by dyspnea, pulmonary edema, and renal damage manifested by azotemia and proteinuria. Other effects develop during the two or three days following

---

* Dr. I. Herbert Scheinberg, Department of Medicine, Albert Einstein College of Medicine, 1300 Morris Park Ave., Bronx, New York 10461, Tel. 212-430-2091.

exposure, e.g., weakness and malaise, anorexia, and nausea. Chronic exposure to cadmium fumes and dusts results primarily in progressive pulmonary emphysema.

Acute cadmium poisoning by the oral route mainly results in severe damage to the liver and kidneys. In addition, damage to the heart occurs. The first symptoms are severe nausea, vomiting, diarrhea, muscular cramps, and salivation. Cardiac damage occurs and death may result from cardiac failure. Chronic poisoning by the oral route results in proteinuria. Elevated renal excretion of the low molecular weight protein beta-2 microglobulin occurs first. At higher levels of exposure, a more generalized proteinuria occurs. A peculiar osteoporotic syndrome has been reported in Japan, with spontaneous fractures and skeletal deformities. This syndrome is thought to result from the combined effects of vitamin D deficiency and cadmium. It is prevalent among older multiparous women.

B. LABORATORY FINDINGS

The organ most sensitive to toxic effects is the kidneys. Elevated urinary excretion of beta-2 microglobulin is highly suggestive of cadmium intoxication. The urinary excretion of cadmium is also helpful in arriving at a diagnosis of cadmium poisoning. Normally, excretion is less than 5 μg./per day.

C. TREATMENT

There is no known effective therapeutic agent that will accelerate the excretion of cadmium without at the same time aggravating the toxic effects.

D. PROGNOSIS

Acute cadmium poisoning caused by inhalation is completely reversible. This conclusion is based on follow-up studies of a limited number of cases. For chronic inhalation toxicity, experience suggests that termination of exposure arrests the progression of respiratory effects but does not result in remission of signs and symptoms. The prognosis for recovery from renal effects of cadmium exposure is not clearly known.

VIII. OTHER METALS

Two categories of metals have been included in this section. The first consists of metals which are familiar as a result of industrial exposure. The second consists of metals for which excessive exposure is a reasonable possibility but poisoning is only infrequently reported.

A. ALUMINUM

A vast literature attests to the low toxicity of aluminum salts by ingestion, inhalation, or application to the skin. The only reason for including aluminum is the possibility that relatively low concentrations in the dialysate of hemodialysis units may be highly toxic and even fatal. Dialysis encephalopathy has been attributed to dialysate concentrations as low as 0.2–1.0 mg. aluminum per liter. The neurological manifestations attributed to aluminum are dementia, muscle twitching, generalized seizures, tremor, and impaired speech. The onset is slow, and the course of the disease is reported to be several weeks, often terminating in death. Symptomatic treatment appears to have little if any beneficial effect.

B. BARIUM

Barium poisoning occurs as a result of the accidental or suicidal ingestion of soluble salts of barium. These are most commonly used in depilatory preparations and rodenticides. The average toxic oral dose for adults is approximately 2.5 gm. The minimal fatal dose may in some cases be less than this. The most consistent and serious effect is muscular weakness progressing rapidly to paralysis. Death is usually due to paralysis of the respiratory muscles. Other major features of toxicity are hypokalemia, cardiac arrhythmia, and respiratory acidosis. Vigorous diuretic therapy may enhance urinary excretion of barium. Recovery under proper therapeutic management is relatively rapid.

C. BERYLLIUM

Beryllium poisoning is an occupational disease. Exposure is generally by inhalation of dusts and fumes generated in the processing of beryllium ores and in the production of beryllium alloys and phosphors. Most of the original cases of beryllium poisoning in this country were in connection with the manufacture of fluorescent lamps in which beryllium phosphors were used in the 1940s. Although this particular use of beryllium is no longer practiced, accelerated uses of beryllium in the manufacture of ceramics, thermal coatings, airplane brakes, nuclear reactors, and rocket motors presents a continuing problem.

Although acute beryllium poisoning may occur, the major concern is chronic, relatively low-level inhalation. In either case the major target organ is the lung. The predominant effect of beryllium inhalation is progressive interstitial pneumonitis with reduction in lung function, often delayed for a number of years after exposure. The delayed onset of pneumonitis may be precipitated by acute stress, e.g., pregnancy, viral infections, and surgery. Heart disease (cor pulmonale) may be a more serious consequence of beryllium exposure than the pulmonary effects of the exposure. Diagnosis is based on x-ray findings, pulmonary function tests, and establishment of beryllium exposure by finding beryllium in urine or lung tissue or by epidemiological evidence. Treatment with steroids is partially effective in suppressing symptoms.

D. BISMUTH

Bismuth salts were at one time used extensively in the treatment of syphilis. More recently, soluble salts have been used orally for the treatment of warts. Insoluble salts such as bismuth subgallate are frequently given orally as gastric and enteric protectives, sometimes for prolonged periods of time. Two forms of toxicity have been reported. Excessive doses of soluble salts of bismuth cause nephropathy, occasionally accompanied by severe liver damage. Treatment is supportive.

Encephalopathy has recently been reported to occur during prolonged oral administration of insoluble salts. The dosage schedules used have been within the accepted therapeutic range. The onset is slow, with ataxia, difficulty performing tasks requiring manual dexterity, and confusion. Myoclonic jerks and tremor also occur. The disease may progress to delirium and grand mal seizures, sometimes with fatal consequences. Withdrawal of bismuth generally results in slow recovery. Nephropathy is not reported to occur. The level of bismuth in blood and urine is elevated.

E. CHROMIUM

The rare cases of nonoccupational poisoning generally result from swallowing chromate salts. Signs and symptoms may be limited to nausea, vomiting, and other signs of acute gastroenteritis. In more severe cases renal damage may occur.

Most of the recent literature concerns the toxic effects from industrial exposure of chromium. The effects are primarily on the respiratory tract and skin. The hexavalent form is far more toxic than the trivalent form. Inhalation of chromate dust causes rhinitis and inflammation of the lungs in proportion to the concentration and duration of exposure. Ulcers may develop in the nasal septum, progressing to perforation. Chromate is also capable of causing ulceration of the skin with prolonged contact. In some people, allergic contact dermatitis may occur.

The most serious effect of chromate seen in industrial exposure is lung cancer. As with most carcinogenic agents, the latency period is quite long, generally more than 10 years. The lung cancers of chromate workers are not of any single histologic cell type.

F. LITHIUM

Lithium carbonate is used in psychiatry to treat manic depressives. The therapeutic index is low, and side effects commonly encountered are loose stools, fine tremor of the hands, lethargy, muscular weakness, polyuria, and polydipsia. More severe signs of toxicity may occur from single large doses, cumulative doses, or reduced lithium excretion. These signs are ataxia, impaired consciousness leading to coma, and epileptiform fits. The eyes are wide open and there is hyperextension of the arms and legs. Toxicity can occur at serum levels > 1.5 mEq./liter.

In spite of widespread use of lithium carbonate, there have been very few reports of severe intoxication. The management of intoxication is support of vital functions and correction of electrolyte and water imbalances. Agents which enhance renal excretion of lithium are sodium salts, acetazolamide, mannitol or urea, and aminophylline.

G. NICKEL

The usual form of nickel toxicity is allergic contact dermatitis. It is most commonly observed as a result of occupational exposure, e.g., in electroplating and in the manufacture of nickel alloys and nickel-cadmium batteries. It also occurs in the general population from jewelry, clothing fasteners, cooking utensils, and tools.

No treatment is known and various means of effecting desensitization have been unsuccessful.

Nickel in various forms has been shown to cause lung cancer and cancer of the nasal cavities from industrial exposure in which high atmospheric concentrations are attained, e.g., ore roasting and smelting. As with many other cancers induced by environmental agents, the latency period is long.

Nickel carbonyl, a compound generated during nickel refining by the Mond process, is the only form which has been known to cause systemic nickel toxicity in humans. Inhalation causes both immediate and delayed effects. Immediate effects are dyspnea, fatigue, nausea, and vertigo. Delayed effects (12 to 36 hours after exposure) are mainly dyspnea with painful inspiration, substernal pain, nonproductive cough, and chills. Muscular pain, sweating, visual disturbances, diarrhea, abdominal pain, muscle cramps, and hypoesthesia occur less commonly.

Chelating agents, notably sodium diethyldithiocarbamate (dithiocarb), appear to be of some benefit in relieving signs and symptoms. The benefits from other chelating agents are equivocal.

H. Selenium

The only hazardous source of selenium for the general population is gun blueing, which contains selenious acid. This form of selenium is highly toxic. The minimum lethal dose in laboratory animals is approximately 1–5 mg./kg. The only other form of selenium likely to be encountered is selenium sulfide, a component of dandruff shampoo. This form is essentially nontoxic.

A case of acute fatal poisoning has been described from swallowing gun blueing compound. The course was rapid and fatal. Signs of poisoning were retching and vomiting progressing rapidly to a comatose state with purposeless body movements. Other prominent signs were cyanosis and a strong garlic odor on the breath. Blood pressure and peripheral pulse were unrecordable on admission to the hospital. At autopsy, widespread focal hemorrhages and edema were observed.

Some nonfatal cases of occupational poisoning have been recorded from inhalation of selenium dioxide or hydrogen selenide dusts and fumes. In these forms selenium is highly irritant to the nasal passages and lungs. The syndrome is best described as a chemical pneumonitis.

There is no specific antidote for selenium. Treatment is symptomatic.

I. Tin

Inorganic salts of tin have been used in toothpastes. Limited data in dogs and cats fed large amounts of tin salts for prolonged periods of time indicate that the likelihood of toxicity is extremely remote. One dog fed stannous chloride at 500 mg./kg. per day for 14 months ultimately died of a paralytic syndrome, probably due to the tin.

Aryl and alkyl tin compounds are considerably more toxic than inorganic compounds, but people are rarely exposed to hazardous amounts. Inhalation or dermal exposure to toxic amounts cause severe headaches and nausea. In the most severe cases of poisoning, bradycardia, hypotension, and abrupt variations in the sinus rhythm of the heart are observed.

BIBLIOGRAPHY

I. Lead

Chisolm, J. J., Jr.: Treatment of acute lead intoxication: choice of chelating agents and supportive therapeutic measures. Clin. Toxicol. *3:*527–540, 1970.

Zielhuis, R. L.: Dose-response relationships for inorganic lead. Int. Arch. Occup. Health, *35:*1–35, 1975.

II. Mercury

Anon.: Methyl mercury in fish: a toxicologic-epidemiologic evaluation of risk. Nord. Hyg. Tidsk., suppl. *4,* 1971.

Al-Damluji, S. F.: Intoxication due to alkylmercury-treated seed: 1971–72 outbreak in Iraq in Conference on Intoxication due to alkylmercury-treated seed. Bull. WHO, *53,* suppl. 1976.

Bakir, F., Al-Khalidi, A., Clarkson, T. W., and Greenwood, R.: Clinical observations on treatment of alkylmercury poisoning in hospital patients. Bull. WHO, suppl. *53,* 1976.

Kark, R. A. P., Poskanzer, D. C., Bullock, J. D., and Boylen, G.: Mercury poisoning and its treatment with n-acetyl-D, L-penicillamine. N. Engl. J. Med., *285:*10–16, 1971.

III. ARSENIC

Jenkins, R. B.: Inorganic arsenic and the nervous system. Brain, *89:*479–498, 1966.

Pinto, S. S., and Nelson, K. W.: Arsenic toxicology and industrial exposure. Ann. Rev. Pharmacol. Toxicol., *16:*95–100, 1976.

Pinto, S. S., Varner, M. O., Nelson, K. W., Labbe, A. L., and White, L. D.: Arsenic trioxide absorption and excretion in industry. J. Occup. Med., *18:*677–680, 1976.

IV. IRON

Green, V. A.: Iron ingestions: the Children's Mercy Hospital. Clin. Toxicol., *4:*245–252, 1971.

Greengard, J.: Iron poisoning in children. Clin. Toxicol., *8:*575–597, 1975.

U.S. Department of Health, Education and Welfare: Handbook of Common Poisonings in Children. HEW Pub. No. (FDA) 76-7004. Washington, D.C., U.S. Government Printing Office, 1976.

V. THALLIUM

Kamerbeek, H. H., Rauws, A. G., ten Ham, M., and van Heijist, A. N. P.: Prussian blue in therapy of thallotoxicosis. Acta Med. Scand. *189:*321–324, 1971.

Stevens, W., van Peteghem, C., Heyndrickx, A., and Barbier, F.: Seven cases of thallium intoxication treated with prussian blue. Int. J. Clin. Pharmacol. *10:*1–22, 1974.

VI. COPPER

Chuttani, N. K., Gupta, P. S., Gulati, S., and Gupta, D. N.: Acute copper sulfate poisoning. Am. J. Med. *39:*849, 1965.

NAS: Copper: Medical and Biologic Effects of Atmospheric Pollutants. Washington, D.C., National Academy of Sciences, 1977.

VII. CADMIUM

Beton, D. C., Andrews, G. S., Davies, H. J., Howells, L., and Smith, G. F.: Acute cadmium fume poisoning: five cases with one death from renal necrosis. Br. J. Ind. Med. *23:*292–301, 1966.

Friberg, L., Piscator, M., and Nordberg, G.: Cadmium in the Environment. Cleveland, CRC Press, 1971.

Wisniewska-Knypl, J. M., Jablonska, J., and Myslak, Z.: Binding of cadmium on metaleothionein in man: an analysis of a fatal poisoning by cadmium iodide. Arch. Toxicol. *28:*46–55, 1971.

VIII. OTHER METALS

Campbell, I. R., Cass, J. S., Cholak, J., and Kehoe, R. A.: Aluminum in the environment of man. A.M.A. Arch. Ind. Health, *15:*359–448, 1957.

Carter, R. F.: Acute selenium poisoning. Med. J. Aust. *1:*525–528, 1968.

Gould, D. B., Sorrell, M. R., and Lupariello, A. D.: Barium sulfide poisoning. Arch. Intern. Med. *132:*891–894, 1973.

Loiseau, P., Henry, P., Jallon, P., and Legroux, M.: Encephalopathies myocloniques iatrogenes aux sels du bismuth. J. Neurol. Sci., *27:*133–143, 1976.

NAS: Medical and Biologic Effects of Environmental Pollutants: Chromium. Washington, D.C., National Academy of Sciences, 1974.

NAS: Medical and Biological Effects of Atmospheric Pollutants: Nickel. Washington, D.C., National Academy of Sciences, 1975.

NIOSH: Occupational Exposure to Beryllium. HSM 72-10268. Washington, D.C., U.S. Government Printing Office, 1972.

NIOSH: Occupational Exposure to Organotin Compounds. DHEW Publ. No. 77-115. Washington, D.C., U.S. Government Printing Office, 1976.

Rozas, V. V., Port, F. K., and Rutt, W. M.: Progressive dialysis encephalopathy from dialysate aluminum. Arch. Intern. Med. *138:*1375–1377, 1978.

Saran, B. M., and Gaind, R.: Lithium. Clin. Toxicol. *6:*257–269, 1973.

Thomsen, K., and Schou, M.: Renal lithium excretion in man. Am. J. Physiol. *215:*823–827, 1968.

Urizar, R., and Vernier, R. L.: Bismuth nephropathy. J.A.M.A., *198:*187–189, 1966.

Wilson, H. M.: Selenium oxide poisoning, N.C. Med. J. *23:*73–75, 1962.

17. CARBON MONOXIDE, CYANIDES, AND SULFIDES

Thomas Elo, M.D.

I. CARBON MONOXIDE

Carbon monoxide (CO) is a colorless, odorless, tasteless gas. It is ubiquitous and of concern because it can be lethal if the inspired air contains as little as 0.1 vol%. It is the result of incomplete combustion of carbonaceous material. Many persons are overcome by the gas because they believe that without smoke there is no danger from carbon monoxide.

Carbon monoxide is derived from many sources, including car exhaust, space heaters, defective fireplace flues, flame-type water heaters, improperly vented gas ranges and furnaces, coal and oil furnaces, poorly ventilated charcoal and gas grills, fires of all types, and methylene chloride in, for example, paint remover.

Of all workers, fire fighters are at greatest risk because smoke from fires contains anywhere from 0.1% to 10% carbon monoxide. Despite the heavy use of portable respirators, over 10,000 fire fighters are intoxicated each year.

A. MECHANISM OF ACTION

The deleterious effects are caused by the strong binding of carbon monoxide with the hemoglobin molecule. Hemoglobin has an affinity for carbon monoxide 210 times greater than for oxygen. It not only competes successfully with oxygen for hemoglobin, but the presence of carboxyhemoglobin (HbCO) greatly impedes the dissociation of oxygen from hemoglobin. This in turn leads to a decreased oxygen partial pressure in the blood and a diminished gradient for oxygen diffusion from the red blood cells to tissue cells. As a result, there is tissue anoxia. A progressive arterial hypoxemia results from any one or all of the following mechanisms:

1. Pulmonary venous admixture of central origin from an uneven ventilation perfusion relationship such as might be caused by disseminated microatelectasis.
2. Decreased oxygenation caused by cardiac dysfunction. Concentrations above 65% carboxyhemoglobin cause marked inhibition of the circulatory system.
3. Direct effects of carbon monoxide on the pulmonary tissue. It adversely affects capillary permeability and can cause pulmonary edema. In addition, it can decrease pulmonary surfactant.
4. Changes in the oxyhemoglobin dissociation curve. Carbon monoxide causes a shift to the left. This increases with increasing concentrations of carboxyhemoglobin (see Fig. 17-1).

A state of equilibrium between the concentration of carbon monoxide in air and blood occurs more slowly in the lower concentrations. The rate of combination is more rapid at first and then slows as equilibrium is approached. Exercise increases the rate of combination and the toxic symptoms of carbon monoxide poisoning.

As with most toxic gases, the systemic effects from carbon monoxide is a product of concentration times the length of exposure (Table 17-1).

Of interest is that every smoker as well as those present in a room with a smoker are exposed to carbon monoxide. Inhaled cigarette smoke contains up to 800 ppm carbon monoxide, and cigar or pipe smoke has considerably more. Smokers blood may reach a concentration of 5% or greater within two hours.

B. CLINICAL FEATURES

There are several symptoms directly related to carbon monoxide intoxication.

177

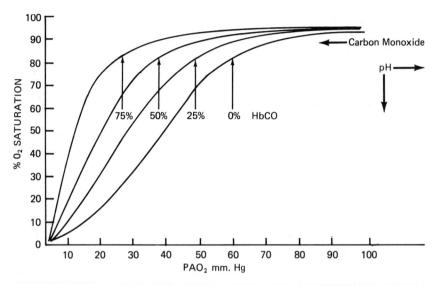

Fig. 17-1. Carbon monoxide and its effect on the oxyhemoglobin dissociation curve.

These correlate with the percentage of carboxyhemoglobin saturation in the blood. Four levels of intoxication can be identified, and treatment is determined by the level (Fig. 17-2).

As can be seen from Figure 17-2 the most common symptoms in the lower levels are headache, nausea, and vomiting. Once higher levels are reached, dizziness, blurred vision, and a syndrome not unlike acute ethanol intoxication occurs. Some clinicians have reported a characteristic cherry red color of the mucous membranes at concentrations of carboxyhemoglobin around 25% which becomes more apparent at 35–40%. This color, however, is rarely seen until higher concentrations are reached. At 60–70% concentration of carboxyhemoglobin, death is almost certain without treatment.

C. LABORATORY FINDINGS

1. Carboxyhemoglobin level must be monitored in anyone suspected of carbon monoxide poisoning.

2. WBC is often elevated in level 2 and above.

3. The hematocrit may rise significantly in the upper-level groups.

4. Urinalysis may show a significant proteinuria.

5. SGOT is usually elevated in the upper levels. A combination of an elevated hematocrit and SGOT is usually a poor prognostic sign.

6. Arterial blood gases—In upper levels there is decreased pH, slightly increased Pa_{O_2} (caused by tachypnea) and decreased Pa_{CO_2}. A low pH and a low base excess indicate a poorer prognosis.

7. A fairly rapid method for carboxyhemoglobin determination in the hospital emergency department is as follows:

a. Look for a cherry red color to the blood.

b. Simultaneously prepare two test tubes: one containing about 15 ml. of distilled water plus one or two drops of a normal person's venous blood; the other containing the same amount of water and one or two drops of the patient's blood. If available, a positive control should be used. To each specimen, add five drops of 30% sodium hydroxide. Quickly cap with the thumb, shake, and observe if the original faint pink color persists or immediately changes to straw yellow.

c. If the blood is negative or contains less than 20% carboxyhemoglobin, the pink color will immediately turn a straw yellow. If the pink color persists for several more seconds, then carbon monoxide is present in excess of 20%. Even at concentrations above 80%, the mixture will eventually turn a straw color (within about 60 seconds).

d. The intensity of the pink color, and its persistence before turning yellow, will give a rough approximation of the concentration of carboxyhemoglobin.

e. The test is specific for carboxyhemoglobin, and only fetal blood behaves similarly.

8. More accurate methods of carboxyhemoglobin determination are spectrophotometry, gas chromotography, and rapid diffusion techniques.

D. Treatment

In the treatment of carbon monoxide poisoning the most important goal is to achieve dissociation of the carboxyhemoglobin molecule and replace the carbon monoxide with oxygen.

The initial treatment requires maintenance of a patent airway and removing the patient from the noxious environment. In level 1 intoxication (0–10% carboxyhemoglobin), no treatment is necessary other than fresh air. In the lower concentrations of level 2 (10–15% carboxyhemoglobin), simple rest and fresh air are usually sufficient. If there is cardiovascular disease or the patient is over 40–45 years old, oxygen therapy is advised. Above 15% carboxyhemoglobin, 100% oxygen therapy is the best treatment available. This high oxygen concentrations can cause dissociation of 50% of the carboxyhemoglobin in 40 minutes. This is compared with 300 minutes for fresh room air.

In the 30–40% range (level 3), oxygen is clearly indicated. It takes 8–10 hours for the carboxyhemoglobin level to fall to

Table 17-1. **Concentrations of Carbon Monoxide and the Time Necessary to Produce Physiological Effects**

Physiological Effect	Vol (ppm)
Several-hour exposure without ill effects	100
1 hour without ill effects	400–500
Some light effects after 1-hour exposure	600–700
Unpleasant effects after 1-hour exposure	1,000–1,200
Dangerous effects after 1-hour exposure	1,500–2,000
Fatal in less than 1-hour exposure	4,000 and above

10% with fresh air alone. Other treatment includes bedrest and judicious use of antiemetics for nausea and vomiting.

For those with greater than 40% carboxyhemoglobin levels, immediate treatment is essential to prevent CNS and cardiac damage. The airway and blood pressure must be maintained and 100% oxygen given. If the equipment is available the patient should be considered for hyperbaric oxygen therapy (OHP) at 2–2.5 atmospheres of pressure. Hyperbaric oxygen acts to correct the tissue hypoxia with extra oxygen dissolved in the plasma. It also accelerates the rate of dissociation of carboxyhemoglobin and shifts the oxyhemoglobin curve to the right. Breathing oxygen at 2 atmospheres pressure can eliminate all detectable carboxyhemoglobin within 90 minutes. Carbon monoxide has been shown to increase the susceptibility to oxygen toxicity when OHP is used at 3 atmospheres or more. Disadvantages of hyperbaric oxygen therapy involve the risk of fire and explosion, and the small space in which to manage the patient both in terms of equipment and personnel.

E. Chronic Intoxication

There is no evidence that long-term exposure to low carbon monoxide concentration produces any deleterious effects upon health and physical well-being.

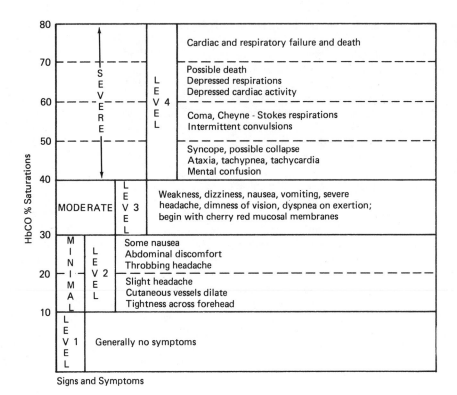

Fig. 17-2. Signs and symptoms of various blood levels of HbCO.

F. PROGNOSIS

Up to 25% of patients who have recovered from level 3 to level 4 intoxication can exhibit permanent cognitive and personality changes or frank neurological abnormalities (such as extrapyramidal signs and spastic hemiplegias). These sequelae can worsen with time or can appear after an apparent uneventful recovery. It is recommended that persons who recover from high level exposures to carbon monoxide undergo periodic medical re-evaluation.

II. CYANIDES

Although not a very common form of poisoning, cyanide can be one of the most rapidly acting of all poisons. If encoun-

tered in the volatile form of hydrocyanic acid, its inhalation can be fatal in a few minutes. Cyanides and their derivatives are produced in large quantities and are used in both the home and industry.

The cyanides and derivatives can be broken down into three classes:

1. Hydrogen cyanide and simple salts (potassium cyanide, sodium cyanide, etc.)
2. Halogenated cyanides such as cyanogen chloride
3. Nitriles such as acrylonitrile and acetonitrile

The cyanides and related compounds are used as fumigants and in chemical synthesis (hydrogen cyanide), in synthetic rubber (acrylonitrile), in fertilizers (cyanamide), and in metal refining and hardening (cyanide salts). In the home they can be found in some furniture polishes and rodenticides (Table 17-2).

Of note is that the seeds of stone fruits (apple, peach, plum, apricot, cherry, and almond), jetberry bush, and toyon contain amygdalin (a cyanogenetic glycoside). These seeds can release cyanide upon ingestion with the reaction occurring more quickly in an alkaline (duodenal) medium. The fatal dose for a small child is somewhere between 4 and 30 seeds. The seeds are only harmful if the capsule is broken. Most will pass through the gastrointestinal tract undigested.

The maximal allowable concentration of hydrocyanic acid vapor is 10 ppm. At higher concentrations (greater than 250 ppm) just a few inhalations of vapor or the ingestion of 50–75 mg. sodium cyanide or potassium cyanide is usually followed by immediate collapse and respiratory arrest.

Cyanide gas (hydrocyanic acid vapor) has a characteristic odor of bitter almonds which can be recognized in the air with concentrations as low as 2–5 ppm.

The cyanides can be inhaled, ingested, or absorbed through the skin to cause their toxic effects.

A. MECHANISM OF ACTION

The free ions of cyanide combine with the trivalent form of iron (Fe^{+3}) in the mitochondrial cytochrome oxidase system according to the formula:

$$CN^{(-)} + \text{cytochrome oxidase} \rightarrow$$
$$\text{cytochrome} - CN \text{ complex (inactive)}$$

Electron transfer is thus prevented along the cytochrome oxidase system, and oxygen uptake in the tricarboxylic acid cycle is blocked. However, cyanide is a relatively nonspecific inhibitor, and there are as many as 42 other enzyme systems it may effect. Many of these contain iron or copper. Because of the inhibition of these enzyme systems, oxygen is not utilized and organ function persists only as long as it

can be sustained by anaerobic metabolism. The end result is cellular anoxia and death.

The conversion of hydroxocobalamin (vitamin B_{12a}) to vitamin B_{12} (cyanocobalamin) and the elimination of hydrocyanic acid vapor through the lungs is the basis for the characteristic odor of bitter almonds on a patient's expired breath.

B. CLINICAL FEATURES

With lesser amounts, ingestion, inhalation, or skin absorption causes dizziness, headache, drowsiness, tachypnea, tachycardia, and hypotension. Generalized convulsions and death occur within three to four hours with all cyanide compounds except nitroprusside.

Inhalation of hydrocyanic acid vapor or ingestion of larger quantities of cyanide is usually associated with a very rapid onset of giddiness, headache, palpitations, and tachypnea. These are followed by convulsions and death, usually within 15 minutes.

Tachypnea is generally thought to occur through anoxic stimulation of the carotid chemoreceptors and the medullary respiratory center. Cyanosis is a grave prognostic sign.

One of the most specific and interesting findings in acute intoxication is the bright red color of venous blood. This occurs because of the inability of tissues to utilize oxygen.

Halogenated cyanide materials such as cyanogen bromide and cyanogen chloride are generally very irritant vesicant gases similar to phosgene. They cause tearing, excessive salivation, and marked pulmonary irritation that frequently leads to pulmonary edema. These effects can be delayed for several hours after exposure.

Other compounds such as the nitriles cause symptoms similar to those of hydrocyanic acid, but the onset is generally slower. In addition, these materials act as marked skin and eye irritants. They may be readily absorbed through intact

Table 17-2. Cyanide-Containing Compounds, Their Forms, Uses, Fatal Doses, and Absorption

Chemical Formula	Name	Commercial Use	Form (liquid, solid vapor)	Fatal Dose (TLV)*	How Absorbed	Comments
HCN	Hydrocyanic acid	Fumigant, in nitriles	Colorless liquid	0.5 mg./kg. (10 ppm)	Ingestion, inhalation	Flammable; charateristic odor
NaCN	Sodium cyanide	Electroplating, organic reactions	White crystalline solid, deliquescent	2 mg./kg.	Ingestion, skin absorption, inhalation	Very common in industry, found in pesticides
KCN	Potassium cyanide	Similar to NaCN	White crystalline solid, deliquescent	2 mg./kg.	Ingestion, skin absorption, inhalation	Very common in industry
Ca(CN)$_2$	Calcium cyanide	Fumigant, pesticide	White powder	5 mg./cu.	Ingestion, inhalation	Similar toxicity to other cyanide salts
CaCN$_2$	Calcium cyanamide	Fertilizer	White crystalline solid	40–50 gm.	Ingestion	Unknown mechanism of toxicity
(CH$_3$)$_2$ NCN	Dimethyl cyanamide	Organic synthesis	Colorless liquid	75 mg./kg.	Ingestion, skin absorption	Hazardous especially by skin absorption
N:CC:N	Cyanogen	Fumigant, blast furnace	Gas	13 ppm	Inhalation, skin absorption	Very readily absorbed through the skin
CNCL	Cyanogen chloride	Organic synthesis	Liquid or gas	13 ppm	Inhalation, ingestion	Very irritating, pulmonary edema
CNBr	Cyanogen bromide	Fumigant	Colorless crystals	13 ppm	Inhalation, ingestion	Penetrating odor, bitter taste
CH$_2$:CHCN	Acrylonitrile	Synthetic fibers and plastic	Volatile liquid	35–90 mg./kg. (20 ppm)	Inhalation, skin absorption	Severe skin and eye irritant; characteristic unpleasant odor
CH$_3$ CN	Acetonitrile	Solvent, extractant	Colorless liquid	120 mg./kg.	Inhalation, ingestion	Ethereal odor, sweetish taste

Formula	Name	Uses	Appearance	TLV*	Route	Notes
$(CH_3)_2C(OH)CN$	Acetone cyanohydrin	—	Colorless liquid	15 mg./kg.	Inhalation, ingestion, skin absorption	Decomposes to HCN
$NA_2[Fe(NO)(CN)_5].H_2O$	Nitroprusside	Rx hypertension, analytical reagent	Red crystals	10 mg./kg.	Ingestion, given I.V.	Converted to SCN, releases nitrite
$K_2Fe(CN)_6$	Potassium ferrocyanide	Metallurgy, photography	Red solid	Slightly toxic	Ingestion	Converted rapidly to ferrocyanide
$K_4Fe(CN)_6.3H_2O$	Potassium ferrocyanide	Metallurgy, graphic arts	Lemon-yellow solid	1,600 mg./kg.	Ingestion	Chemical reagent
$KOCN$	Potassium cyanate	Weed killer, chemical intermediate	White solid	1,000 mg./kg.	Ingestion	Less toxicity than most cyanides

*TLV = threshold limit value.

skin. Skin absorption is not limited to the nitriles; hydrocyanic acid and its soluble salts can also be absorbed in this manner.

C. LABORATORY FINDINGS

Laboratory findings are not specific for cyanide poisoning. Blood gas analyses are generally normal. Cyanide blood levels can be obtained, but this requires special laboratory equipment usually not available in the average hospital. For levels that are obtained, Table 17-3 gives the correlation between the cyanide levels and the symptoms of intoxication.

Serial ECG changes have been described. These are due to progressive hypoxia of the myocardial cells and include premature ventricular contractions, heart block, and ischemic changes.

D. TREATMENT

Without rapid medical treatment, cyanide poisoning is universally fatal at or above the LD_{50}.

General measures to maintain airway and blood pressure should be undertaken. In addition, a nasogastric tube should be inserted and lavage performed if the cyanide is ingested. Activated charcoal instilled through the nasogastric tube is beneficial.

Fortunately, specific antidotes for cyanide poisoning provide a good chance of survival. Antidotal treatment is based on two reactions:

1. Hemoglobin + nitrite →
$$\text{methemoglobin}$$
Methemoglobin + cyanide →
$$\text{cyanmethemoglobin}$$
Cytochrome oxidase-cyanide complex
+ methemoglobin → cytochrome oxidase
+ cyanmethemoglobin

2. Thiosulfate +
$$\text{cyanide} \underset{\substack{\text{thiocyanate} \\ \text{oxidase} \\ \text{or methylene blue}}}{\overset{\text{rhodanese}}{\rightleftarrows}} \text{thiocyanate}$$

Thiosulfate + cytochrome −
$$\text{CN complex} \rightleftarrows \text{thiocyanate} + \text{active cytochrome oxidase}$$

In the first reaction, Fe^{+3} is created in methemoglobin. This pool of ferric ions competes with cytochrome for cyanide (CN^-). Methemoglobin is produced through the use of amyl nitrite perles and I.V. injection of sodium nitrite. Dosages of the nitrites are as follows:

1. Amyl nitrite perles: 1 ampule (0.2 ml.) inhaled every three to five minutes. Make sure the patient is well oxygenated. As soon as an I.V. line is inserted, discontinue the amyl nitrite and administer sodium nitrite.
2. Sodium nitrite (3% solution): Dosage depends on weight of the patient and hemoglobin level. Give 0.19 ml./kg. at a 7 gm./100 ml. hemoglobin to 0.39 ml./kg. at a 14 gm./100 ml. hemoglobin. Another way to administer the drug is to use 6–8 ml./cu.m. of body surface area or 300 mg. I.V. above 25 kg. and 10 mg./kg. below 25 kg. body weight.

The production of methemoglobin should be monitored closely. Methemoglobin shifts the oxyhemoglobin curve to the left and can further decrease the amount of tissue oxygenation. The objective is to obtain about 25% methemoglobin and avoid levels of over 40%.

In the second reaction, thiocyanate is formed and is readily excreted through the kidneys. A 25% solution of sodium thiosulfate should be given I.V. at a dose of 50 mg./kg. for those persons under 25 kg., and 12.5 gm. (50 ml.) for those over 25 kg. at a rate of 2.5 to 5.0 ml. per minute. This can be repeated in an hour at half the original dose if symptoms recur or persist.

Oxygen therapy: A necessary adjunct in treatment is 100% oxygen therapy because of the oxygen debt incurred in moderate to severe cyanide poisoning managed with nitrites and thiosulfate.

The following compounds also have

been used in the treatment of cyanide intoxication and are beneficial especially if used in conjunction with the nitrites and thiosulfate:

1. Dicobalt EDTA (Co$_2$ EDTA): 600 mg. I.V. rapidly in adults; 10mg./kg. in persons under 25 kg. Cobalt salts exert their effect by combining directly with the cyanide ion as a chelate. Hypertonic glucose (50 ml. of 50%) should be given after the Co$_2$ EDTA to decrease the direct toxicity of the cobalt salt itself.
2. Hydroxocobalamin (vitamin B$_{12a}$): Hydroxocobalamin changes into cyanocobalamin (vitamin B$_{12}$) upon contact with cyanide. This compound holds the cyanide in a tight bond. It works well if given before or slightly after the cyanide exposure.

E. SEQUELAE AND CHRONIC POISONING

Sequelae are rare from acute cyanide poisoning; the patient either succumbs or makes an uneventful recovery. However, chronic poisoning may occur if very low concentrations of cyanide are inhaled for extended periods (a year or longer). Dizziness, hoarseness, vague weakness, decreased appetite and weight loss, coryzalike symptoms, and some mental deterioration have been reported. Chronic ingestion of cyanide has not been reported.

III. SULFIDES

Sulfide poisonings in general are due to hydrogen sulfide (H$_2$S), carbon disulfide (CS$_2$), and the mercaptans. Sulfide salts such as ammonium and sodium sulfides release hydrogen sulfide when in contact with water.

Hydrogen sulfide is a very toxic gaseous material approaching hydrocyanic acid. It is commonly found in sewers, petroleum refineries, tanneries, in the production of rubber, rayon, glue, and in wells, caissons, and tunnels. Fortunately, poisonings are fairly infrequent.

Hydrogen sulfide is a colorless gas with a characteristic "rotten egg" odor. It is also a primary irritant. The odor can be

Table 17-3. **Correlation Between Blood Cyanide Levels and Symptoms of Intoxication**

Mild Levels (0.5 MG./ LITER)	Moderate Levels (1.0–2.5 MG./ LITER)	Severe Levels (2.5 MG./LITER OR GREATER)
Flushing	Responsive to	Unresponsive
Tachycardia	stimuli	Hypotension
Headache	Tachycardia	Tachycardia
Dizziness	Tachypnea	Slow respirations
Patient	Probable	Cyanosis at
conscious	severe	higher levels
	headache	Bulging eyeballs
		Dilated pupils
		Death imminent
		unless treated

detected as low as 0.025 ppm and is intense and offensive at 3–5 ppm. With higher concentrations, the odor is pungent and pronounced, and the sense of smell quickly fatigues.

Carbon disulfate, by contrast, is a liquid that boils at 46°C and ignites at 100° C. It is a colorless fluid with a sweetish aromatic odor. Industrial grades generally have a yellowish color and smell like decaying cabbage. The vapors of carbon disulfate can be highly explosive. It is used in the rayon industry as a solvent, and in the manufacture of rubber accelerators, floatation agents, plywood adhesive, disinfectants, and pesticides.

The mercaptans are generally gases formed in the petroleum refining processes. They include ethyl mercapten (C$_2$H$_5$ SH) and methyl mercaptan (CH$_3$SH).

Carbonyl sulfide (COS) is a gaseous, colorless, almost odorless agent found in the distillation of coal and petroleum refining. It is frequently (if not always) present in association with hydrogen sulfide or carbon disulfide. Its toxicity and treatment are the same as those for hydrogen sulfide and carbon disulfide.

After ingestion, sulfur and some of the soluble sulfide salts will release varying amounts of hydrogen sulfide through the reactions with gastric acid and colonic bacteria.

Table 17-4. **Features of Some Sulfide Compounds**

Material	TLV* (ppm)	MAC† (ppm)	Fatal Dose	Comments
Hydrogen sulfide	10	20	1,000 ppm (rapidly fatal)	
Carbon disulfide	20	20	30–60 ml. or 1 gm.	Fat-soluble
Methyl mercaptan	0.5	1.0	?50–100 ppm	Very toxic
Ethyl mercaptan	0.5	1.0	?50–100 ppm	Very toxic
Carbonyl sulfide	?500	—	?	Associated with H_2S or CS_2
Lead sulfide	—	—	10 gm./kg.	Lower toxic potential
Potassium sulfide	—	—	100 mg./kg.	Fairly high toxicity
Sulfur	—	—	—	10–20 gm. produce GI irritation and renal injury

*Threshold limit values.
†Maximum allowable concentrations.

Table 17-4 lists the threshold limit values, the maximal allowable concentrations, and the fatal doses of some of the sulfides.

Systemic poisoning occurs by:

1. Inhalation (the most common)
2. Ingestion of liquids and salts
3. Absorption through the skin, especially carbon disulfide

A. MECHANISM OF ACTION

Hydrogen sulfide is very similar to cyanide. It inhibits the cytochrome oxidase system, thereby producing severe tissue hypoxia. The hydrosulfide anion (HS^-) complexes with ferric (Fe^{+3}) heme and forms a compound, sulfmethemoglobin. Sulfmethemoglobin undergoes a slow autoreduction to hemoglobin polysulfides, thiosulfate, or sulfate. Hydrogen sulfide also has a direct effect on the chemoreceptors of the carotid bodies, producing a hyperpnea. It also has a direct central nervous system effect in that it rapidly produces paralysis of the respiratory center. Sulfur, sulfide salts, and the mercaptans act similarly.

The exact mechanism of action of carbon disulfide is not clearly defined. However, it does react with a variety of nucleophilic functional groups:

1. Amino → dithiocarbamic acids
2. Mercapto → trithiocarbamic acids
3. Hydroxyl → xanthogenic acids

The metabolic products of carbon disulfide interfere with the oxidation of acetaldehyde in the same manner as disulfiram (Antabuse), and produce similar symptoms. The thiocarbamic acid groups will chelate metal ions to interfere with the energy metabolism of cells and also prevent the incorporation of amino acids. Some of the carbon disulfide is converted to hydrogen sulfide. Carbon disulfide produces its toxic effects in the following organs and organ systems:

1. Skin: It is the most irritant of all the organic solvents.
2. Peripheral and central nervous system: Carbon disulfide is a potent neurotoxin that can cause paralysis, large pupils, paresthesias, spasmodic tremor, extrapyramidal signs, and psychiatric symptoms.
3. Cardiovascular: It causes diffuse vascular changes throughout all organs (mostly atheromata and fatty infiltrations of vessel walls).

All sulfides undergo fairly rapid metabolic degradation. The products are slowly excreted by the kidneys. There is some release of gaseous hydrogen sulfide through the lungs in most sulfide poisonings. Small amounts of carbon disulfide and hydrogen sulfide are directly excreted through the kidneys.

B. CLINICAL FEATURES

Table 17-5 shows the various concentrations and the allowable time before symptoms occur for hydrogen sulfide and carbon disulfide.

1. Hydrogen Sulfide Intoxication

a. Acute intoxication causes painful conjunctivitis, photophobia, excessive lacrimation, rhinitis, cough, and pulmonary edema. It also may cause bronchopneumonia, erythema, giddiness, headache, vertigo, amnesia, confusion, and coma, and tachypnea, tachycardia, sweating, weakness, and muscle cramps.

b. High concentrations (above 700 ppm) produce sudden collapse and unconsciousness. Respiratory paralysis and death occur within 30–60 minutes.

c. After sublethal exposure, recovery can be slow with persistent cough, peripheral neuritis, albuminuria and amnesia. Recovery is generally complete without residua.

d. Chronic intoxication causes persistent hypotension, nausea, anorexia with weight loss, conjunctivitis, corneal opacity, chronic cough, and impaired gait and balance.

2. Carbon Disulfide Intoxication

a. Acute intoxication causes headache, fatigue, weakness in the legs, vertigo, unsteady gait, skin irritation with vesicle formation (absorption can occur through the skin), garlic breath, nausea, vomiting, occasional abdominal pain, weak pulse, palpitations, mania, hallucinations, CNS depression with respiratory paralysis. Death may occur after a convulsion.

b. Chronic intoxication causes tremors, weakness, paralysis, peripheral neuritis,

Table 17-5. Various Concentrations of H_2S and CS_2 and Their Effects

Concentration	Time for Symptoms to Appear
H_2S	
MAC = 20 ppm	Prolonged exposure
50–150 p pm	Several hours
150–300 ppm	About 1 hour
300–700 ppm	15 minutes to 1 hour
> 700 ppm	Almost immediate collapse
CS_2	
MAC = 20 ppm	Prolonged exposure
100–250 ppm	Slight or no effect
250–400 ppm	Slight symptoms after several hours
400–550 ppm	After 30 minutes
550–1,100 ppm	Serious symptoms after 30 minutes
1,100–4,000 ppm	Life-threatening after 30 minutes
> 4,500 ppm	Fatal within 30 minutes

MAC = maximum allowable concentration

absence of corneal reflex, emotional instability (mild neurasthenia to psychosis), hypertension, atherosclerosis, and cardiac dilatation. Recovery, although very slow (months or years), may occur, but paralysis is frequently permanent.

c. Women are more sensitive to the neurotoxic effects.

3. Mercaptan Intoxication

Ethyl and methyl mercapten in the higher concentrations produce tremors, cyanosis, headache, fever, hemolytic anemia, coma, and occasionally irreversible depression of cerebral function.

C. LABORATORY FINDINGS

1. Albumin, casts, and red blood cells may be present in the urine.

2. There is a decrease in blood polymorphonuclear leucocytes, and an increase in lymphocytes and monocytes, and possibly eosinophiles.

3. ECG changes in carbon disulfide poisoning include both nonspecific and ischemic changes.

4. Serum cholinesterase may be decreased in carbon disulfide intoxication.

5. Serum cholesterol and beta-lipoprotein are elevated after chronic carbon disulfide exposure.

6. Specific urine tests to detect carbon disulfide are based on the iodine-azide reaction.

7. Lead acetate paper can detect hydrogen sulfide in the air.

D. TREATMENT

Because hydrogen sulfide produces its major toxic effects through mechanisms similar to that of cyanide, the treatment of acute intoxication is virtually the same as for cyanide. It is based on the production of methemoglobin by the nitrites that then combine with the hydrosulfide anion (HS^-) molecule to form sulfmethemoglobin which is then excreted through the kidneys or gradually metabolized to various nontoxic products. One difference in the therapy is the deletion of the sodium thiosulfate injection. As in cyanide therapy, cobaltous chloride can also be used. Of course, removing the person from the source of the intoxication is essential. In addition:

1. Provide high flow oxygen or artificial respiration.

2. Keep the patient calm and quiet.

3. Perform gastric lavage or emesis for those who ingested a hydrogen sulfide solution, soluble salts, or a product which contains sulfur.

4. Give atropine (0.4–0.6 I.M. or I.V.) for symptomatic relief but withhold if cyanosis is present.

5. Treat conjunctivitis with an antibiotic ointment, warm compresses, and if indicated, topical epinephrine.

6. Give antibiotics for pneumonitis.

7. Treat pulmonary edema by the standard methods.

The treatment of carbon disulfide poisoning is more difficult because there is no known antidote. Symptomatic treatment is as follows:

1. Remove the patient from the source of intoxication.

2. Provide high flow oxygen therapy or artificial ventilation.

3. Gastric lavage or emesis if the material is ingested.

4. A trial of large parenteral doses of pyridoxine (vitamin B_6) because of similarities between B_6 deficiencies and carbon disulfide poisoning.

5. For severe delirium, use tranquilizers.

6. Hospitalization for a minimum of three to four days at complete bedrest for observation.

BIBLIOGRAPHY

I. CARBON MONOXIDE

Abbott, D. F.: Slow recovery from carbon monoxide. Postgrad. Med. J., *48*:639–642, 1972.

Agostini, J., Ruben, G. R., Solomon, N. A., et al.: Successful reversal of lethal carbon monoxide intoxication by total body asanguineous hypothermic perfusion. Surgery, *75*(2):213–219, 1974.

Carbon monoxide. Lab. Med. *37*, 1972.

Dinman, B. D.: The management of acute carbon monoxide intoxication. J. Occup. Med., *16*:662–664, 1974.

Larking, M. K., Brahos, G. H., and Moylan, J. A.: Treatment of carbon monoxide poisoning: prognostic factors. J. Trauma, *16*(2):111–114, 1976.

Mayer, B. W., Smith, D. S., and Hayden, M. J.: Acute smoke inhalation in children. Am. Fam. Physician, *7*(4):80–84, 1973.

Ogawa, H. T., Katsurado, K., Sugimoto, T., et al.: Respiratory changes in carbon monoxide poisoning with reference to hyperbaric oxygenation. Med. J. Osaka Univ., *22*(3):251–258, 1972.

Patty, F. A.: Carbon monoxide. *In* Industrial Hygiene and Toxicology. 2nd ed., pp. 924–936. New York, Wiley-Interscience, 1962.

Polk, L. D.: Carbon monoxide poisoning and other hazards of the energy crisis. Clin. Ped., *14*(3):219–220, 1975.

Sone, S., Toburo, H., Takeshi, K., et al.: Pulmonary manifestations in acute monoxide poisoning. Am. J. Roentg. Radium Ther. Nucl. Med. *120*(4):865–871, 1974.

Stewart, R. D., Stewart, R. S., Stamin, W.; and Seelen, R. P.: Rapid estimation of carboxyhemoglobin level in fire fighters. J.A.M.A. *235*:390–392, 1976.

Zarem H. A., Ratenborg, C. C., and Harmel, M. H.: Carbon monoxide toxicity in human fire victims. Arch. Surg. *197:*851–853, 1073.

II. CYANIDES

Arena, J: Cyanide. *In* Poisoning, Toxicology, Symptoms, Treatments. 3rd ed., pp. 182–184. Springfield, Ill., Charles C Thomas, 1973.

Dalerup, L. M.: Cyanide intoxication. Lancet, *6:*25, 1973.

Isom, G., and Way, J. L.: Effect of oxygen arcyanide intoxication. J. Pharm. Exp. Ther., *189* (1): 235–243, 1974.

————: Cyanide intoxication: protection with cobaltous chloride. Toxicol. Appl. Pharmacol. *24:* 449–456, 1973.

Naughton, M.: Acute cyanide poisoning. Anesth. Intensive Care, *2*(4):351–356, 1974.

Patty, F. A.: Cyanides and nitriles. *In* Industrial Hygiene and Toxicology. 2nd. ed., pp. 1991–2036. New York, Wiley-Interscience, 1962.

Smith, R. P.: Cobalt salts: effects in cyanide and sulfide poisoning and on methemoglobinemia. Toxicol. Appl. Pharmacol., *15:*505–516, 1969.

Stewart, R.: Cyanide poisoning. Clin. Toxicol., *7* (5):561–564, 1974.

III. SULFIDES

Arena, J.: Sulfide and derivatives. *In* Poisoning, Toxicology, Symptoms, and Treatments. 3rd ed., pp. 184–185. Springfield, Ill., Charles C Thomas, 1973.

Davidson, M., and Manning, F.: Carbon disulfide poisoning: a review. Am. Heart J., *83:*100–114, 1974.

Gleason, M. D., Gosselin, R. E., Hodge, H. C., and Smith, R. P.: Hydrogen sulfide, carbon disulfide. *In* Clinical Toxicology of Commercial Products: Acute Poisoning. 4th ed. Baltimore, Williams & Wilkins, 1976.

Patty, F. A.: Sulfides. *In* Industrial Hygiene and Toxicology. 2nd ed., pp. 896–905. New York, Wiley-Interscience, 1962.

Smith, R.: Sulfide poisoning. *In* Blood, F. (ed.): Essays in Toxicology. Vol. 1, pp. 87–91, 1969.

Tolonen, M.: Vascular effects of carbon disulfide—a review. Scan. J. Work Envir. Health, *1:*63–77, 1975.

18. PESTICIDES

Donald P. Morgan, M.D., Ph.D.

I. ORGANOCHLORINE PESTICIDES

This class includes chemicals in which chlorine has been substituted for hydrogen in various aromatic, aliphatic, and complex hydrocarbon structures. Highly soluble in fat and organic solvents, these insecticides are essentially insoluble in water. They exhibit low vapor pressures. They are resistant to degradation in human tissue and in the environment. After absorption, some are excreted in days or weeks; others require months or even years for elimination. To some extent, all undergo some storage in body fat until they are excreted.

Commonly used organochlorine pesticides (approximately in order of decreasing toxicity) are as follows:

1. Highly toxic: endrin (Hexadrin), a stereoisomer of dieldrin
2. Moderately toxic: aldrin (Aldrite, Drinox), endosulfan (Thiodan), dieldrin (Dieldrite), toxaphene (Toxakil, Strobane-T), lindane (Isotox, Gammexane), benzene hexachloride (BHC, HCH), DDT (Chlorophenothane), heptachlor, kepone, terpenepolychlorinates (Strobane), chlordane (Chlordan), dicofol (Kelthane), chlorobenzilate (Acaraben), mirex, methoxychlor (Marlate)

Solid organochlorine pesticides are absorbed by the gut, across the skin, and, to a limited extent, by transport across the pulmonary membrane. They interfere with axonic transmission of nerve impulses, and therefore disrupt the function of the nervous system, principally that of the brain. This results in behavioral changes, sensory and equilibrium disturbances, involuntary muscle activity, and depression of vital centers, particularly respiration. They also increase the irritability of the myocardium and cause degenerative changes in the liver. In many cases of poisoning, the toxicity of the hydrocarbon solvent vehicle (notably respiratory depression) is superimposed on that of the active pesticidal ingredient.

A. CLINICAL FEATURES

These include apprehension, excitability, dizziness, headache, disorientation, weakness, paresthesias, muscle twitching, tremor, tonic and clonic convulsions (often epileptiform), and coma. Soon after ingestion, nausea and vomiting are often prominent. When the chemicals are absorbed by parenteral routes, apprehension, twitching, tremors, and convulsions may be the first symptoms. Pallor occurs in moderate to severe poisoning. Cyanosis may result as respiratory depression deepens and as convulsive activity interferes with respiratory excursions.

B. LABORATORY FINDINGS

Pesticides and their metabolites can almost always be identified in blood or urine by gas-liquid chromatography of samples taken within 72 hours of poisoning. Some chlorinated hydrocarbon pesticides persist in the serum for weeks or months after absorption. Treatment of acute poisoning cannot be delayed pending confirmatory analysis of blood. Qualitative identification of chlorinated hydrocarbon residues in blood or tissues does not, of itself, indicate poisoning; actual concentrations must be taken into consideration.

C. TREATMENT

1. Establish clear airway and tissue oxygenation by aspiration of secretions, and, if necessary, by assisted pulmonary ventilation with oxygen.
2. Control convulsions. The anticon-

vulsant of choice is diazepam—(Valium). For adults (including children over 6 years of age, or 23 kg. in weight), inject 5–10 mg. (1–2 ml.) slowly intravenously (no faster than 1 ml. per minute), or give total dose intramuscularly (deep). Repeat in two to four hours if needed to control seizures. For children (under 6, or less than 23 kg.), inject 0.1–0.2 mg./kg. (0.02 –0.04 ml./kg.) slowly intravenously (no faster than one-half total dose per minute), or give total dose intramuscularly (deep). Repeat in two to four hours if needed. Slow injection is necessary to avoid irritation of vein, occasional hypotension, and slowing of respiration.

Because of a greater tendency to cause respiratory depression, barbiturates are probably of less value than diazepam. The one used successfully in the past is pentobarbital (Nembutal). The maximum safe dose is 5 mg./kg. body weight. If possible, inject solution intravenously, at a rate not exceeding 1 ml. per minute until convulsions are controlled. If intravenous administration is not possible, give total dose rectally, not exceeding 5 mg./kg. body weight.

Caution: Assist pulmonary ventilation mechanically if respiration is depressed. Keep the patient in a quiet environment.

3. If the pesticide has been ingested in quantity sufficient to cause poisoning, the stomach must be emptied. If the patient is alert and respiration is not depressed, give syrup of ipecac to induce vomiting (30 ml. for adults; 15 ml. for children under 12 years). Observe the patient closely after administering ipecac. If consciousness level declines, or if vomiting has not occurred in 20 minutes, proceed immediately to intubate the stomach.

After emesis, have patient drink a suspension of 30 gm. activated charcoal in 3–4 oz. water to limit absorption of toxicant remaining in the gut.

If patient is not fully alert, empty the stomach immediately by intubation, aspiration, and lavage, using isotonic saline or 5% sodium bicarbonate. Because most pesticides are dissolved in petroleum distillates, emesis and intubation of the stomach involve a serious risk that solvent will be aspirated, leading to chemical pneumonitis. For this reason:

a. If the patient is unconscious or obtunded, and if facilities are at hand, insert an endotracheal tube (cuffed, if available) prior to gastric intubation.

b. Keep the patient's head below the level of the stomach during intubation and lavage (Trendelenburg, or left lateral decubitus, with head end of table tipped downward). Keep the head turned to the left.

c. Aspirate pharynx as regularly as possible to remove gagged or vomited stomach contents.

After aspiration of gastric contents and washing of stomach, instill 30 gm. activated charcoal in 3–4 oz. water by way of stomach tube to limit absorption of remaining toxicant. Do not instill milk, cream, or other substances containing vegetable or animal fats, because these enhance absorption of chlorinated hydrocarbons.

If patient is fully conscious, give sodium sulfate as a cathartic. Adult dose is 30 gm. in 6–8 oz. water. For children under 12, give 0.2 gm./kg. body weight in 1–6 oz. water.

4. If poisoning has occurred because of contamination of skin and hair, bathe and shampoo the patient vigorously with soap and water.

5. Do not give epinephrine or other adrenergic amines, because of the myocardial irritability produced by chlorinated hydrocarbons. Avoid the use of opiates and other respiratory depressants.

6. During convalescence, enhance carbohydrate, protein, and vitamin intake by diet or parenteral therapy to minimize toxic injury to the liver.

The chemical endrin is more hepatotoxic than the other chlorinated hydrocarbons in common use. Bilirubinemia and elevated blood enzyme activities occur commonly in poisoning. Special measures should be taken to minimize liver injury by supplying ample nutrients.

7. Except in endrin poisoning, the likelihood of recovery from poisoning by chlorinated hydrocarbon pesticides is generally good, even when convulsions occur. Fatalities occur as a result of massive doses. The prognosis in endrin poisoning is somewhat more guarded.

II. ORGANOPHOSPHATE PESTICIDES

Nearly all organophosphates are malodorous, strongly lipid-soluble insecticides that are commonly applied in spray, dust, emulsion, or granular formulations. In the environment, and in mammalian tissues, an interchange of oxygen with the divalent sulfur commonly occurs, yielding the much more toxic "oxon" analogs. Organophosphates are readily degraded in the environment and metabolized in mammals by hydrolytic cleavage between the "leaving group" and alkyl phosphate (or alkyl phosphorothioate) moieties. Urinary excretion of these metabolites can be used to detect excessive absorption of organophosphates. Some of these chemicals are "systemic" insecticides, i.e., they are taken up by the plant roots and translocated into foliage and sometimes into the flower and fruit.

Commonly used organophosphate pesticides (approximately in order of decreasing toxicity) are as follows:

1. Highly toxic: TEPP, phorate (Thimet), mevinphos (Phosdrin), fensulfothion (Dasanit), demeton* (Systox), disulfoton* (Disyston), sulfotepp (Bladafume, Dithione), counter, ethyl parathion (Parathion, Thiophos), fonofos (Dyfonate), EPN, azinphos-methyl (Guthion), methyl parathion (Dalf), monocrotophos (Azodrin), dicro-

tophos (Bidrin), methamidophos (Monitor), carbophenothion (Trithion), phosphamidon (Dimecron)
2. Moderately toxic: famphur (Warbex, Bo-Ana, Famfos), ethoprop (Mocap), methidathion (Supracide), coumophos (Co-Ral), demeton-methyl* (Metasystox), dichlorvos (DDVP, Vapona), dioxathion (Delnav), crotoxyphos (Ciodrin), phosalone (Zolone), chlorpyrifos (Lorsban, Dursban), ethion, fenthion (Baytex, Entex), diazinon (Spectracide), dimethoate (Cygon), naled (Dibrom), trichlorfon (Dylox, Dipterex, Neguvon), crufomate (Ruelene), ronnel (Korlan), malathion (Cythion)

Toxicants of this class can be absorbed by inhalation, ingestion, and skin penetration. They irreversibly phosphorylate varying amounts of the acetylcholinesterase enzyme of tissues, allowing accumulation of acetylcholine at cholinergic neuroeffector junctions (muscarinic effects), and at skeletal muscle myoneural junctions and in autonomic ganglia (nicotinic effects). They also impair CNS function. Phosphorylating action extends to other esterase enzymes of the body, including the acetylcholinesterase of red blood cells and the pseudocholinesterase of plasma.

A. CLINICAL FEATURES

Symptoms of acute poisoning develop during organophosphate exposure or within 12 hours of contact. These include headache, dizziness, extreme weakness, ataxia, miosis, blurred or "dark" vision, muscle twitching, tremor, convulsions, mental confusion, incontinence, unconsciousness, nausea, vomiting, abdominal cramps, diarrhea, tightness in chest, bradycardia, wheezing, productive cough, and sometimes pulmonary edema (up to 12 hours after poisoning), sweating, rhinorrhea, tearing, salivation. Severe poisoning may cause sudden unconscious-

---

*Systemic insecticides.

*Systemic insecticides.

ness, or produce a toxic psychosis which resembles acute alcoholism. Extreme bradycardia and heart block have been observed. Respiratory depression is caused by the toxicant and also the hydrocarbon solvent. Continuing absorption at intermediate dosage may cause an influenzalike illness characterized by weakness, anorexia, and malaise.

B. LABORATORY FINDINGS

Depression of plasma or RBC cholinesterase activity is the most satisfactory and generally available evidence of excessive absorption of organophosphates. Depression of plasma cholinesterase often persists from 1 to 3 weeks; depression of RBC acetylcholinesterase persists up to 12 weeks, depending on magnitude of initial depression.

Test values below the lower limits of normal plasma and red cell cholinesterase activities of human blood usually indicate excessive absorption of a cholinesterase-inhibiting chemical. The red cell activity test is more specific for organophosphate inhibition than the plasma assay; plasma cholinesterase is depressed by liver injury from a variety of causes. Also, about 3% of the population has a genetically determined deficiency of plasma cholinesterase activity caused by generation of an atypical enzyme by the liver.

For these reasons, and because of the wide natural range of blood cholinesterase activities, comparison of a "test" sample measurement with a "preexposure" value offers the best confirmation of organophosphate action. A depression of 25% or more is strong evidence of excessive organophosphate absorption.

Metabolites of organophosphates are commonly detectable in the urine of poisoning victims from 12 to 48 hours after absorption and can be found when dosage was insufficient to depress blood cholinesterase activities.

Caution: If diagnosis is probable, do not delay treatment until it is confirmed by blood or urine tests.

C. TREATMENT

1. Persons attending the patient must avoid contamination with vomitus and other sources of toxicant. Rubber gloves should be worn while decontaminating the patient.

2. Establish clear airway and tissue oxygenation by aspiration of secretions and, if necessary, by assisted pulmonary ventilation with oxygen. Do not proceed with atropine administration until a satisfactory level of oxygenation has been achieved. Atropine may induce ventricular fibrillation if patient is severely hypoxic.

3. Administer atropine sulfate intravenously, or intramuscularly if I.V. injection is not possible. Atropine protects the end-organs from excessive concentrations of acetylcholine. It does not reactivate cholinesterase, and effects of unmetabolized toxicant may appear as atropinization wears off.

   a. In moderately severe poisoning, the adult dose (including children over 12 years) is 0.4–2.0 mg. (1.0–5.0 ml. of 0.4 mg./ml. solution) repeated every 15–30 minutes until atropinization is achieved (tachycardia, flushing, dry mouth, mydriasis). Maintain atropinization by repeated doses for 2–12 hours (or even longer) depending on severity of poisoning. Watch the patient closely for relapse as atropinization wears off.

   b. The child's dose (to 12 years) is 0.05 mg./kg. body weight (0.125 ml./kg. of 0.4 mg./ml. solution) repeated every 15–30 minutes until atropinization is achieved. Maintain atropinization by repeated doses.

   c. In severe poisoning, use twice the dosage of atropine recommended above.

4. Administer pralidoxime (Protopam-Ayerst, 2-PAM) in those cases of severe poisoning by organophosphate pesticides in which muscle weakness and twitchings persist despite atropine therapy. When

administered early (less than 36 hours after poisoning) pralidoxime is of value in relieving the nicotinic effects of severe poisoning that are not reversed by atropine. It is of no value in poisonings by cholinesterase-inhibiting carbamate compounds.

a. The adult dose (including children over 12 years) is 1.0 gm. intravenously, at no more than 0.5 gm. per minute, repeating dose in 1 hour if muscle weakness has not been relieved. In severe poisoning, dosage may be doubled.

b. The child's dose (under 12 years) is 20–50 mg./kg. (depending on severity) intravenously, injecting no more than 50% of the total dose per minute. This dosage amounts to 0.4 ml.–1.0 ml./kg. of a 5% solution. Repeat every 10–12 hours as needed, up to three times. Intramuscular administration may be used if intravenous injection is not possible.

5. Observe patient closely at least 24 hours to ensure that symptoms do not occur as atropinization wears off.

6. Give bath and shampoo if there is contamination of skin and hair.

7. If pesticide has been ingested in quantity sufficient to cause poisoning, the stomach must be emptied. If patient is alert and respiration is not depressed, give syrup of ipecac to induce vomiting (30 ml. for adults; 15 ml. for children under 12 years). Observe the patient closely after administering ipecac. If consciousness level declines, or if vomiting has not occurred in 20 minutes, proceed immediately to intubate the stomach.

Following emesis, have victim drink a suspension of 30 gm. activated charcoal in 3–4 oz. water to bind toxicant remaining in the gut.

If patient is obtunded or respiration is depressed, empty the stomach by intubation, aspiration, and lavage, using isotonic saline or 5% sodium bicarbonate. Because many pesticides are dissolved in petroleum distillates, emesis and intubation of the stomach involve a serious risk that solvent will be aspirated, leading to chemical pneumonitis. For this reason:

a. If the victim is unconscious or obtunded and if facilities are at hand, insert an endotracheal tube (cuffed, if available) prior to gastric intubation.

b. Keep the patient's head below the level of the stomach during intubation and lavage (Trendelenburg, or left lateral decubitus, with head end of table tipped downward). Keep patient's head turned to the left.

c. Aspirate pharynx as regularly as possible to remove gagged or vomited stomach contents.

After aspiration of gastric contents and washing of stomach, instill 30 gm. activated charcoal in 3–4 oz. water by way of stomach tube to limit absorption of remaining toxicant.

If patient is fully conscious, give sodium sulfate as a cathartic. The adult dose is 30 gm. in 6–8 oz. water. For children under 12, give 0.2 gm./kg. body weight in 1–6 oz. water.

8. Do not give morphine, aminophylline, phenothiazines, or reserpine.

9. If intractable convulsions (unresponsive to antidotes) occur in severe poisoning, causes unrelated to direct organophosphate action may be responsible: head trauma, cerebral anoxia, mixed poisoning. Although not thoroughly tested in these circumstances, diazepam (Valium) (5–10 mg. for adults; 0.1–0.2 mg./kg. for children under 6 years or 23 kg.) is probably the safest and most reliable anticonvulsant to use. Be prepared to intubate and assist pulmonary ventilation mechanically if respiration is depressed. Diazepam may be given slowly intravenously or by deep intramuscular injection. Hypotension and respiratory depression may occur.

10. Persons who have been clinically poisoned by organophosphate pesticides should not be reexposed to cholinesterase-inhibiting chemicals until symptoms and signs have resolved completely and blood

cholinesterase activities have returned to at least 80% of prepoisoning values. If no measurements of blood cholinesterase were made prior to poisoning, activities should reach at least minimum-normal levels before the victim is returned to a pesticide-contaminated environment.

11. It is neither practical nor medically sound to administer atropine or pralidoxime prophylactically to workers exposed to organophosphate pesticides.

III. CHOLINESTERASE-INHIBITING CARBAMATE INSECTICIDES

Chemicals of this class are degradable insecticides. Some have significant water solubility, but most are marketed in organic solvents or adsorbed on dust or granules. Particular carbamate insecticides are "systemic," i.e., they are translocated from the soil into the foliage and sometimes the fruit of the plant. Carbamate insecticides are to be distinguished from the carbamate herbicides, which do not have cholinesterase-inhibiting properties.

Commonly used carbamate insecticides (approximately in order of decreasing toxicity) are as follows:

1. Highly toxic: aldicarb* (Temik), oxyamyl* (Vydate), carbofuran (Furadan), aminocarb (Matacil), methomyl (Lannate, Nudrin), mexacarbate (Zectran), methiocarb (Mesurol)
2. Moderately toxic: propoxur (Baygon), Landrin, carbaryl (Sevin), metalkamate (Bux)

Insecticides of this class cause reversible carbamylation of the acetylcholinesterase enzyme of tissues, allowing accumulation of acetylcholine at cholinergic neuroeffector junctions (muscarinic effects) and at skeletal muscle myoneural junctions and in autonomic ganglia (nico-

---

*Systemic insecticides.

tinic effects). The toxin also impairs CNS function. The carbamyl-enzyme combination dissociates more readily than the phosphorylated enzyme produced by organophosphate insecticides. This lability of the enzyme-inhibitor complex not only tends to mitigate the toxicity of carbamates but also limits the usefulness of blood enzyme measurements in the diagnosis of poisoning. Carbamates are absorbed by inhalation, ingestion, and dermal penetration, are metabolized by the liver, and the degradation products are excreted by the liver and kidney.

A few carbamate insecticides are formulated in methyl (wood) alcohol. In cases of ingestion of these formulations, the toxicology of the methanol must be taken into consideration: severe gastroenteric irritation, acidosis, and CNS injury.

A. CLINICAL FEATURES

Symptoms of acute poisoning develop during carbamate exposure or within 12 hours (usually less) of absorption of the toxicant. They include headache, dizziness, weakness, ataxia, miosis, blurred or "dark" vision, muscle twitching, tremor, convulsions, mental confusion, incontinence, unconsciousness, nausea, vomiting, abdominal cramps, diarrhea, tightness in chest, slow heartbeat, wheezing, productive cough, occasionally pulmonary edema, sweating, rhinorrhea, tearing, salivation. Severe poisoning may cause sudden unconsciousness or a toxic psychosis. Respiratory depression may result from actions of the toxicant and solvent. Continuing absorption at intermediate dosage may cause protracted weakness, anorexia, and malaise.

B. LABORATORY FINDINGS

Depression of plasma or RBC cholinesterase activity is sometimes useful in detecting excessive absorption of toxicants of this class. However, because enzyme activities commonly revert to normal within minutes or a few hours, they are not reliable detectors of carbamate poisoning: intoxication may exist when enzyme activities are normal. The rapid methods for cholinesterase estimation (Acholest, ChE-TEL, Merck-O-Test, Voss-Sachsse) are more likely to detect depressions than methods requiring dilution of the sample and much time for analysis.

When test values are below lower limits of normal plasma and red cell cholinesterase activity levels of human blood, excessive absorption of a cholinesterase-inhibiting carbamate should be suspected. Blood cholinesterase activities vary over wide ranges in persons having no known exposures to inhibitors. The plasma cholinesterase is depressed by a variety of agents damaging the liver. Also, about 3% of the population has a genetically determined deficiency of plasma enzyme. For these reasons, a comparison of the test sample activity with a preexposure value actually offers the best confirmation of excessive carbamate absorption. A depression of 25% is strong evidence of excessive exposure.

Some carbamates yield metabolites that are measurable by gas-liquid chromatography in the urine of poison victims up to 48 hours after absorption of significant quantities.

Caution: If diagnosis is probable, do not delay treatment until diagnosis is confirmed by blood enzyme or urine metabolite tests.

C. TREATMENT

1. Persons attending the patient must avoid contamination with vomitus and other sources of toxicant. Rubber gloves should be worn while decontaminating the patient.

2. Establish clear airway and tissue oxygenation by aspiration of secretions, and if necessary, by assisted pulmonary ventilation with oxygen. Do not proceed with atropine administration until a satisfactory level of oxygenation has been achieved. Atropine may induce ventricular fibrillation if patient is severely asphyxic.

3. Administer atropine sulfate intravenously, or intramuscularly if I.V. injection is not possible. Atropine protects the end-organs from excessive concentrations of acetylcholine. It does not reactivate cholinesterase, and effects of unmetabolized toxicant may appear as atropinization wears off.

a. In moderately severe poisoning, the adult dose (including children over 12 years) is 0.4–2.0 mg. (1.0–5.0 ml. of 0.4 mg./ml. solution) repeated every 15–30 minutes until atropinization is achieved (tachycardia, flushing, dry mouth, mydriasis). Maintain atropinization by repeated doses for 2–12 hours, depending on severity of poisoning.

b. The child's dose (to 12 years) is 0.05 mg./kg. body weight (0.125 ml./kg. of 0.4 mg./ml. solution) repeated every 15–30 minutes until atropinization is achieved.

c. In severe poisoning, use twice the dosage of atropine recommended above.

4. Do not give praladoxime. It is of no value in carbamate poisonings.

5. Observe patient closely at least 24 hours to ensure that symptoms (possibly pulmonary edema) do not occur as atropinization wears off.

6. Give bath and shampoo if skin or hair have been contaminated.

7. If pesticide has been ingested in quantity sufficient to cause poisoning, the stomach must be emptied. If patient is alert and respiration is not depressed, give syrup of ipecac to induce vomiting, (30 ml. for adults; 15 ml. for children under 12 years).

Caution: Observe the patient closely after administering ipecac. If consciousness level declines, or if vomiting has not occurred in 15 minutes, proceed immediately to intubate the stomach.

After emesis, have patient drink a suspension of 30 gm. activated charcoal in

3–4 oz. water to limit absorption of toxicant remaining in the gastrointestinal tract.

If patient is obtunded or respiration depressed, empty the stomach by intubation, aspiration, and lavage, using isotonic saline or 5% sodium bicarbonate. To minimize the risk of pneumonitis from aspiration of toxicant and petroleum distillate solvent, take every possible precaution to keep stomach contents out of the airway: (1) endotracheal intubation (cuffed tube) before gastric intubation of unconscious patients; (2) Trendelenburg or left lateral decubitus position, with head low and turned to left; (3) frequent aspiration of the pharynx.

After aspiration of gastric contents and lavage, instill 30 gm. activated charcoal in 3–4 oz. water by way of stomach tube to limit absorption of remaining toxicant.

If bowel movement has not occurred in four hours and if patient is fully conscious, give sodium sulfate as a cathartic. The adult dose is 15 gm. in 6–8 oz. water. For children under 12, give 0.2 gm./kg. body weight in 1–6 oz. water.

8. Do not give morphine, aminophylline, phenothiazines, or reserpine.

9. If intractable convulsions (unresponsive to antidotes) occur in severe poisoning, causes unrelated to direct carbamate action may be responsible: head trauma, cerebral anoxia, mixed poisoning. Although not thoroughly tested in these circumstances, diazepam (5–10 mg. for adults, 0.1–0.2 mg./kg. for children under 6 years or 23 kg.) is probably the safest and most reliable anticonvulsant to use. Be prepared to intubate and assist pulmonary ventilation mechanically if respiration is depressed.

10. Persons who have suffered clinical poisoning by carbamate insecticides should not be reexposed to cholinesterase-inhibiting chemicals in an occupational environment until symptoms and signs have resolved completely and blood cholinesterase activities have recovered. Ac-

tivities should have reached 80% of the preexposure normal, or, if this is not known, activities should approximate minimum normal values.

IV. HALOCARBON AND SULFURYL FUMIGANTS

Commonly used halocarbon and sulfuryl fumigants are as follows:

1. Aliphatic: chloroform, carbon tetrachloride, methyl bromide (Brom-O-Gas, Fumigant-1, Kayafume, Me Br, Meth-O-Gas, Pestmaster, Profume); chloropicrin (Acquinite, Chlor-O-Pic, Pic-clor, Picfume, Trichlor); ethylene dichloride (EDC); ethylene dibromide (EDB, Bromofume, Celmide, Dowfume W-85, Kopfume, Nephis, Pestmaster EDB-85, Soilbrom); dichloropropene and dichloropropane (Telone, D-D); dibromochloropropane (DBCP, Nemagon, Fumazone, Nemafume). The Dowfume series of fumigants manufactured by the Dow Chemical Company are mixtures of halocarbons, mainly EDC, EDB, carbon tetrachloride, Me Br, and chloropicrin, formulated to meet specific needs.
2. Aromatic: paradichlorobenzene (PDB, Paracide, Paradow).
3. Sulfuryl: sulfuryl fluoride (Vikane).

Except for the solid paradichlorobenzene moth crystals, these chemicals are either gases or are highly volatile liquids at room temperature. A remarkable capacity for penetration is essential for their effectiveness as fumigants. Some, especially the bromine compounds, pass readily through human skin and rubber protective gear, thus complicating the protection of exposed workers. In varying degrees, they irritate the skin, eyes, and respiratory tract. When held on the skin by an occluding cover, such as contaminated gloves, the irritant action is accentuated, causing acute dermatitis and vesiculation. Repeated contact with the liquid halocarbons defats the skin, leading to chronic dermatitis. All are capable of producing pulmonary edema and hemorrhage in persons heavily exposed by inhalation, ingestion, or dermal absorption. Death following exposure to the halocarbon fumigants is usually due either to pulmonary edema or to respiratory depression.

Inhalation of pyrolysis products of these fumigants has caused massive necrosis of respiratory tract linings in exposed firefighters.

Toxic action on the central nervous system is generally depressant, causing unconsciousness, seizures, and general muscle weakness, including weakened respiratory effort. The neurotoxic action of methyl bromide apparently also includes the basal ganglia, causing not only sensory and motor impairment but also behavioral and affective disturbances. These may or may not progress to epileptiform seizures and coma. In some cases, behavioral and neurological manifestations have first appeared several hours or even days after exposure and have then persisted for days to months.

The chlorocarbons (notably chloroform) increase myocardial irritability and impair contractile strength. Large inhalation dosages may cause death by inducing ventricular fibrillation.

In varying degree, these fumigants damage the liver and kidney. In laboratory animals and in autopsy specimens from fatal human cases, this is commonly manifest as fatty degeneration. More severe poisoning causes centrilobular necrosis of the liver and acute tubular necrosis of the kidney.

Methyl bromide and ethylene dichloride (and possibly other chemicals of this series, by analogy) are alkylating agents in mammalian tissues. As such, they are capable of inhibiting multiple enzyme systems, including the sulfhydryl enzymes and hexokinases. This may be a major mechanism of toxicity of this series of chemicals.

Paradichlorobenzene is substantially less toxic to humans than the gaseous and liquid fumigants. It has neither the hemolytic nor the cataractogenic properties of

naphthalene fumigant, which it has largely displaced.

A. CLINICAL FEATURES

Headache, dizziness, nausea and vomiting are prominent early symptoms of the poisonings produced by these fumigants. Irritants, especially methyl bromide and the 3-carbon chlorocarbons often produce tearing, rhinorrhea, pharyngitis, cough, and dyspnea. These symptoms may progress to pulmonary edema, with coughing of frothy sputum.

Drowsiness, tremors, ataxia, diplopia, muscle twitchings and weakness, and Jacksonian seizures are the major early manifestations of central nervous system injury. Twitching and regional myoclonic movements may progress to general and severe epileptiform seizures, coma, and death in respiratory failure.

Delayed manifestations have characterized some poisonings by methyl bromide. Convulsions or pulmonary edema may appear up to 48 hours after exposure. Bizarre myotonic states, behavioral and emotional disturbances, impaired speech, and awkward gait have developed after repeated, relatively low-level occupational exposures, which have persisted for weeks or months.

Heavy accidental exposures to the chloropropanes and chloropropenes have occasionally led to protracted neurological manifestations, including headache, irritability, fatigue, poor memory, and personality changes.

Ingestion of acutely toxic amounts of liquid halocarbons is likely to be followed by pulmonary edema, seizures, and shock. Because toxic dosages and individual susceptibilities vary widely, cases of ingestion should be treated vigorously, irrespective of estimated dosage.

Paradichlorobenzene has caused occasional dermal sensitization. Tremors and liver injury produced by extreme doses in laboratory animals have occurred rarely, if ever, in humans.

Sulfuryl fluoride may cause muscle twitchings, then convulsions, on acute exposure. Because pulmonary and renal damage may develop on repeated contact, every attempt should be made to minimize exposure.

B. LABORATORY FINDINGS

Although there are methods available for measuring gaseous halocarbons in expired air, they are only available in anesthesiology research units or industrial plants. Paradichlorobenzene concentrations can be measured in the blood.

Blood bromide concentrations have some value in identification of poisonings by methyl bromide (and possibly ethylene dibromide), provided it can be established that the person exposed to the fumigant has not recently taken inorganic bromide medication. A level of organic bromide of more than 5 mg./100 ml. indicates excessive absorption of fumigant. A blood concentration of more than 10 mg./100 ml. of organic bromide represents a serious threat to health. A blood level of more than 15 mg./100 ml. endangers life.

C. TREATMENT

1. Flush contaminating fumigant from the eyes with copious amounts of water.

2. Wash liquid fumigant from the skin with soap and water. Severe inflammation and vesiculation will require medical management.

3. Remove victims of fumigant inhalation to fresh air. If respiration is depressed, resuscitate by mechanical intermittent positive pressure breathing (IPPB) with 100% oxygen, if available. Otherwise use intermittent mouth-to-mouth resuscitation.

4. Pulmonary edema must be treated initially by vigorous IPPB with 100% oxygen. Keep patient at complete bedrest to limit activity.

5. Control convulsions. Although there is no published experience to document its value in these poisonings, diazepam is probably the drug of choice to control seizures caused by the halocarbon fumigants. Give 0.1–0.2 mg./kg. by slow intravenous injection, stopping with the lowest effective dose. Deep intramuscular injection can be used if seizures preclude intravenous administration. Administer slowly I.V. to avoid irritation of the vein, hypotension, and respiratory depression.

6. Severe seizures caused by methyl bromide have been controlled with barbiturates. A maximum dosage of pentobarbital of 5 mg./kg. body weight may be given slowly I.V. until convulsions are controlled, and repeated in 4–6 hours if necessary. If I.V. administration is not possible, the total 5-mg./kg. dose can be administered rectally.

Caution: Be prepared to assist pulmonary ventilation mechanically, if respiration is depressed. In methyl bromide poisoning, it may be necessary to give diazepam or pentobarbital orally for some time after the acute convulsive episode to control involuntary motor activity.

7. Ingested fumigant liquids must be removed. Because of the strong likelihood of respiratory depression shortly after ingestion, it is probably best to avoid use of ipecac, and to undertake gastric intubation, aspiration, and lavage immediately. To avoid aspiration of gastric contents: (1) place the patient in left lateral Trendelenburg position; (2) if the patient is unconscious, insert a cuffed endotracheal tube prior to gastric intubation; (3) if the patient is conscious, or if it is not possible to accomplish endotracheal intubation for other reasons, aspirate the pharynx as regularly as possible during gastric intubation.

Aspirate the stomach as completely as possible. Then lavage the stomach with 2 liters of 0.9% sodium chloride, or 5% sodium bicarbonate, containing a slurry of 60–90 gm. activated charcoal. After lavage, instill 30 gm. activated charcoal into the stomach before withdrawing the tube, to absorb remaining toxicant.

8. In poisonings by methyl bromide and ethylene dichloride (and possibly by other chemicals of this series, by inference), there may be some therapeutic value in the administration of dimercaprol (BAL, dimercaptopropanol), especially if it can be given within a few minutes of absorption of the toxicant. Administered in vegetable oil intramuscularly, the usually recommended dosage is 3 mg./kg. body weight every 6 hours for 8 doses in the first 2 days; then 3 mg./kg. every 12 hours for 2 doses during day 3; then 3 mg./kg. every 24 hours for 10 doses during succeeding 10 days.

Caution: Dimercaprol may cause troublesome side effects (hypertension, tachycardia, nausea, headache, paresthesia, pain, lacrimation, sweating, anxiety, and restlessness). Although usually not so severe as to stop treatment, these manifestations may require antihistamine therapy for adequate control.

9. Monitor poisoning victims closely for recurrent pulmonary edema and secondary bronchopneumonia. Fluid balance should be charted and the urine sediment should be examined regularly to detect incipient tubular necrosis. Measure serum alkaline phosphatase, GOT, GPT, LDH, and bilirubin to assess liver injury. Administer intravenous fluids cautiously to avoid exacerbating the pulmonary edema.

10. Protracted neurological manifestations of poisoning may require several days or weeks of sedative therapy. Pulmonary function tests should be done after resolution of acute symptoms to evaluate the degree of permanent lung damage, if any.

V. ANTICOAGULANT RODENTICIDES

Commonly used commercial rodenticides of these classes are as follows:

1. Coumarin type: warfarin (Kypfarin, Warf-42, D-Con, Warficide, Prolin), coumafuryl (Fumarin), Dethmor, Rax

2. 1,3-Indandione type: diphacinone, or diphenadione (Ramik), chlorophacinone (Drat, Caid, Liphadione, Microzul, Ramucide, Rotomet, Raviac, Topitox), pindone (Pivalyn, Pivacin, Tri-ban, Pival), valone (PMP)

These materials are commonly added to baits or dissolved in small amounts of water for pest rodents to drink. One hundred grams of the prepared commercial baits must be ingested to yield 25 mg. of anticoagulant. Rodenticide "drinks" are made by adding dry concentrate (0.54 gm. active ingredient per 100 gm. powder) to specified volumes of water. The poison in the concentrate is coated on sugar or sand to facilitate measurement and handling.

Gastrointestinal absorption of these toxicants is efficient, beginning within minutes of ingestion, and continuing for two to three days afterward.

Both types of anticoagulant depress the hepatic synthesis of substances essential to normal blood clotting: prothrombin (Factor II) and Factors VII, IX, and X. The antiprothrombin effect is best known and provides the basis for detection and assessment of clinical poisoning. Direct damage to capillary permeability occurs concurrently. In rare instances not related to excessive dosage, coumarin-type anticoagulants have caused ecchymosis and extensive skin necrosis in humans.

Unlike the coumarin anticoagulants, the indandiones cause symptoms and signs of neurological and cardiopulmonary injury in laboratory rats; these often lead to death before hemorrhage occurs. These actions may account for the somewhat greater toxicity of this class of anticoagulants. Cardiopulmonary and neurological symptoms and signs have not been reported in human poisonings.

Lengthened prothrombin time from a toxic dose can be expected to appear within 24 hours of toxicant ingestion and reach a maximum in 36 to 72 hours.

Without intervention, hypoprothrombinemia may persist 10–15 days, depending on the agent and dosage. Prothrombin depression will occur in response to doses that are much lower than those necessary to cause hemorrhage.

A. CLINICAL FEATURES

In most instances of accidental ingestion of anticoagulant baits, persons remain asymptomatic because the dosage has been small. Even in cases involving ingestion of substantial doses, hypoprothrombinemia occurs without symptoms of poisoning. Hemorrhage appears only when extraordinary amounts have been absorbed. In these cases, the anticoagulants were either taken deliberately, were absorbed over long periods out of neglect of elementary hygienic standards, or were ingested by starving indigents who used rodent bait for food.

Large doses produce hematuria, nosebleed, hematomata, bleeding gums, and melena. Abdominal pain and back pain probably reflect abdominal and retroperitoneal hemorrhage. Weakness occurs as a result of anemia. Renal colic often complicates severe hematuria. Nasal and gastrointestinal hemorrhages have caused death from exsanguination.

B. LABORATORY FINDINGS

Increase of the prothrombin time reflects a reduction in serum prothrombin concentration. This test offers a sensitive and reliable diagnostic method for detection of the toxic effects of these compounds. Readily detectable change in prothrombin time appears within 24–48 hours of ingestion of anticoagulant.

Methods are available in a few laboratories for measurement of warfarin and its metabolites in human urine.

C. TREATMENT

1. If it is known or suspected that anticoagulant rodenticide has been ingested recently, but the total amount is less than 0.25 mg./kg. body weight, administer a single dose of the specific antidote, phytonadione, intramuscularly, 25 mg. I.M. (adults); 0.4 mg./kg. body weight (children). Phytonadione (vitamin K_1, Mephyton, Aquamephyton, Konakion) specifically is required. Vitamin K_3 (menadione, Hykinone) and vitamin K_4 (menadiol) have little or no antidotal effect. This represents adequate treatment for cases in which the total amount of toxicant ingested is known not to have exceeded the limits stated above, and in which no preexisting liver injury or blood clotting disease is present.

2. If anticoagulant rodenticide has been ingested within the preceding 2–3 hours in amounts that may have exceeded 0.25 mg./kg., induce vomiting with syrup of ipecac: adult dose, 30 ml; children's dose, 15 ml. After emesis, give 30 gm. activated charcoal in 4–6 oz. water to limit absorption of rodenticide still in the gut.

3. If anticoagulant rodenticide may have been ingested in amounts exceeding 0.25 mg./kg. at any time in the preceding 15 days, or if there is reason to suspect preexisting liver or bleeding disease, determine the prothrombin time. Then administer phytonadione intramuscularly (25 mg. for adults; 0.4 mg./kg. for children). Subsequent treatment will depend on the degree of lengthening of prothrombin time and on the estimated dosage and time of toxicant ingestion. High dosage or lengthening of the prothrombin time by more than 10 seconds over the control may dictate administration of a second dose of phytonadione (as above) and another measurement of prothrombin time 24 hours after the first. In some cases, reversal of prothrombin time requires as long as 3 days, irrespective of antidote dosage. Doses of phytonadione in excess of 25 mg. may be hepatotoxic, and should be given only when lower doses have not been effective. Doses in excess of 50 mg. involve significant hazard and are of doubtful benefit.

4. If the patient shows symptoms or signs of poisoning (bleeding, anemia, hematomata) in addition to hypoprothrombinemia, it may be necessary to give phytonadione intravenously. Aquamephyton may be administered in this way at doses of 25 mg. in adults or 0.4 mg./kg. in children, repeating this amount once in 24 hours if bleeding is still not controlled. Inject at rates not exceeding 1 mg. per minute (proportionately slower in children). To achieve slow intravenous injection, dilute the phytonadione in either 0.9% saline or 5% glucose solution. Control of bleeding usually occurs within three to six hours of intravenous infusion. Adverse reactions, some fatal, have occurred from intravenous phytonadione injections, even when recommended dosage limits and injection rates were observed. For this reason, the intravenous route should be used only in cases of severe poisoning. Flushing, dizziness, hypotension, dyspnea, and cyanosis have characterized adverse reactions.

5. Antidotal therapy in cases of severe poisoning should be supplemented with transfusions of fresh blood or fresh frozen plasma. Use of fresh blood or plasma represents the most rapidly effective method for stopping hemorrhage due to the anticoagulants. Determine prothrombin times (and hemoglobin concentrations, if appropriate) every 6–12 hours to assess effectiveness of antidotal and antihemorrhagic measures.

6. Give ascorbic acid (vitamin C) orally or intramuscularly in mild and severe poisonings (adult dose, 100 mg.; children's dose, 50–100 mg.). Ascorbic acid is thought to limit capillary injury caused by the anticoagulants.

7. Following restoration of normal blood coagulability in cases that have suffered internal hemorrhages, it may be advisable to drain large hematomata.

8. Ferrous sulfate may be appropriate in the recuperative period to rebuild lost erythrocyte mass.

Common commercial pesticide products are as follows:

Vacor Rat Killer (2% RH-787 in vehicle resembling corn meal); DLP-787 Bait (2% RH-787 in vehicle resembling corn meal); DLP-787 House Mouse Tracking Powder (10% RH-787 in a light green powder vehicle). Compound RH-787 is the active ingredient of both formulations.

Acute oral LD_{50} values for RH-787 in the dog and Rhesus monkey are 2,000–4,000 mg./kg. LD_{50} ratings of the diluted formulations ingested by rodents are as follows:

	Rats	Mice
Vacor Rat Killer or Bait	580 mg./kg.	4,120 mg./kg.
DLP-787, 10% Tracking Powder	—	1,050 mg./kg.

The minimum lethal dose in humans is not known. The exact mechanism of RH-787 toxicity is not known. It has no anticoagulant action, and is therefore entirely different from the coumarin-indandione rodenticides. One established effect in rats is interference with nicotinamide metabolism. Symptoms and signs in poisoned animals suggest toxic actions on the brain, the peripheral nerves, myoneural junctions, the pancreas (including islet tissues), the autonomic nervous system, and the conducting tissues of the heart. Abnormalities of renal and vascular function may be due to direct toxic effects or may reflect metabolic and autonomic nervous system disturbances (hypotension).

If absorbed in adequate dosage by rats or by humans, RH-787 can induce persistent diabetes mellitus, which manifests as hyperglycemia, glycosuria, and ketoacidosis. This has occurred in humans following ingestion of one 30-gm. package of Vacor.

A. CLINICAL FEATURES

Human poisonings have occurred only after deliberate ingestions of RH-787. Symptoms vary, depending on dose and individual susceptibility.

Symptoms may appear 4–48 hours after ingestion of the formulated rodenticide. Early symptoms include nausea, vomiting, abdominal cramping, chills, and mental confusion.

Later clinical manifestations are aching and fine tremors of the extremities, dilated pupils, peripheral neuropathy (plantar hyperesthesia), muscle weakness, dysphagia, chest pain, postural hypotension, anorexia, constipation or diarrhea, urinary bladder dystonia (urinary retention), hypothermia, and the consequences of diabetes mellitus: glycosuria, polyuria, ketoacidosis, and dehydration.

Abnormal laboratory findings include hyperglycemia, glycosuria, ketosis (acidosis and electrolyte disturbances), and elevation of serum amylase and lipase activities.

Death may result from respiratory failure, cardiovascular collapse, or ketoacidosis.

Late and persistent manifestations of poisoning are postural hypotension and diabetes mellitus.

B. LABORATORY FINDINGS

Analysis of blood, urine, and tissues for RH-787 is difficult and is not done routinely. In cases of poisoning requiring chemical confirmation, contact the Health Effects Monitoring Branch, Technical Services Division, Office of Pesticide Programs, Environmental Protection Agency.

C. TREATMENT

1. If no more than 12 hours have elapsed since toxicant ingestion, evacuate the stomach by induced emesis and lavage. Induce emesis with syrup of ipecac (30 ml. for adults and children over 12 years; 15 ml. for children under 12) only if vomiting has not already occurred and if the patient is fully alert. If consciousness declines after ipecac administration, proceed immediately with gastric intubation.

Intubate the stomach, aspirate contents, and lavage with 2–3 liters of isotonic saline or 5% sodium bicarbonate solution. To avoid aspiration of stomach contents, put the patient in left lateral Trendelenburg position, aspirate the pharynx frequently, and, in unconscious patients, intubate the trachea with a cuffed tube prior to gastric intubation.

After gastric lavage, instill 30 gm. activated charcoal in 3–4 oz. water through the stomach tube to limit absorption of the toxicant.

2. Administer niacinamide (nicotinamide) intravenously (slowly) or intramuscularly. In adults and in children over 12 years or 30 kg. body weight, give 500 mg. immediately, then repeat injections of 200–400 mg. every four hours for 10–12 doses. Select the proper dosage on the basis of body weight and estimated quantity of Vacor or DLP-787 ingested. If symptoms and signs of rodenticide toxicity appear, administer nicotinamide by continuous I.V. infusion at a rate of 400 mg. every four hours. Avoid total dosage of nicotinamide above 3,000 mg. per day. Dosage for children under 12 years, or less than 30 kg. body weight, is approximately half that needed in adults. When the patient is able to take medication by mouth, give 100 mg. nicotinamide orally four times daily for two weeks.

3. Monitor blood and urine sugar concentrations, serum alkaline phosphatase, amylase, LDH, and GOT activities, urine ketone concentrations, blood electrolytes and BUN. Examine the electrocardiogram for arrhythmias.

4. Unless the patient is able to void easily, insert a catheter to monitor urine flow.

5. Infuse electrolyte solutions intravenously to correct errors in specific ion concentrations. If ketoacidosis appears, use bicarbonate or Ringer's lactate to control acidosis.

6. If diabetic ketoacidosis appears (ketonuria, metabolic acidosis, hyperglycemia), administer enough regular insulin to control the acidosis and hyperglycemia, as in naturally occuurring diabetic ketosis. The diabetes resulting from RH-787 tends to be brittle and difficult to control.

7. In all cases of ingestion of Vacor or DLP-787 (whether or not acute poisoning occurs), follow the patient's clinical status carefully for at least six months. Look for indications of diabetes mellitus and for consequences of autonomic nervous system disorders: orthostatic hypotension, urinary retention, constipation, diarrhea, or abdominal cramping.

BIBLIOGRAPHY

I. ORGANOCHLORINE PESTICIDES

California Bureau of Occupational Health: Diagnosis and Treatment of Phosphate Ester Pesticide Poisoning. Technical Bulletin for Physicians, 1971.

Davies, J. E.: Recognition and management of pesticide toxicity. Adv. Int. Med., *18*:23, 1972.

Durham, W. F., and Hayes, W. J., Jr.: Organic phosphorus poisoning and its therapy. Arch. Envir. Health, *5*:21, 1962.

Hayes, W. J., Jr.: Toxicology of Pesticides. Baltimore, Williams & Wilkins, 1975.

————: Clinical Handbook on Economic Poisons: Emergency Information for Treating Poisoning. Washington, D.C., U.S. Public Health Service, 1963.

Milby, T. H.: Prevention and management of organophosphate poisoning. J.A.M.A., *216*(13): 2131, 1971.

Trainor, D. C.: Agricultural Chemicals: A Synopsis of Toxicity and a Guide to Treatment. New South Wales, Ministry for Health, 1967.

II. CHOLINESTERASE-INHIBITING CARBAMATE INSECTICIDES

Hayes, W. J., Jr.: Toxicology of Pesticides. Baltimore, Williams & Wilkins, 1975.

————: Clinical Handbook on Economic Poisons: Emergency Information for Treating Poisoning. Washington, D.C., U.S. Public Health Service, 1963.

Trainor, D. C.: Agricultural Chemicals: A Synopsis of Toxicity and a Guide to Treatment. New South Wales, Ministry for Health, 1967.

III. HALOCARBON AND SULFURYL FUMIGANTS

Conway, E. J.: Microdiffusion Analysis and Volumetric Error. 3rd ed. London, Crosby Lockwood, 1950.

IV. ANTICOAGULANT RODENTICIDES

Lange, P. F., and Terveer, J.: Warfarin Poisoning, U.S. Armed Forces Med. J., *5*(6):872, 1954.

Nalbandian, R. M., Mader, I. J., Barrett, J. I., Pearce, J. F., and Rupp, E. C.: Petechiae, ecchymoses, and necrosis of skin induced by coumarin congeners. J.A.M.A., *192*(7):603, 1965.

O'Reilly, R. A., Aggeler, P. M., and Leong, L. S.: Studies on the coumarin anticoagulant drugs: the pharmacodynamics of warfarin in man. J. Clin. Invest., *42*(10):1542, 1963.

19. HERBICIDES

Donald P. Morgan, M.D., Ph.D.

I. ARSENICALS

Commonly used compounds and commercial preparations are as follows:

1. Trivalent inorganics: Arsenic trioxide (sodium arsenic), potassium arsenite, sodium arsenite (Acme Weed Killer, Atlas A, Penite, As-655 Weed Killer, Kill All), copper arsenite (Paris Green), copper ammonium arsenite (Chemonite)
2. Pentavalent inorganics: Arsenic acid (Zotox Crabgrass Killer, Dessicant L-10, Lincks Liquid Di-met, Pax Total, Purina Top Grass and Weed Killer)
3. Pentavalent organics:
   a. MSMA (monosodium methyl arsonate) (Ansar 170, Bueno, Weed-E-Rad, Ansar 529, Broadside, Crabgrass Dallis Grass Killer, Daconate, Fertilome Nutgrass and Weed Killer, Mad, Nutgrass Spray, Selector #1, Spot Grassy Weed Killer)
   b. DSMA (disodium methyl arsonate) (ANSAR 8100, Biochecks, Burpee Crabgrass Killer, Chipco Crab Kleen, Clout, D Krab R + Prills, DMA, E Krab R, Greenfield Crabgrass and Dandelion Killer, Sears Liquid Crabgrass Killer, Lawn Weed Killer, Proturf Monocot Weed Control, Arsinyl)
   c. Cacodylic acid (dimethyl arsinic acid) (Silvisar 510)
   d. Sodium cacodylate (sodium dimethyl arsinate) (Phytar 560, Acme Weed Killer)
   e. Ammonium methane arsonate (AMA, Ansar 157, Super Crab E-Rad, C-4000, Antrol Crabgrass Killer, Crabgrass Broadleaf Killer, Systemic Crabgrass and Broadleaf Killer)
   f. Methane arsonic acid (MAA, Ortho Crabgrass Killer)
   g. Arsanilic acid (feed additive)

The pentavalent (organic and inorganic) arsenicals are generally less toxic than the trivalent compounds, especially triox-ide and arsenite. Even so, there is enough reduction of pentavalent arsenicals to trivalent forms in the gut and tissues to require that all poisonings by arsenic-containing substances be regarded as serious threats to life and health.

Although some absorption of solid arsenical compounds may occur by dermal or pulmonary routes, the great majority of poisonings occur as a result of ingestion. Intestinal absorption is generally efficient. Most absorbed arsenic is excreted by way of the kidneys, a lesser proportion by the liver and gut.

Trivalent arsenicals bind critical sulfhydryl-containing enzymes in tissues. When taken up from the gut, they injure the splanchnic vasculature, causing colic and diarrhea. Once absorbed, they produce injury to the liver, kidney, bone marrow, brain, and peripheral nerves. Liver injury is manifest as hepatomegaly, jaundice, and increase in circulating hepatocellular enzymes LDH and GOT. Renal damage is reflected in albuminuria, hematuria, pyuria, cylindruria, and azotemia. Acute tubular necrosis may occur in severe poisoning. Injury to blood-forming tissues can take the form of agranulocytosis, aplastic anemia, thrombocytopenia, or pancytopenia. Toxic encephalopathy may be manifest as speech and behavioral disturbances. Peripheral neuropathy occurs in both acute and chronic forms. Inhalation of large amounts of arsenic dusts may cause bronchitis or pneumonitis.

Sequelae of arsenic poisoning include cirrhosis of the liver, hypoplastic bone marrow, renal insufficiency, and peripheral neuropathy. Excessive exposures to arsenicals have caused cancers of skin and various epithelial tissues.

A. CLINICAL FEATURES

1. Arsenic Poisoning

Colic, burning abdominal pain, vomiting, and watery or bloody diarrhea are the primary manifestations of ingestion. More severe symptoms follow ingestion of inorganic arsenicals than result from the pentavalent compounds. Symptoms sometimes do not appear for minutes or even hours after ingestion. Headache, dizziness, muscle spasms, delirium, and sometimes convulsions reflect direct injury to the central nervous system plus extracellular electrolyte disturbances and shock. A garlic odor to the breath and feces helps to identify the responsible toxicant. Shock, toxic nephrosis, hepatitis (hepatomegaly and jaundice), and neurological injury (delirium, paralysis, respiratory depression) may progress to a fatal outcome.

2. Subacute Arsenic Poisoning

Dosages less than those necessary to produce severe acute symptoms are known to cause chronic headache, abdominal distress, salivation, low-grade fever, and persistent symptoms of upper respiratory irritation. Stomatitis and garlic breath are characteristic.

3. Chronic Arsenic Poisoning

Prolonged low-level intakes of arsenic cause peripheral neuropathy (paresthesias, pain, anesthesia, paresis, ataxia), encephalopathy (apathy), varied dermatological disorders (keratoses, pigmentation, eczemas, brittle nails, loss of hair), and toxic hepatitis (hepatomegaly, sometimes progressing to cirrhosis with ascites). Weakness and vulnerability to infections may result from bone marrow depression. Local edema (frequently eyelids) is characteristic of some chronic poisoning cases.

B. LABORATORY FINDINGS

Measurement of 24-hour urinary excretion of arsenic probably represents the most satisfactory means of confirming excessive arsenic absorption, although methods for measuring blood arsenic concentration are available. Persons on ordinary diets usually excrete less than 20 μg. per day, but diets rich in seafood may generate as much as 200 μg. per day. Excretions in excess of 100 μg. per day should be viewed with suspicion, and repeat determinations made. Excretions in excess of 200 μg. per day should be regarded as indicative of absorption of potentially toxic amounts.

The qualitative Gutzeit test for arsenic in the urine is available in most hospital laboratories and is useful in promptly identifying acute poisonings.

Chronic storage of arsenic can be detected by analysis of hair and fingernails.

C. TREATMENT

1. Wash contaminated eyes and skin with copious amounts of fresh water.

2. In cases of poisoning by recently ingested (up to six hours) arsenicals:

    a. Intubate the stomach, aspirate, and lavage with 3 liters of isotonic saline or 5% sodium bicarbonate. Use all available precautions to avoid aspiration of vomitus: (1) insert an endotracheal tube (cuffed, if available) if patient is obtunded or unconscious, prior to gastric intubation; (2) keep patient's head below level of the stomach during intubation (Trendelenburg or left lateral decubitus position, with head end of table tipped downward) and head turned toward left; and (3) aspirate the pharynx as frequently as possible to remove gagged or vomited stomach contents.

    b. After lavage, instill 60 gm. activated charcoal in 6–8 oz. water (as little as necessary to deliver the charcoal).

    c. Give sodium sulfate as a cathartic. For adults, give 30 gm. in 6–8 oz. of water; for children under 12, give 0.2 gm./kg. body weight in 1–6 oz. water.

    d. Administer intravenous electrolyte and glucose solutions to maintain hydration. Combat shock with transfusions of whole blood and inhalation of 100% oxygen. Monitor fluid balance, body weight, and central venous pressure to guard against fluid overload resulting from acute tubular necrosis (anuria).

e. Promptly begin administration of dimercaprol (BAL, British antilewisite, dimercaptopropanol) intramuscularly, as a 10% solution in vegetable oil. This antidote effectively neutralizes the toxic action of arsenicals. Recommended dosage schedule is:

	Mild Poisoning	*Severe Poisoning*
Days 1 and 2	2.5 mg./kg. q6h × 8 doses	3.0 mg./kg. q4h × 12 doses
Day 3	2.5 mg./kg. q12h × 2 doses	3.0 mg./kg. q6h × 4 doses
Succeeding 10 days	2.5 mg./kg. q24h × 10 doses	3.0 mg./kg. q12h × 20 doses

Dimercaprol is capable of causing troublesome side effects (hypertension, tachycardia, nausea, headache, paresthesias, pain, lacrimation, sweating, anxiety, and restlessness). Although usually not so severe as to handicap treatment, these manifestations may require antihistamines, ephedrine, or both, for control.

f. Intense abdominal pain may require morphine (4–15 mg. for adults; 0.1–0.2 mg./kg. for children).

g. Severe poisonings (especially when renal function is impaired) may require hemodialysis to remove arsenic combined with dimercaprol from the blood.

3. If ingestion of arsenical occurred more than 48 hours prior to treatment, or if excessive absorption has occurred over an extended period, treatment should probably be limited to administration of dimercaprol (as described above) plus nutritional supplements (glucose and vitamins) to restore metabolic functions to normal as promptly as possible.

II. PENTACHLOROPHENOL

Pentachlorophenol (or its sodium salt) is used as a weed killer, defoliant, wood preservative, germicide, fungicide, and molluskicide. It is an ingredient of many formulated mixtures sold for one or more of these purposes. Pentachlorophenol is a volatile compound.

Commonly used commercial products are as follows:

PCP, Dowicide-7, Penchlorol, Pentacon, Penwar, Weedone, Veg-I-Kill, Wood Preserver, Wood Tox 140, Purina Insect Oil Concentrate, Gordon Termi Tox, Usol Cabin Oil, Certified Kiltrol-74 Weed Killer, Ciba-Geigy Ontrack OS 3, 4 or 5, Ortho Triox Liquid Vegetation Killer, Black Leaf Grass, Weed and Vegetation Killer Spray

Pentachlorophenol is irritating to the skin, eyes, and upper respiratory mucous membranes. It is efficiently absorbed across the skin, the lung, and the gastrointestinal lining. Like the nitrophenolic compounds, it stimulates oxidative metabolism of tissue cells by uncoupling oxidative processes from the normal phosphorylation reactions. In common with other phenols, it is toxic to the liver, kidney, and central nervous system.

The majority of severe poisonings have occurred in workers exposed to hot environments. However, poisoning has occurred in infants who absorbed PCP from treated diapers. Dehydration and metabolic acidosis are important features of poisoning in children.

Albuminuria, glycosuria, and elevated BUN reflect renal injury. Liver enlargement has been observed in some cases. Anemia and leukopenia have been found in chronically exposed workers, but leukocytosis is more commonly found in acute poisoning.

A. Clinical Features

Irritation of nose, throat, eyes, and skin is the most common symptom of exposure to PCP. Severe or protracted exposure may result in a contact dermatitis. Intensive occupational exposure has resulted in chloracne, which is probably due to impurities in the chemical formulation.

Profuse sweating, headache, weakness, and nausea are the most consistent presenting symptoms of systemic poisoning by absorbed PCP. Fever is usually present but may be minimal or absent. Tachycardia, tachypnea, and pain in the chest and abdomen are often prominent. Declining mental alertness may progress to stupor and convulsions. Protracted exposure results in weight loss from increased basal metabolic rate.

B. Laboratory Findings

PCP can be measured in blood, urine, and adipose tissue by gas-liquid chromatography. A few parts per billion can usually be found in the blood and urine of persons having no known exposure. Based on studies of persons occupationally exposed to PCP, symptoms of systemic toxicity probably do not appear in adults until blood and urine concentrations reach about 1 ppm (0.1 mg./100 ml., or 1,000 ppb).

If poisoning is strongly suspected on grounds of exposure, history, symptoms, and signs, do not postpone treatment until diagnosis is confirmed.

C. Treatment

1. Wash contaminated skin promptly with soap and water.
2. Flush chemical from eyes with copious amounts of clean water.
3. In event of systemic poisoning:
   a. Reduce body temperature by physical means. Sponge baths and cooling blankets probably offer the best opportunity for survival of poisoning by PCP. In fully conscious patients, administer cold, sugar-containing liquids by mouth, as tolerated.

   b. Administer oxygen continuously by mask to minimize tissue anoxia.

   c. Administer intravenous fluids at maximum tolerated rates to enhance urinary excretion of toxicant and to support physiological mechanisms for heat loss. Monitor blood electrolytes and sugar, adjusting I.V. infusions to achieve stability of electrolyte concentrations.

   d. Administer sedatives if necessary to control apprehension and excitement. Amobarbital or pentobarbital, 100–200 mg. I.M. or slowly I.V., every four to six hours may be needed (children's dosage: 5 mg./kg.). Diazepam, 10 mg. I.M. should be useful, although it has not been employed in this type of poisoning (children's dosage: 0.1–0.2 mg./kg). Be prepared to assist pulmonary ventilation mechanically in the event of respiratory depression.

   e. If toxicant has been ingested, the stomach must be emptied. If patient is alert and respiration is not depressed, give syrup of ipecac to induce vomiting (30 ml. for adults, 15 ml. for children under 12 years). Observe the patient closely after administering ipecac. If consciousness level declines, or if vomiting has not occurred in 20 minutes, proceed immediately to intubate the stomach.

   Following emesis, have patient drink a suspension of 30 gm. activated charcoal in 3–4 oz. water to bind toxicant remaining in the gastrointestinal tract.

   If patient is not fully alert, empty the stomach immediately by intubation, aspiration, and lavage, using isotonic saline or 5% sodium bicarbonate. To minimize the risk of pneumonitis from aspiration of toxicant and petroleum distillate solvent, take every possible precaution to keep gastric contents out of the airway: (1) endotracheal intubtion (cuffed tube) before gastric intubation of unconscious patients; (2) Trendelenburg or left lateral decubitus position, with the head low and turned to the left; (3) frequent aspiration of the pharynx.

After aspiration of gastric contents and washing of stomach, instill 30 gm. activated charcoal in 3–4 oz. water by way of stomach tube to limit absorption of remaining toxicant. Do not instill milk, cream, or other materials containing vegetable or animal fats, as these are likely to enhance absorption.

Give sodium sulfate as a cathartic. For adults (over 12 years of age), give 30 gm. in 6–8 oz. water. For children under 12, give 0.2 gm./kg. body weight in 1–6 oz. of water.

f. Do not administer aspirin or other antipyretics to control fever.

g. During convalescence, administer high-calorie, high-vitamin diet to facilitate repletion of body fat and carbohydrate stores.

h. Discourage subsequent contact with the toxicant for at least four weeks to allow full restoration of normal metabolic processes.

III. NITROPHENOL AND NITROCRESOL

These yellow aromatic substances are formulated in petroleum solvents or are converted to sodium salts when an aqueous solution is required. Less volatile than halophenols, they are usually applied in spray form as contact herbicides.

Commonly used chemicals of this class are as follows:

Dinitrophenol (Chemox PE), dinitro-orthocresol (DNOC, DNC, Sinox) Dinoseb (DNBP, DN-289), dinosam (DNAP), DN-111 (DNOCHP), dinoprop, dinoterbon, dinoterb, dinosulfon, binapacryl (Morocide,

Endosan, Ambox, Mildex) dinobuton, dinopenton

Nitrophenols and nitrocresols are highly toxic to humans. They are efficiently absorbed from the gastrointestinal tract, across the skin (especially when toxicant is contained in petroleum distillate), and by the lung (when very fine droplets are inhaled). Except in a few persons, they are only moderately irritating to the skin and mucous membranes. They usually produce a yellow stain wherever contact occurs. In common with other phenols, they are toxic to the liver, kidney, and nervous system. Basic mechanism of toxicity affecting all cells is a stimulation of oxidative metabolism in cell mitochondria, by interference with the normal coupling of carbohydrate oxidation to phosphorylation reactions. Increased oxidative metabolism depletes body carbohydrate and fat stores and leads to pyrexia, tachycardia, and dehydration. Most severe poisonings by these compounds have occurred in workers exposed to hot environments, wherein extreme body temperatures have resulted from increased production of body heat with inadequate mechanisms for its dissipation. Direct action on the brain causes cerebral edema, manifest clinically as a toxic psychosis and sometimes convulsions. Liver parenchyma and renal tubules show degenerative changes. Albuminuria, pyuria, hematuria, and increased BUN are often prominent signs of renal injury. Fatal agranulocytosis has occurred following large doses of dinitrophenol. Cataracts have occurred in some chronically poisoned laboratory species. This is a possible, but as yet unconfirmed, hazard in humans. Death in nitrophenol poisoning is followed promptly by intense rigor mortis.

A. CLINICAL FEATURES

Yellow staining of skin and hair signify contact with a chemical of this class.

Staining of the sclerae and urine indicates absorption of potentially toxic amounts. Profuse sweating, headache, thirst, malaise, and lassitude are the common early symptoms of poisoning. Warm, flushed skin, tachycardia, and fever characterize a serious degree of poisoning. Apprehension, restlessness, anxiety, manic behavior, or unconsciousness reflect severe cerebral injury. Cyanosis, tachypnea, and dyspnea occur as a consequence of extreme stimulation of metabolism, pyrexia, and tissue anoxia. Weight loss occurs in persons who are chronically poisoned at lower dosage levels.

B. LABORATORY FINDINGS

Unmetabolized nitrophenols and nitrocresols can be identified spectrophotometrically in the serum and urine at concentrations well below those necessary to cause poisoning. In addition, many laboratories can measure these compounds by gas-liquid chromatography. If poisoning is probable, do not await confirmation before commencing treatment.

C. TREATMENT

1. Wash contaminated skin promptly with soap and water.
2. Flush chemical from eyes with copious amounts of clean water.
3. In the event of systemic poisoning:

a. Reduce body temperature by physical means. Sponge baths and cooling blankets probably offer the best opportunity for survival of poisonings by these agents. In fully conscious patients, administer cold, sugar-containing liquids by mouth, as tolerated.

b. Administer oxygen continuously by mask to minimize tissue anoxia.

c. Administer intravenous fluids at maximum tolerated rates to enhance urinary excretion of toxicant and to support physiological mechanisms for heat loss (insensible water loss, sweat, and circulatory transport of heat from deep tissues to skin). Monitor blood electrolytes and sugar, adjusting I.V. infusions to achieve stability of electrolyte concentrations.

d. Administer sedatives if necessary to control apprehension and excitement. Amobarbital or pentobarbital, 100–200 mg. I.M. or slowly I.V., every four to six hours may be needed. Diazepam, 10 mg. I.M. may be useful, although it has not been used in this type of poisoning. Be prepared to assist pulmonary ventilation mechanically in the event of respiratory depression.

e. If toxicant has been ingested, the stomach must be emptied. If patient is alert and respiration is not depressed, give syrup of ipecac to induce vomiting (30 ml. for adults, 15 ml. for children under 12 years). Observe patient closely after administering ipecac. If consciousness level declines, or if vomiting has not occurred in 20 minutes, proceed immediately to intubate, aspirate, and lavage the stomach.

After emesis, have patient drink a suspension of 30 gm. activated charcoal in 3–4 oz. water to limit absorption of toxicant remaining in the gut.

If patient is not fully alert, empty the stomach immediately by intubation, aspiration, and lavage, using isotonic saline or 5% sodium bicarbonate. To minimize the risk of pneumonitis from aspiration of toxicant and petroleum distillate solvent, take every possible precaution to keep gastric contents out of the airway: (1) endotracheal intubation (cuffed tube) before gastric intubation of unconscious patients; (2) Trendelenburg or left lateral decubitus position, with the head low and turned to the left; (3) frequent aspiration of the pharynx.

After aspiration of gastric contents and washing of stomach, instill 30 gm. activated charcoal in 3–4 oz. water by way of stomach tube to limit absorption or remaining toxicant. Do not instill milk, cream, or other materials containing vegetable or animal fats, as these are likely to enhance absorption.

Give sodium sulfate as a cathartic. For adults (over 12 years of age), give 30 gm. in 6–8 oz. of water. For children under 12, give 0.2 gm./kg. body weight in 1–6 oz. water.

f. Do not administer aspirin or other antipyretics to control fever. Animal tests indicate that aspirin enhances, rather than reduces, the toxicity of nitrophenolic and nitrocresolic compounds.

g. During convalescence, adminiser a high-calorie, high-vitamin diet to facilitate repletion of body fat and carbohydrate stores.

h. Discourage subsequent contact with the toxicant for at least four weeks, to allow full restoration of normal metabolic processes.

IV. PARAQUAT AND OTHER DIPYRIDYLS

Paraquat, diquat, and morfamquat are three dipyridyl compounds that are effective as contact herbicides. Paraquat is used worldwide in agricultural practice as a defoliant and weed killer, and is formulated at low concentration for use in lawn and garden weed control. Diquat is used to kill water weeds. Morfamquat has not been used commercially in the United States. All of these compounds are highly polar and water soluble. Their virtue as herbicides lies in their strong adsorption to plant tissues and soil particles, limiting herbicidal effect to treated areas.

Commonly used products of this class are as follows:

1. Paraquat: Paraquat Cl, Dual Paraquat, EM-7217, Gramoxone S, Weedol, and Dextrone X are all concentrates containing 20% paraquat ion. Preeglone extra and Gramonol are concentrate mixtures with other herbicides. Ortho Spot Weed and Grass Killer contains 0.2% paraquat ion.

2. Diquat: Aquakill, Aquacide, Heavy Duty Weed Control, Aquatate, Aquatic Weed Killer, Reglone, Vegetrole, Watrol, and Di-Kill Vegetation Killer are all packaged as concentrates. Preeglone extra is a concentrate mixture with paraquat.
3. Morfamquat: Morfoxone, PP-745.

The toxicology of paraquat has been more thoroughly studied than that of the other dipyridyls. Diquat appears to be substantially less toxic than paraquat. Little is known about effects of morfamquat.

Dipyridyl compounds injure the epithelial tissues of skin, nails, eyes, nose, mouth, and respiratory and gastrointestinal tracts. Concentrated solutions cause inflammation and sometimes ulceration of mucosal linings.

Dermal absorption of paraquat is minimal unless the application site is occluded. Direct pulmonary absorption is also minimal in the course of exposure to ordinarily used sprays. Ingestion of paraquat concentrate (which accounts for nearly all of the serious morbidity and mortality caused by dipyridyls) generates a unique series of pathophysiological events. For 1 to 5 days, demonstrable toxicity is often limited to irritation (sometimes ulceration) of mouth and gastrointestinal linings; 2 to 4 days after ingestion, evidence of renal and hepatic toxicity appears, which is usually reversible. From 3 to 14 days after ingestion, because of selective uptake of paraquat by lung tissue, a diffuse tissue reaction occurs, consisting of intraalveolar edema and hemorrhage, proliferation of bronchiolar epithelium, focal atelectasis, and rapid growth of fibrous connective tissue within alveoli. Progressive impairment of gas exchange often, but not always, leads to death. Fibrosis persists for months in surviving patients. Electrocardiographic evidence of a toxic myocarditis is often observed.

Cranial nerve palsies have rarely been reported as toxic manifestations of exposure to paraquat.

A. Clinical Features

Skin irritation, drying, and cracking follow untreated skin contact with paraquat. Discoloration and irregularity of fingernails commonly occur in workers whose hands are exposed to paraquat concentrates. Delayed conjunctivitis and keratitis develop 12–48 hours after contact of the chemical with the eye. Inhalation of spray droplets irritates the nose and throat, and sometimes causes nosebleed.

After ingestion of paraquat concentrate, the earliest symptoms and signs are due to mucosal irritation and ulceration of the gastrointestinal tract. Pain (oral, substernal, abdominal), vomiting, and diarrhea (sometimes melena) occur. Generalized muscle aching is reported. Early symptoms are sometimes so mild that vigorous treatment is delayed.

From 48–96 hours, albuminuria, hematuria, pyuria, and elevated BUN and creatinine are likely to appear. Oliguria from acute tubular necrosis may develop in cases of severe poisoning; jaundice and elevations of serum GOT, GPT, alkaline phosphatase, and LDH reflect hepatocellular injury. The effects on liver and kidney are generally reversible.

Usually, from 3–14 days after ingestion, indications of lung injury appear. Cough, dyspnea, and tachypnea often progress in the manner of a diffuse pneumonitis causing impairment of gas exchange. In some cases, severe pulmonary edema occurs and persists for several days. In most cases, the lung disease, characterized finally by extensive pulmonary fibrosis, progresses to death.

B. Laboratory Findings

Qualitative and quantitative methods for paraquat and diquat in urine are available at some toxicology laboratories and at the Chevron Environmental Health Center, 225 Bush Street, San Francisco, California 94104, telephone (415) 233-3737.

C. Treatment

1. Skin contamination by dipyridyls must be flushed away with copious amounts of water. Material splashed in the eye must be removed by prolonged irrigation with water. Eye contamination should thereafter be treated by an ophthalmologist.

2. Ingestion of any dipyridyl should be treated promptly and vigorously by measures to limit absorption from the gastrointestional tract and accelerate excretion of material already absorbed. Because the absorption of dipyridyls from the gut is relatively slow, measures to minimize absorption offer the most promising opportunity to save the patient. They must be undertaken even though the patient is essentially free of signs of systemic toxicity, and even when, by all accounts, the ingested dose was probably small, and was taken as long as 72 hours prior to treatment.

3. Lavage the stomach with at least 2 liters normal saline or 5% sodium bicarbonate solution. With stomach tube still in place, introduce a slurry of 8–10 oz. adsorbent. Suitable adsorbents are, in order of effectiveness: Fuller's Earth*, 30% suspension; Bentonite (or Montmorillonite), 7% suspension; activated charcoal, 15% suspension. These agents effectively bind dipyridyls with which they come in contact in the gut. In 15–30 minutes, administer sodium sulfate as a cathartic. For adults; give 30 gm. in 6–8 oz. water. For children under 12, give 0.2 gm./kg. body weight in 1–6 oz. water. Repeat the dosage of Fuller's Earth (or other adsorbent

---

*Optimal mesh 100–200. Sources of adsorbents are as follows: Sigma Chemical Co., 3500 Dekalb Street, St. Louis, Missouri 63178; Robinson's Bentonite U.S.P., Cat. No. 1138, Robinson Laboratories, Inc., San Francisco, California 94104; Robinson's Fuller's Earth U.S.P., Cat. No. 1343, Robinson Laboratories, Inc., San Francisco, California 94104; U.S.P. Volclay Bentonite, American Colloid Co., Skokie, Illinois; Emathlite VPM 600, Mid-Florida Mining Co., Lowell, Florida 32663.

if Fuller's Earth is not available) by mouth every four hours for at least 12 complete doses. Repeat the saline catharsis if continuing bowel movements do not occur.

4. If at all possible, remove the patient to a treatment facility where hemodialysis and hemoperfusion can be used if needed. The following treatment regimens are recommended:

a. Produce a diuresis. Put a retention catheter in place to ensure accurate monitoring of urine output. Examine the urine sediment and serum creatinine to determine whether dipyridyl nephrotoxity with reduction of renal function already exists. Insert central venous pressure catheter to monitor intravascular volume. In the absence of contraindications, infuse intravenously, in rotation, at a rate of about one liter every 3 hours, either 5% dextrose, 0.9% sodium chloride, or 5% mannitol. As time progresses, alternative electrolyte solutions will be required to maintain normal extracellular fluid composition. Give parenteral furosemide (Lasix), 20–40 mg. adult dose, every two to six hours, slowly intravenously, to sustain diuresis. Monitor fluid balance and blood electrolyte concentrations regularly, and look for signs of fluid overload (basilar rales, venous distention, high central venous pressure) that would warn of excessive fluid accumulation. Discontinue infusion if signs of severe fluid accumulation appear.

b. If circumstances do not permit vigorous forced diuresis, undertake peritoneal dialysis, extracorporeal hemodialysis, or hemoperfusion. These measures are mandatory in patients not able to tolerate high rates of intravenous fluid infusion, either because of preexisting heart disease or renal disease or acute tubular injury (anuria) by paraquat. Hemodialysis with ultrafiltration is reported to effectively remove paraquat from the circulating blood. Measure dipyridyl in urine to estimate levels of remaining toxicant.

5. Do not administer supplemental oxygen, unless Pa_{O_2} drops below 60–70 mm. Hg. Increased levels of alveolar oxygen accelerate the pathologic process caused by dipyridyls.

6. Superoxide dismutase (Truett Laboratories) is an enzyme from bovine erythrocytes which, by virtue of its free radical scavenging property, represents a rational antidote for dipyridyl poisoning. Tests of antidotal power in rats have yielded promising results. The value of the material in treating human poisonings has not yet been reported. It can be given both by aerosol and I.V. and appears to be nontoxic.

7. Corticosteroids have usually been administered in human poisoning cases but are of questionable value. Immunosuppressive drugs have been tried in a few cases without apparent benefit.

8. There is some evidence that expectorants (especially ammonium chloride and potassium iodide) may be of therapeutic value in minimizing the reduction in lung surfactant activity that is characteristic of paraquat poisoning.

V. CHLOROPHENOXY COMPOUNDS

Commonly used herbicides of this class are as follows:

2,4-D (Weedone), 2,4,5-T, 2,4,5-TP, Silvex (Kuron), 2,4-DB (Butyrac, Butoxone), erbon, Fenac, 2,4-DEP, MCPA, MCPB, MCPP (Mecoprop), Weedestron, Esteron, Estone, Dacamine, Weed-B-Gon, Weed-No-More, Weed-Out, Ded-Weed, Weed or Brush-Rhap, Broadleaf Weed Killer, Dandelion Killer, Vegetation Killer, Chickweed, and Clover Killer. There are several hundred commercial herbicide preparations which include one or more chlorophenoxy compound. They can usually be identified in the active ingredient description on the product label.

The chlorophenoxy acids, salts, and esters are mildly to severely irritating to skin, eyes, and respiratory and gastrointestinal linings. They are absorbed across the gut wall, the lung, and skin. They are not significantly stored in fat: excretion occurs within hours or, at most, days, primarily in the urine.

These compounds apparently have very low toxic potential for most persons. Human subjects have tolerated 0.5-gm. ingested doses daily for two to four weeks without adverse effects. Even so, isolated cases of peripheral neuropathy have been reported in workers after seemingly minor exposures to 2,4-D. Whether these persons were peculiarly predisposed or were exposed concurrently to other unidentified neurotoxic materials is not known.

A. CLINICAL FEATURES

Irritation of the skin follows excessive contact with many of these compounds. Protracted inhalation of spray is likely to irritate the nose, eyes, throat, and bronchi, causing local burning sensations and cough. Prolonged inhalation has also caused dizziness and ataxia, usually of a transient nature. When ingested, these compounds irritate the mouth and throat, and usually cause enough gastrointestinal irritation to induce prompt emesis. Chest pain from esophagitis is common. Abdominal pain and tenderness and diarrhea usually ensue. Absorption of large quantities of chlorophenoxy herbicide may produce fibrillary muscle twitching, skeletal muscle tenderness, and myotonia.

B. LABORATORY FINDINGS

Gas-liquid chromatographic methods are available for detecting and measuring many of the chlorophenoxy compounds in urine. These analyses are useful in confirming and assessing the magnitude of toxicant absorption. Urine samples should be collected as soon as possible after exposure because these materials may be almost completely excreted in 24–72 hours (depending on dose). The analyses can be done at special laboratories oper-

ated by states, agricultural research facilities, commercial chemical companies, and by the Environmental Protection Agency. Treatment should not be delayed pending confirmation of the causative agent, if there is a strong circumstantial basis for the diagnosis.

C. TREATMENT

1. Wash with soap and water to remove chemical contamination of the skin. Persons with chronic skin disease or with a tendency to become sensitive to chemicals should either avoid use of these herbicides, or should avoid direct contact.

2. Flush contaminating chemicals from the eyes, using copious amounts of clean water for 10–15 minutes.

3. If symptoms of illness occur during or following inhalation of spray, remove the patient from contact with the material for at least two days. Allow subsequent use of the chlorophenoxy compounds only if effective respiratory protection is practiced.

4. When chemicals of this class have been ingested, spontaneous emesis usually occurs and may empty the stomach as effectively as intubation and lavage. If vigorous emesis has not occurred, and the patient is fully alert, induce emesis with syrup of ipecac (adult dose, 30 ml.; 15 ml. for children under 12 years).

a. If consciousness level is depressed, an effect of the solvent petroleum distillates or other pesticides should be suspected. In this case, empty the stomach by intubation, aspiration, and lavage, using all available means to avoid aspiration of vomitus: Trendelenburg or left lateral decubitus position, frequent aspiration of the pharynx, and, in unconscious patients, tracheal intubation (using a cuffed tube) prior to gastric intubation.

b. After emesis or aspiration of the stomach and washing with isotonic saline or sodium bicarbonate, administer or instill 30 gm. activated charcoal in 3–4 oz. water to limit absorption of remaining toxicant.

c. Give sodium sulfate (Glauber's Salts) as a cathartic. For adults, give 30 gm. in 6–8 oz. water. For children under 12, give 0.2 gm./kg. body weight in 1–6 oz. water.

d. If absorption of as much as 0.5 gm. may have occurred in an adult (or about 0.02 gm./kg in children under 12 years), administer glucose and electrolyte solutions intravenously to accelerate excretion of toxicant. Observe the patient for renal irritation (albuminuria, hematuria), liver injury (serum bilirubin, alkaline phosphatase, serum LDH, GOT, and GPT), gastrointestinal ulceration (melena), leukopenia (WBC and differential), myalgia and myotonia (manifested by stiffness and incoordination), and peripheral neuropathy (paresthesia, pain, hypesthesia, and paresis of the extremities).

VI. ORGANONITROGEN

Classes of organonitrogen herbicides and common commercial products are as follows:

1. Urea-based compounds: Monuron (Monurex, Telvar), diuron (Di-on, Diurex, Karmex, Vonduron), linuron (Hoe 2810, Afalon, Lorox, Sarclex)
2. Uracil-based compounds: Bromacil (Hyvar X-L, Hyvar-X, Borea, Borocil IV, Urox HX or B, Isocil), terbacil (Sinbar)
3. Acetanilide-based compounds: Propachlor (Ramrod), allachlor (Lasso), propanil (DPA, Propanex, Stam F-34)
4. Acetamide compounds: Allidochlor (Randox, CDAA)
5. s-Triazine compounds: atrazine (Aatrex, Atranex, Gesaprin, Primatol A), simazine (Princep, Primatol S, Simanex, Gesatop), propazine (Milogard, Gesomil, Primatol P), prometone (Pramitol, Gesafram, promaton) atraton (Atratone), prometryn (Caparol, Gesagard, Primatol O, Prometrex), amatryn (Evik, Ametrex, Gesapax), desmetryne (Semeron), terbutryn (Igran, Shortstop E), cyanazine (Bladex, Scogal), cyprazine (Outfox)
6. Picolinic acid compounds: Picloram, Borolin
7. Carbamate compounds: Chlorpropham (Chloro IPC, CIPC, Furloe)

Adverse effects have occurred only rarely as a result of human or animal contact with these herbicides.

Certain of these chemicals, however, are irritating to skin and mucous membranes (uracil, acetanilide, acetamide, and picolinic acid compounds), and some can actually cause sensitization (acetanilides and acetamides).

When administered to experimental animals at extreme dosage levels, certain of these chemicals are capable of causing injury to the nervous system, liver, kidney, and capillary membranes. Large doses of triazines have caused anemia and impaired adrenal function. None of these effects have been observed in persons exposed to the herbicides occupationally or by reason of accidental ingestion. Absorbed herbicide is not stored in the body; excretion of the parent compound and metabolites is primarily by way of the urine. Ingestion of large quantities of any of these materials is likely to cause gastrointestinal irritation. In such cases, the hazard of the petroleum distillate solvent may equal or exceed the hazards presented by the active herbicidal ingredients.

A. CLINICAL FEATURES

Irritant effects on skin and mucous membranes are the most commonly reported adverse reactions to contact with these chemicals. Ingestions of large amounts can be expected to result in nausea, vomiting, abdominal distress, and diarrhea. Sensitization (to acetanilides or acetamides) can result in protracted dermatitis.

B. LABORATORY FINDINGS

Particular industrial, university, and government laboratories can detect some of these compounds or their metabolites in the urine of persons who have absorbed significant amounts. These laboratories can be reached through health departments or poison control centers.

C. TREATMENT

1. Flush the chemical from the eyes with copious amounts of clean water. Severe contamination may require specialized ophthalmologic attention.

2. Wash contaminating herbicide from the skin with soap and water. Severe irritation may require medical attention, and persons who become sensitized may require management with anti-inflammatory agents. Thereafter they will need to take special precautions to avoid contact with the sensitizing agent.

3. Considering the low inherent toxicities of these herbicides, and the risk of hydrocarbon pneumonitis that is unavoidable when the stomach is intubated or emesis is induced, ingestions of these chemicals known to involve less than 10 mg./kg. body weight are probably treated best by administration of 30–60 gm. activated charcoal in 5–10 oz. water. If diarrhea has not already developed, follow the charcoal administration in four hours with sodium sulfate catharsis. For adults (over 12 years of age), give 30 gm. in 6–8 oz. water; for children under 12, give 0.2 gm./kg. in 1–6 oz. water.

4. Ingestions of more than 10 mg./kg. body weight (especially when ingestion occurred less than an hour prior to treatment) should be managed by evacuation of the stomach.

5. If patient is alert, and respiration is not depressed, give syrup of ipecac: 30 ml. for adults; 15 ml. for children under 12 years. Observe the patient closely. If consciousness level declines, or if vomiting has not occurred in 20 minutes, proceed immediately to intubate, aspirate, and lavage the stomach with isotonic saline or sodium bicarbonate solution.

After emesis, have patient drink a suspension of 30 gm. activated charcoal in 3–4 oz. of water to limit toxicant absorption.

If patient is not fully alert, or if respiration is depressed, empty the stomach immediately by intubation, aspiration, and lavage, using isotonic saline or 5% sodium bicarbonate. Because these herbicides are usually dissolved in petroleum distillates, emesis and intubation of the stomach involve a serious risk of chemical pneumonitis if the solvent is aspirated. For this reason:

a. If the patient is either unconscious or obtunded, and if the facilities are at hand, insert an endotracheal tube (a cuffed tube if one is available) prior to gastric intubation.

b. Keep the victim's head below the level of the stomach during intubation and lavage (Trendelenburg, or left lateral decubitus position, with head end of table tipped downward). Keep the head turned to the left.

c. Aspirate pharynx as regularly as possible to remove gagged or vomited stomach contents.

After aspiration of gastric contents and washing of stomach, instill 30 gm. activated charcoal in 3–4 oz. water by way of stomach tube to limit absorption of remaining toxicant. Do not instill milk, cream or other substances containing vegetable or animal fats, because they may enhance toxicant absorption. If bowel movement has not occurred in four hours, and if patient is fully conscious, give sodium sulfate as a cathartic.

VII.
DIMETHYLDITHIOCARBAMATE AND ETHYLENE *BIS*-DITHIOCARBAMATE

Commonly used chemicals of these classes are as follows:

1. Tetramethyl thiuram disulfide: Thiram (Arasan, Thiramad, Thirasan, Thylate, Tirampa, Pomasol forte, TMTDS, Thiotex, Fernasan, Nomersan, Tersan, TUADS)
2. Metallodimethyldithiocarbamates: Ziram

and Pomasol Z forte (Zinc), Ferbam (Iron), Vapam (Sodium)

3. Metallo - ethylene - *bis*- dithiocarbamates (EBDC compounds): Zineb (Zinc), (Dithane Z78), Maneb (Manganese) (Dithane-M22 Special), Naban (Na) (Dithane-D14)

These compounds are absorbed by the gut (slowly) and probably by the skin and lung. They exhibit low acute systemic toxicities for mammals. Many are irritants, and some (notably thiram) are sensitizers.

Thiram and the metallodialkyldithiocarbamates are metabolized in mammals to dialkylamine and carbon disulfide. The intermediate dialkyl dithiocarbamate inhibits sulfydryl enzymes in the liver and CNS. Carbon disulfide is neurotoxic. To this extent, the toxicology of these fungicides can be expected to resemble that of the medicinal disulfiram (Antabuse), the ethyl analog of thiram. In laboratory animals, thiram is more toxic than disulfiram but produces qualitatively similar toxic effects.

Systemic effects of the dialkyldithiocarbamates must be considered in two categories: (1) those following absorption of toxicant alone, and (2) those resulting from ingestion of alcohol following absorption of a dithiocarbamate compound.

Given to laboratory animals in extreme doses, medicinal disulfiram causes gastrointestinal irritation, demyelinization of the central nervous system, and necrosis of the liver, spleen, and kidney parenchyma. Functional and anatomical CNS damage has been demonstrated in rats on high chronic dietary intakes of iron and zinc dimethyldithiocarbamates. Peripheral neuropathy and psychotic reactions have occurred in alcohol-abstinent persons on disulfiram regimens (ingestion of several hundred milligrams daily). A possible role of the metabolite carbon disulfide has been suspected in these neurotoxic reactions.

Illness following combined intake of di-sulfiram and alcohol is due primarily to inhibition of liver enzymes necessary for oxidation of acetaldehyde to acetic acid. Peripheral vasodilatation is the main pathophysiological feature of the disulfiram-alcohol reaction, presumably as a result of high tissue levels of acetaldehyde. This may occasionally lead to shock and even more rarely to myocardial ischemia, cardia arrhythmias, congestive failure, and death. Animal experimentation has supported certain other biochemical mechanisms of toxicity involving reaction products of ethanol and disulfiram.

The EBDC fungicides are metabolized to ethylene thiourea. Either the native fungicides or their metabolites are goitrogenic, probably by blocking thyroxine synthesis, thus stimulating thyrotropic hormone production.

A. Clinical Features

1. Dialkyldithiocarbamates

Itching, redness, and eczematoid dermatitis have resulted when sensitive or predisposed persons come in contact with these compounds. Persons excessively exposed to air-borne dust formulations have suffered upper respiratory congestion, hoarseness, and cough. When large amounts have been ingested, nausea, emesis, and diarrhea ensue. Hypothermia and ataxia are characteristic. Muscle weakness, progressing to a condition of ascending paralysis and finally respiratory paralysis, can be anticipated from animal toxicological studies based on extreme dosage.

2. Dialkyldithiocarbamates and Alcohol

The reaction to ethanol that follows absorption of disulfiram is characterized by flushing, sweating, pounding headache, sensation of warmth, weakness, congestion of upper respiratory and conjunctival membranes, dyspnea, hyperpnea, chest pain, tachycardia, palpitation, and hypotension. The respiratory distress may resemble asthma, and, in some instances, respiratory depression has been life-threatening. Emesis commonly occurs. Severe reactions may result in shock, unconsciousness, and convulsions. It must be emphasized that absorption of sufficient fungicidal compounds to cause a severe reaction to ethanol would occur only under exceptional circumstances.

3. EBDC Compounds

These fungicides may cause irritation of skin, respiratory tract, and gut.

B. LABORATORY FINDINGS

The native pesticides are too rapidly metabolized in the body to permit detection in blood or urine. There are biochemical methods for measuring blood acetaldehyde to confirm an ethanol-dithiocarbamate reaction. There are also sensitive methods for detecting compounds in the urine that yield carbon disulfide on acid digestion (dithiocarbamates and related substances).

C. TREATMENT

1. Wash contaminating fungicide from the skin with soap and water. Atopic persons and those specifically sensitive to thiuram disulfide compounds (recognized as "rubber sensitive") should be permanently removed from contact with chemicals of this nature.

2. Flush the contaminating fungicide from the eyes with fresh water for 10 to 15 minutes.

3. Treatment for ingestion of dimethyl-dithiocarbamate compounds, not complicated by alcohol ingestion:

a. If dialkyldithiocarbamate compounds have been ingested, it is first essential that the person not take any form of alcoholic beverage for at least three weeks. (Gastrointestinal absorption of some compounds is protracted, and effects on critical enzymes are slowly reversible.)

b. If vigorous emesis has not already

occurred and if patient is fully alert and respiration normal, give syrup of ipecac to induce vomiting (30 ml. for adults, 15 ml. for children under 12 years). Observe the patient closely after administering ipecac. If consciousness level declines, or if vomiting has not occurred in 20 minutes, proceed to empty the stomach by intubation, aspiration, and lavage.

c. After emesis, administer 30 gm. activated charcoal in 3–4 oz. water to bind toxicant remaining in the gut.

d. If consciousness level or respiration is depressed, empty the stomach by intubation, aspiration, and lavage, using all available means to avoid aspiration of vomitus: left lateral Trendelenburg position, frequent aspiration of the pharynx, and, in unconscious persons, tracheal intubation (using a cuffed tube) prior to gastric intubation.

e. After aspiration of the stomach and washing with isotonic saline or sodium bicarbonate, instill 30 gm. activated charcoal in 3–4 oz. water by way of stomach tube to limit absorption of remaining toxicant.

f. Give sodium sulfate as a cathartic. For adults, give 30 gm. in 6–8 oz. water. For children under 12, give 0.2 gm./kg. body weight in 1–6 oz. water.

4. Treatment for a reaction to ethanol ingestion after absorption of a dialkyldithiocarbamate compound:

a. Administer 100% oxygen for as long as the reaction continues. If respiration is depressed, administer the oxygen by an intermittent positive pressure breathing device and monitor the patient closely to assure optimum pulmonary ventilation in case of apnea.

b. If the fungicide was ingested no more than four hours prior to treatment and vigorous emesis has not occurred, evacuate the stomach by intubation, aspiration, and lavage, observing precautions cited above.

c. Irrespective of time interval since ingestion of fungicide, administer 30 gm.

activated charcoal in 3–4 oz. of water to limit absorption of toxicant remaining in the gut. Absorption of these compounds is slow.

d. Inject 1.0 gm. ascorbic acid (vitamin C) intraveneously at a rate not exceeding 0.2 gm. per minute. As a "hydrogen-donor," ascorbic acid may have significant antidotal action against absorbed dithiocarbamate compound.

e. For severe or protracted reactions, infuse 5% glucose in water.

f. Administer sodium sulfate for catharsis.

g. If the patient has myocardial insufficiency, diabetes, neuropathy, cirrhosis, or other severe chronic disease, observe carefully for 48 hours to ensure that complications (especially myocardial infarction, toxic psychosis, and neuropathy) are treated promptly.

5. Because EBDC compounds have low acute systemic toxicity for mammals, there may be greater risk from aspiration of hydrocarbon solvent in the course of gastric emptying than there is from the toxicity of the fungicides themselves. Therefore, if dosage was definitely less than 10 mg./kg., it is probably best simply to administer 30–60 gm. activated charcoal, followed by sodium sulfate catharsis. If dosage may have exceeded 10 mg./kg., empty the stomach, administer activated charcoal, then cathartic, as indicted in the full series of instructions above.

BIBLIOGRAPHY

II. PENTACHLOROPHENOL

Bergner, H., Constantinidis, P., and Martin, J. H.: Industrial pentachlorophenol poisoning in Winnipeg. Can. Med. Assoc. J, 92:488, 1965.

Deichmann, W., Machle, W., Litzmiller, K. V., and Thomas, G.: Acute and chronic effects of pentachlorophenol and sodium pentachlorophenate upon experimental animals. J. Pharmacol., 76:104, 1942.

Gordon, D.: How dangerous is pentachlorophenol? Med. J. Aust., 2:485, 1956.

Robson, A. M., Kissane, J. M., Elvick, N. H., and Pundavela, L.: Pentachlorophenol poisoning in a nursery for newborn infants. I, Clinical features and treatment. Pediatr. Pharm. Ther., 75:309, 1969.

III. NITROPHENOL AND NITROCRESOL

Harvey, D. G.: On the metabolism of some aromatic nitro compounds by different species of animal. III, The toxicity of the dinitrophenols, with a note on the effects of high environmental temperature. J. Pharm. Pharmacol., 11:462, 1959.

Harvey, D. G., Bidstrup, P. L., and Bonnell, J. A. L.: Poisoning by dinitro-ortho-cresol: some observations on the effects of dinitro-ortho-cresol administered by mouth to human volunteers. Br. Med. J., 2:13, 1951.

Spencer, H. C., Rowe, V. K., Adams, E. M., and Irish, D. D.: Toxicological studies on laboratory animals of certain alkyldinitrophenols used in agriculture. J. Ind. Hyg. Toxicol., 30:807, 1948.

Sproull, D. H.: A comparison of sodium salicylate and 2:4-dinitrophenol as metabolic stimulants in vitro. Biochem. J., 66:527, 1957.

Wolfe, H. R., Durham, W. F., and Batchelor, G. S.: Health hazards of some dinitro compounds. Arch. Envir. Health, 3:468, 1961.

IV. PARAQUAT AND OTHER DIPYRIDYLS

Bullivant, C. M.: Accidental poisoning by paraquat: report of two cases in man. Br. Med. J., 1:1272, 1966.

Clark, D. G., McElligott, T. F., and Hurst, E. W.: The toxicity of paraquat. Br. J. Ind. Med.; 23:126, 1966.

Fairshter, R. D., and Wilson, A. F.: Paraquat poisoning: manifestations and therapy. Am. J. Med. 59:751, 1975.

Fisher, H. K., Humphries, M., and Bails, R.: Paraquat poisoning: recovery from renal and pulmonary damage. Am. Rev. Resp. Dis., 107:246, 1973.

Kerr, F., Patel, A. R., Scott, P. D. R., and Tompsett, S. L.: Paraquat poisoning treated by forced diuresis. Br. Med. J., 3:290, 1968.

McKean, W. I.: Recovery from paraquat poisoning. Br. Med. J., 3:292, 1968.

Sinow, J., and Wei, E.: Ocular toxicity of paraquat. Bull. Envir. Contam. Toxicol., 9(3):163, 1973.

Smith, L. L., Wright, A., Wyatt, I., and Rose, M. S.: Effective treatment for paraquat poisoning in rats and its relevance to treatment of paraquat poisoning in man. Br. Med. J., 4:569, 1974.

V. CHLOROPHENOXY COMPOUNDS

Berkley, M. C., and Magee, K. R.: Neuropathy following exposure to a dimethylamine salt of 2,4-D. Arch. Int. Med. 111:351, 1963.

Berwick, P.: 2,4-Dichlorophenoxyacetic acid poisoning in man. J.A.M.A., *214*(6):1114, 1970.

Bucher, N. L. R.: Effects of 2,4-dichlorophenoxyacetic acid on experimental animals. Proc. Soc. Exp. Biol. Med., *63*:204, 1946.

Desi, I., Sos, J., Olasz, J., Sule, F., and Markus, V.: Nervous system effects of a chemical herbicide. Arch. Envir. Health, *4*:95, 1962.

Seabury, J. H.: Toxicity of 2,4-dichlorophenoxyacetic acid for man and dog. Arch. Envir. Health, *7*:202, 1963.

VI. ORGANONITROGEN

Dinerman, A. A., and Larrent'eva, N. A.: Toxicity of the herbicides propazine and prometryn. Gigiena i Sanit, *34*(3):94, 1969. (Abstr. Health Asp. Pesticides, *2*(10), no. 69–1245).

Johnson, A. E., Van Kampen, K. R., and Binns, W.: Effects on cattle and sheep of eating hay treated with the triazine herbicides, atrazine and prometone. Am. J. Vet. Res., *33*:1443, 1972.

Palmer, J. S., and Radeleff, R. D.: The toxicologic effects of certain fungicides and herbicides on sheep and cattle. Ann. N.Y. Acad. Sci. *3*:729, 1964.

Schlicher, J. E., and Beat, V. B.: Dermatitis resulting from herbicide use: a case study. J. Iowa Med. Soc., *62*(8):419, 1972.

Weed Science Society of America. Herbicide Handbook. 3rd Ed. Springfield, Ill., Charles C Thomas, 1974.

Yelizarov, G. P.: Occupational skin diseases caused by simazine and propazine. Vestn. Dermatol. Venerol., *46*(2):27, 1972. (Abstr., Health Asp. Pesticides, *6*(2), no. 73–0352).

VII. DIMETHYLDITHIOCARBAMATE AND ETHYLENE *BIS*-DITHIOCARBAMATE

Child, G. P., and Crump, M.: The toxicity of tetraethylthiuram disulphide (Antabuse) to mouse, rat, rabbit and dog. Acta Pharmacol. Toxicol., *8*: 305, 1952.

Hodge, H. C., Maynard, E. A., Downs, W. L., Coye, R. D., Jr., and Steadman, L. T.: Chronic oral toxicity of ferric dimethyldithiocarbamate (Ferbam) and zinc dimethyldithiocarbamate (Ziram). J. Pharmacol. Exp. Ther., *118*:174, 1956.

Hodgson, J. R., Hoch, J. C., Castles, T. R., Helton, D. O., and Lee, C. C.: Metabolism and disposition of Ferbam in the rat. Toxicol. Appl. Pharm., *33*:505, 1975.

Ivanova-Chemishanska, L., Markov, D. V., Milanov, S., et al.: Effect of subacute oral administration of zinc ethylene bis (dithiocarbamate) on the thyroid gland and adenohypophysis of the rat. Food Cosmet. Toxicol., *13*:445, 1975.

Shelley W. B.: Golf-course dermatitis due to thiram fungicide: cross-hazards of alcohol, disulfiram, and rubber. J.A.M.A., *188*:415, 1964.

20. TOPICAL AGENTS

Edward A. Emmett, M.B., B.S., M.S., F.R.A.C.P.

Toxic skin reactions may be produced by a large variety of chemical agents. They most commonly arise as a result of inadvertent or deliberate exposures directly to the skin. Adverse reactions may thus arise from cosmetics and toiletries, household and consumer products, from materials used in industry contacted through occupation or materials used in hobbies or avocations. Drug reactions manifested on the skin also are common, but this chapter will primarily deal with ill effects of nontherapeutic agents. Skin damage may also be from systemic absorption of an agent that enters the body by ingestion, inhalation, or injection. The skin is frequently an important route of absorption of toxic materials that cause adverse systemic effects, although this possibility is frequently overlooked. Some metabolism of xenobiotics (e.g., the potentially carcinogenic polycyclic aromatic hydrocarbons) takes place within the skin. To a varying extent, there is some excretion from the skin and its appendages including the apocrine and eccrine sweat, and in milk, hair, nails, and desquamation of the superficial layers. In a limited number of instances foreign materials may alter systemic metabolism in such a way as to induce the overproduction of potentially harmful endogenous substances that may secondarily cause skin disease, e.g., the induction of the cutaneous bullae of porphyria cutanea tarda secondary to hexachlorbenzene ingestion.

Materials contacting the skin may produce local effects or, after absorption, systemic effects. The latter may occur in the absence of any skin injury as in percutaneous poisoning with substances such as organic phosphate insecticides, tetraethyl lead, or aniline dyes. Both cutaneous and systemic effects occur with, for example, hydrofluoric acid and phenol. Generally, the barrier to absorption lies in the outermost thin stratum corneum layer of the skin, which is composed of metabolically dead cells. Percutaneous absorption occurs by passive absorption and is influenced by a number of factors. These can conveniently be grouped as factors related to the chemical, the vehicle, or the state of the skin. Table 20-1 summarizes these influences. The possible effects of percutaneous absorption must always be considered when the adverse effects of topically contacted materials are considered.

There are a number of different ways of classifying toxic reactions to drugs or foreign chemicals affecting the skin. In practice it is often most useful to categorize these according to the morphological type of reaction observed. An appropriate differential diagnosis can then be formulated, and the known types of chemicals or adverse effects that may produce this reaction should be considered. The number of chemicals that may adversely affect the skin is very large. However, the number of ways in which damage to the skin is manifest, whether by toxic substances, microorganisms, immunological damage, or any other cause, is limited. Conversely we must recognize that any particular pattern of response, for example, an eczematous eruption, may have multiple causes. The major types of cutaneous response to toxic chemicals are indicated in Table 20-2. These reactions range from almost immediate responses to injury such as corrosion to long-delayed effects such as carcinogenesis.

Table 20-1. **Selected Factors That Enhance Percutaneous Absorption**

1. Nature of Chemical
   Lipid solubility
   Slight water solubility
   Low molecular weight
   Nonionized form of weak acid or base
   True gas (not vapors)

2. Nature of Vehicle
   High solubility in stratum corneum compared
      with solubility in vehicle
   Presence of surface-active agents (detergents,
      etc.)
   "Solvent" damage to skin
   pH keeps weak acid or base in nonionized
      form

3. State of the Skin
   Region (e.g., relative poor barrier of skin of
      dorsum of hands, scrotum, etc.)
   Loss of physical integrity of skin
   Hydration and occlusion (enhances
      penetration of water-soluble materials)
   Increased temperature

I. CORROSION AND ULCERATION

A. CHEMICAL BURNS

A number of substances, including strong acids and alkalies, are corrosive and can cause severe ulceration following sufficient exposure. A list of some representative materials in this group is shown in Table 20-3. Minor transient skin contact with these materials can result in a first-degree burn characterized by erythema and edema. More severe or prolonged contact results in a second-degree burn characterized by vesicles and bullae. More exposure will result in a third-degree chemical burn where the skin may be either pale gray from ischemia, purple or brown from extravasation or blood, or some other color depending on the specific nature of the material. Severe burns from acids usually cause a dry crust from coagulation necrosis of the tissue. Burns from sulfuric acid are gray black; from hydrogen chloride, sapphire gray; from nitric acid, a deep yellow; and from organic acids such as trichloracetic acid, a greenish gray. Chemical burns from alkalies tend to be softer. The lesions are often extremely painful. Some substances such as phenol may cause local anesthesia so that pain may be absent after a period. Burns from many corrosive materials differ from thermal burns in that the action of the chemical may continue indefinitely unless it is removed by copious washing. In some cases, as with alkyl mercury compounds, removal of the blister fluid may help reduce extension of the lesion.

The effects of systemic absorption from a potentially toxic material should always be borne in mind. The effect will depend

Table 20-2. **Major Patterns of Cutaneous Response to Toxic Chemicals**

Corrosion and Ulceration

Eczematous Dermatitis
   Irritant dermatitis
   Cumulative irritant dermatitis
   Allergic contact dermatitis
   Phototoxic dermatitis
   Photoallergic dermatitis

Fiberglass Dermatitis

Urticaria
   Immunological
   Nonimmunological

Granuloma

Acne of Chemical Origin

Folliculitis

Damage to Hair

Pigmentary Changes
   Depigmentation
   Hyperpigmentation

Skin Tumors
   Keratoses
   Squamous cell carcinoma
   Basal cell epithelioma
   Bowen's disease

on the specific material. For example, oxalic acid and hydrofluoric acid will produce systemic hypocalcemia; white phosphorus, kidney and liver injury. Systemic absorption will be greater the longer the material is allowed to remain in contact with the skin.

Severe chemical burns are frequently occupational and may be complicated by trauma, thermal burns, or forceful injury. Particularly severe injuries may be associated with the injection under pressure of hot material through the skin. Some chemical burns such as white phosphorus burns are more frequently observed in wartime. The cause of a chemical burn is usually obvious, although the extent of the injury may be underestimated on initial evaluation. This is particularly true of hydrogen fluoride, mustard gas, and nitrogen mustard burns.

B. Treatment

With the exception of quicklime (CaO), rapid removal of the corrosive substance with copious quantities of water or irrigation is the most important step. Although there are occasional studies reported to show that removal with certain solvents is superior to water, such studies are often based on experiments where the skin was swabbed with water or on other procedures where an inadequate quantity of water was used for washing. In practice, water should be readily available in large quantities close to most sites where chemical burns are likely to occur. It is most important that clothing, including shoes, be removed to ensure that irrigation is adequate and that material under fingernails and in the hair is not overlooked. If there is any question of eye involvement, the eye should be immediately irrigated with water or an isotonic eye wash for at least 15 minutes. After adequate first aid, consideration should be given to special characteristics of the specific substance causing the burn such as those described in the next section. If necessary, treat-

Table 20-3. Corrosive or Ulcerogenic Substances

Strong Acids
  Sulfuric, nitric, hydrochloric
  Trichloracetic, acetic, carboxylic

Alkalies
  Calcium oxide (quicklime)*
  Sodium hydroxide, potassium hydroxide
  Sodium carbonate, potassium carbonate
  Hydrogen fluoride, fluorine
  Phosphorus
  Phenol
  Demethyl sulfate
  Titanium tetrachloride
  Alkyl mercury
  Alkyl tins
  CS (orthochlorobenzene malonitrile)
  Mustard gas (*bis* (2-chloroethyl) sulfide)
  Nitrogen mustard
  Hexavalent chromium
  Arsenic
  Zinc chloride
  Cement

*Important: Do not attempt initial removal with water.

ment should be given for pain and routine measures instituted for the prevention of shock and infection. Generally, the later treatment of chemical burns is similar to that of thermal burns. Excision and grafting may be necessary, and there will be a need for intensive rehabilitation in cases of severe disfigurement. As a rule, there is a paucity of information on chemical burns, and there are many gaps in our knowledge about optimal treatment methods.

C. Prevention

The majority of cases of chemical burns occur in industry, where considerable attention to prevention should be given. It is particularly important that corrosive materials be carefully identified and handled. Personnel exposed to these materials should have appropriate training, both in practices necessary to avoid burns and in emergency management. Burns tend to occur when containers break or at the sites of transfer operations in industry.

Particular attention should be given to making these processes safe. Corrosive substances should be stored in metal or other unbreakable containers whenever possible. It is vitally important to have operating water faucets near sites where chemical burns might occur.

D. CORROSIVE SUBSTANCES

1. Quicklime

The reaction of quicklime with water is highly exothermic, and the solution of 1 gm. of calcium oxide in water generates over 18,000 calories. The surface of the burn caused by quicklime should be cleaned mechanically and then washed with olive oil or a light liquid paraffin before the lime is wetted. The only alternative is removal using such a rapid copious stream of water under pressure that it mechanically removes the particles.

2. Other Alkalies

Generally, chemical burns from alkalies produce deep caustic burns that should be irrigated copiously until all soapiness disappears. A weak acid could then be used for neutralization.

3. Hot Tar or Asphalt

No attempt should be made to remove the tar until it has hardened. Immediate immersion in cold or ice water will harden the tar and shrink it from the skin. Removal should be attempted when the tar peels away easily.

4. Mustard Gas and Nitrogen Mustard

The reaction to these materials may be delayed. A reaction with erythema after a few hours may herald later edema and vesiculation with the subsequent development of ulcers that are slow to heal. Sites of contact should be washed copiously with water. Avoid scrubbing or trauma because there may subsequently be poor healing. The use of 2% chloramine solution has been suggested as an antidote, as

has the use of 2% sodium bicarbonate dressings.

5. Vesicant War Gases

Of the so-called lacrimators, CS, or orthochlorbenzene malonitrile, is the most likely to cause third-degree burns. These particularly occur in areas of moisture and occlusion such as body folds.

6. Alkyl Mercury Burns

It is important to evacuate the fluid in the vesicles and bullae which result from burns with this material in order to halt progression.

7. Resins and Thermoplastics Including Polymerized Methacrylates

Burns from these materials should be treated by immediate cooling in cold or ice water prior to any attempted removal. In general, when the resin can be easily peeled away, removal should be undertaken. In certain cases, an appropriate solvent, which will vary according to the nature and solubility of the particular resin, may be used to remove the cooled material. The solvent should then be removed as completely as possible with a mild soap and water.

8. Phosphorus

White phosphorus, which burns in air, produces both severe thermal and chemical injury. This material may also reignite as it dries after inadequate washing. Phosphorus is initially luminescent in the dark, which may help in identification. The recommended treatment is to wash copiously, then perform debridement (under water to prevent spontaneous ignition), and apply a 1% copper sulfate solution to convert the phosphorus to copper phosphide. The copper sulfate solution is left on the skin for only a brief time before being removed with copious irrigation. The particles of copper phosphide salt may then be removed with an instrument. It is most important not to leave high concentrations of copper sulfate in contact with large areas of the skin for long periods, as this appears to be associated with massive hemolysis and other manifestations of systemic copper poisoning. Debridement of all embedded particles of phosphorus is most important.

9. Hydrogen Fluoride

Contact with hydrofluoric acid may initially cause a slight reaction which progresses to a more severe burn with blanching and edema, followed by vesiculation and extensive necrosis which heals extremely slowly. Necrosis may progress slowly for several days. Hydrofluoric acid under the nails can produce severe lesions. The burn is often extremely painful. Hydrogen fluoride precipitates intracellular calcium, and hypocalcemia appears both to contribute to the local injury and to have the potential for causing profound systemic hypocalcemia. Treatment consists of prolonged irrigation with copious quantities of water and injection of 10% calcium gluconate until the pain is relieved. Topical calcium gluconate gel has been reported as useful in less severe burns. It is most important that the calcium gluconate be given promptly. If the eyes are involved, they should be irrigated with copious amounts of water followed by a few drops of calcium gluconate.

10. Arsenic

Arsenic trioxide (white arsenic) can lead to eczematous eruptions, folliculitis, furunculosis, and ulcerative lesions of the extremities and nasal septum. In mining communities these changes may occur both in workers (smelter's itch) and exposed community members. Ulceration appears to be facilitated by sweat, excoriations, and wounds, so that the prompt cleansing of these lesions is important.

11. Hexavalent Chromium

Hexavalent chromium is ulcerogenic, whereas trivalent chromium is not. Ulcers ("chrome holes") occur independently of allergic or other reactions to chromium and are generally seen in persons exposed to industrial processes such as tanning, electroplating, and chrome production. Although they generally occur on the exposed skin, ulceration of the nasal septum may occur. The lesions are crusted, painless ulcers that appear punched out after removal of the crust with indurated and undermined borders. Prompt washing with water or sodium pyrosulfite has been shown to reduce the subsequent ulceration. Ascorbic acid cream, 10%, applied to the nasal septum may prevent nasal perforation.

II. ECZEMATOUS DERMATITIS

Perhaps the most common adverse cutaneous reaction from chemical agents is the development of eczematous contact dermatitis. An eczematous dermatitis is characterized at some stage in its development by the development of intraepidermal vesiculation seen either microscopically or macroscopically. An eczematous eruption of any severity usually goes through the clinically observable stages of erythema, edema or papules, vesiculation, weeping, and crusting. Under appropriate circumstances, lichenification may occur. Eczema is a reaction pattern of the skin and, as such, represents a symptom complex with somewhat similar manifestations whatever the cause—constitutional, fungal, bacterial, and external contacting chemical. Between 10% and 25% of all patients seen in skin clinics have an eczematous eruption. Of these, up to 60% are considered to be due to contact dermatitis. Thus, such eruptions constitute one of the most common adverse effects of chemical agents.

A. TYPES OF CONTACT DERMATITIS

There are five major categories of contact dermatitis: irritant dermatitis, cumulative insult dermatitis, allergic contact

Table 20-4. **Selected Cutaneous Irritants**

Strong detergents
Alkalies including sodium silicate and trisodium
  phosphate
Petroleum distillates
Organic solvents: toluene, benzene, perchlorethlyene
Permanent wave solutions (thioglycolates)
Coolants and cutting fluids (including semisynthetic
  and synthetic types)
Feces, urine, colostomy fluids
Formaldehyde
Plant juices: onion, garlic
Tear gas (including mace)
Hydrogen peroxide and other peroxides

dermatitis, phototoxic dermatitis, and photoallergic dermatitis.

Irritant dermatitis is caused by contact with a strongly irritating substance. In its most severe form, the reaction is that of a corrosive dermatitis. Usually the reaction is erythematous and edematous, and vesicles and bullae may occur. This type of dermatitis is particularly likely to occur from contact with strong acids or alkalies, solvents, and many other materials. The diagnosis is usually straightforward because a good history of contact with the injurious substance can generally be obtained. A list of selected irritating substances is given in Table 20-4.

A more subtle form of dermatitis is cumulative insult dermatitis, which results from more prolonged or repeated applications of one or more substances that are usually only mildly irritating. Such substances are often referred to as marginal irritants. This form of dermatitis is often multifactorial in origin and may take a prolonged period of time to develop. It may be more prone to occur under circumstances where there are repeated wetting and drying cycles. Cumulative insult dermatitis is common in housework and those occupations which use semisynthetic coolants. A single cause is often very difficult to isolate. However, exposures to soaps, detergents, cosmetics, plant substances (orange peel, pineapple juice), repeated friction, wetting and drying cycles,

irritating local applications, and home remedies are frequently implicated. Although this form of dermatitis tends to develop slowly, it also tends to resolve slowly with treatment and to recur unless causal factors are eliminated.

In contrast to irritant dermatitis and cumulative insult dermatitis, allergic contact dermatitis depends on a specific immunological reaction to a causal material. Allergic reactions of this type are manifestations of type IV cell-mediated immunity; circulating antibodies are not involved. After the first exposure to a potential allergen, an incubation period of 7 to 10 days or more is necessary before sensitization occurs. Once a person is sensitized, the reaction occurs with a characteristic delay of 36 to 48 hours after reexposure. A list of common cutaneous allergens is given in Table 20-5. Definitive diagnosis depends on patch testing. In the case of allergic contact dermatitis, cross reactions may occur with molecules which are structurally closely related. Occasionally, an eczematous eruption can recur in a sensitized person upon the systemic administration of the same or of an immunochemically related drug. For example, persons sensitized to topical neomycin may suffer a recurrence of dermatitis in previously affected areas of the body on being treated with streptomycin

Table 20-5. **Common Causes of Allergic Contact Dermatitis**

Rhus (poison ivy, oak, or sumac)
Rubber additives (accelerators and antioxidants)
Paraphenylenediamine and related hair dyes
Nickel
Chromate salts
Formaldehyde
Ammoniated mercury and other topical mercurials
Ethylenediamine and paraben preservatives in
  topical preparations
Tetracaine, procaine, benzocaine (local anesthetics)
Neomycin
Topical antihistamines
Epoxy resins monomers (resin or hardeners)
Uncured acrylate monomers (of various types)

or kanamycin; those with a topical allergy to tetramethylthiuram used as an additive in rubber may suffer a reaction on being given disulfiram.

More rarely, contact dermatitis results from a substance producing photosensitization whereby the person becomes abnormally sensitive to ultraviolet radiation from sunlight. There are two major categories of such reactions: phototoxic reactions which do not have an immunological basis and photoallergic reactions which, like contact dermatitis, depend on cell-mediated immunity to the inciting substance. Selected causes of phototoxic and photoallergic reactions are given in Table 20-6.

B. DIAGNOSIS

A diagnosis of dermatitis is made on morphological grounds. The distribution of the eruption and a careful history of exposures at work, home, hobbies, use of cosmetics, and so forth may indicate the likelihood of contact dermatitis. The distribution of the dermatitis is particularly important. Contact dermatitis of the hands tends to develop on the dorsal surface of the hands, the dorsal and lateral aspects of the fingers, and the volar surface of the wrists and may be particularly severe under watchbands and rings. Dermatitis from shoes or materials impregnating shoes should always be suspected where an eczematous dermatitis of the feet spares the intertriginous spaces. Photosensitivity eruptions tend to occur on exposed areas and to spare shaded areas such as under the eyelids and chin, whereas dermatitis from airborne substances may be quite severe in those fold areas where foreign materials accumulate.

Because there is no definitive diagnostic test for irritant dermatitis, diagnosis must depend on an appreciation of the irritant qualities of the material, considerations of dose, concentration, and time and circumstances of contact. In contrast, the cause of allergic contact dermatitis may be

Table 20-6. **Selected Chemical Causes of Photosensitivity Eruptions**

Phototoxic Reactions
  Furocoumarins (psoralens)
  Tetracyclines
  Sulfonamides
  Chlorpromazine
  Halogenated xanthene dyes
  Nalidixic acid
  Polycyclic aromatic hydrocarbons (tars, pitches, etc.)

Photoallergic Reactions
  Halogenated salicylanilides and related agents used as topical germicides
    Tetrachlorosalicylanilide
    Bithional
    Tribromosalicylanilide and dibromosalicylanilide
  Sulfonamides
  4,6-Dichlorophenylphenol
  Quinoxaline 1,4-di-N-oxide (animal food growth promoter)
  Phenegan (topically applied)
  Chlorpromazine
  Compositae family of plants (ragweed)

established by diagnostic patch testing. However, it is critical that the latter procedure be performed and interpreted by experts under standard conditions, using nonirritant concentrations of the material applied in an appropriate solvent. Standard diagnostic trays can be provided by the International Contact Dermatitis Research Group for testing with a limited number of allergens. The confirmation of a diagnosis of photosensitivity may require the specialized procedure of photopatch testing where skin, which has been appropriately exposed to the potential causal substance in an appropriate solvent and dilution, is further irradiated with ultraviolet radiation.

C. TREATMENT

As in other types of eczema the choice of topical therapy depends on the clinical stage of the dermatitis. In an acute stage when there is vesiculation and weeping, cool wet dressings of aluminum acetate solution can be used, and acutely inflamed areas of skin should be immobilized. Soothing baths with colloidal oatmeal in lukewarm water can be given if the eruption is widespread. In a less acute stage, topical steroids are appropriate. The use of potent (e.g., fluorinated) topical steroids on areas such as the face should be minimized because of the danger of subsequent atrophic changes in the skin. Chronic, dry, lichenified eruptions may respond to intralesional steroids or the application of coal tar derivative preparations. Systemic antibiotics should be given for any bacterial superinfection. Systemic steroids in doses up to the equivalent of 60 mg. of prednisone daily are important in severe and extensive eruptions. A short course should be sufficient provided the causal agent is eliminated. Sedatives such as tranquilizers or antihistamines are useful. Antihistamines have no specific immunological effect in eczematous contact dermatitis. It is important to avoid the use of irritating or sensitizing medications and also to ensure that the patient does not apply strongly irritating home remedies.

Further treatment and prevention will depend on the specific cause of the dermatitis. The patient must be instructed to meticulously avoid all identifiable etiological factors. Recurrences should be regarded as a failure of preventive management, the reason for the recurrence carefully established, and the preventive regime modified accordingly. The patient must be instructed that the skin will be less tolerant than usual of irritants for several months and that for allergic reactions the sensitization will remain indefinitely.

III. FIBERGLASS DERMATITIS

In persons occupationally exposed to fiberglass, dermatitis is particularly likely to occur in the skin creases. There is marked itching and pinpoint-sized papules that are often excoriated or petechial. There may be urticaria and linear erosions, often secondary to scratching. The likelihood that a particular fiberglass will produce dermatitis is directly related to the fiber diameter and inversely proportional to the length. The source of fiberglass dermatitis may be less obvious; for example, minor epidemics have occurred in persons who have worn clothing that has been inadvertently washed with fiberglass curtains. These episodes tend to be characterized by intense pruritus with only a transient macular eruption or no visible eruption. Microscopic examination of cellophane tape strippings of the skin may reveal fibers in such cases, as may skin scrapings with 20% sodium hydroxide solution. The condition usually resolves rapidly after removal of the cause.

IV. URTICARIA

Urticarial responses are common, have many causes, and may be multifactorial. When caused by foreign materials, they usually result from ingestion but also can result from inhalation or other routes of administration. They often result from a type I immunological reaction but may be caused by a variety of substances which directly release histamine and other mediators. Such substances are found in shellfish, aspirin, and quinine. There are numerous other causes not related to toxic chemicals, including certain internal diseases, infections, physical modalities, and psychic stresses. Angioedema, asthma, and anaphylaxis may accompany urticarial responses.

In a relatively small number of instances urticaria results from direct contact with certain substances after a delay of from a few to thirty minutes. The number of substances causing such reactions is probably quite large; a partial list appears in Table 20-7. Some of these substances, including dimethyl sulfoxide and nettle plant extract, appear to release histamine and other vasoactive substances directly; others, such as potato extracts and phenyl-mercuric propionate, release mediators as part of an immunologic response. In still other cases the mechanism is not clear. The diagnosis of contact urticaria should be suggested by the history and the site of urticarial lesions. Open patch testing and scratch testing of the skin with observation for relatively immediate reactions can be confirmatory but should be performed with great care if anaphylaxis appears to be part of the syndrome. Passive transfer tests and the radioallergosorbent test (RAST) may be helpful.

Long-term management and prevention depend on identifying and eliminating the cause. Antihistamines provide symptomatic therapy. In an emergency that threatens respiratory obstruction, intramuscular epinephrine and intravenous hydrocortisone are the treatment of choice, and tracheostomy equipment should be available. Systemic steroids should rarely be necessary except in severe acute episodes.

V. CUTANEOUS GRANULOMAS

Contact with a number of foreign materials can produce cutaneous granulomas. These may present as slightly erythematous and more or less flesh-colored firm papules which can be grouped and may be associated with inflammatory changes. They are generally confined to sites of contact or inoculation with the causal agents. Zirconium, beryllium, and chromium salts (in tatoos) appear to cause granulomas on an immunological basis. In these cases intracutaneous testing or patch testing may confirm the hypersensitivity. Other foreign materials such as talc and silica introduced subcutaneously appear to cause granulomas in the absence of immunological hypersensitivity. A biopsy can confirm the presence of a granuloma. Specialized stains, polarized light, phase microscopy, and other techniques may allow foreign materials to be visualized and identified.

Table 20-7. **Selected Causes of Contact Urticaria**

Cosmetics (nailpolish, hair sprays, etc.)
Formaldehyde, ammonia
Wood dusts
Horse serum
Streptomycin, penicillin, neomycin
Chlorpromazine
Aspirin
Tetanus antitoxin
Phenylmercuric proprionate; dimethysulfoxide
Nettles, cacti, marine plants
Potato, wheat, carrots, flour
Fish, lamb, turkey skin
Spices
Wool, silk
Animal saliva and danders
Arthropods

VI. ACNE OF CHEMICAL ORIGIN

A number of chemical agents are known to precipitate acne; a partial list appears in Table 20-8. A number of chlorinated hydrocarbons encountered in industry are strongly acnegenic. The acne may occur on areas such as the forearms and anterior surface of the thighs—areas which are not generally affected by acne vulgaris. Pinpoint or larger comedones and varying degrees of inflammatory pustules, cysts, and abscesses are seen, and mutilating scars may result. Although outbreaks have occurred with a variety of manufacturing processes, the precise causal compounds have not always been identified. Frequently, chlorinated debenzodioxins and dibenzofurans present as contaminants of other chlorinated hydrocarbons have been particularly suspect. In some instances, acquired porphyria, hepatotoxicity, neurotoxicity, and teratogenesis have also been observed. Only small amounts of these acnegens are necessary to provoke lesions, and family members of affected workers have also developed acne. The condition is generally difficult to treat. The only really effective measure is removal from the environment, and even so lesions may persist many years.

Table 20-8. **Chemical Causes of Acne**

Chloracne
  2,4-D (2,4-dichlorophenoxyacetic acid)
  2,4,5-T (2,4,5-trichlorophenoxyacetic acid)
    manufacture
  3,4,3,4-tetrachloroazoxybenzene
  2,3,7,8-tetrachlorodibenzo-*p*-dioxin (TCDD)
  2,6-dichlorobenzonitrile manufacture
  DDT manufacture
  Chlorinated biphenyls, chlorinated napthalenes,
    dibenzodioxins, dibenzofurans, and others

Yusho
  Cooking oil that contains polychlorinated
    biphenyls

Acne Cosmetica
  Numerous weakly comedogenic cosmetic
    components

Other Industrial Materials
  Cutting oils
  Coal tar derivatives
  Asbestos
  Crude petroleum oils

Agents that Exacerbate Preexisting Acne
  Topical and systemic adrenocortical steroids
  Androgens
  Diphenylhydantoin
  Trimethadone

Drug-induced Acne
  Iodides
  Bromides
  Isoniazid
  Quinine
  Chloral hydrate
  Thiourea

Antibiotics and other measures tend to be less effective than in acne vulgaris. The use of local acne preparations containing sulphur and/or vitamin A acid to produce mild peeling may be helpful. Acne surgery has been the most beneficial single measure. Systemic steroids may be necessary in severe inflammatory cases.

An epidemic of "Yusho" was reported from Japan due to the ingestion of rice oil contaminated with polychlorinated biphenyls (particularly tetrachlorobiphenyl). Symptoms included nausea, lethargy, subcutaneous edema of the face and upper eyelids, acneiform lesions, pigmentation of the nails and skin, and conjunctival hyperemia. The disorder appears more often in children, adolescents, and young adults.

Acneiform eruptions appear to be precipitated by local preparations applied to the skin, including topical adrenocortical steroids and a number of cosmetic preparations.

VII. FOLLICULITIS

Certain foreign substances lead to superficial folliculitis manifested by small, itchy, follicular or perifollicular papules and pustules which may rupture and heal without scarring. Causal agents include oils, greases, and certain coal tar pitches and their derivatives. Lesions are more prone to occur on areas of contact where there is also friction and pressure such as the buttocks, back, and thighs and forearms. Treatment consists of removal of causal factors and the use of mildly astringent topical preparations. A more severe and deeper inflammatory pustular folliculitis has been described from contact with sharp needles of sugar cane bark. In this case, follicular atrophy and permanent hair loss may occur.

VIII. DAMAGE TO HAIR

Chemical agents can produce two major types of damage to hair.

A. KERATOLYTIC DAMAGE

Alkalies, thioglycollates, and oxidizing agents such as peroxides and perborates produce keratolysis when they contact the hair shaft locally. This leads to softening, matting, and increased fragility of hair. Either local patches or the entire scalp may be involved depending on the extent of exposure. Treatment consists of removing the offending exposure. Because the hair matrix cells that produce hair are not usually damaged, the long-term prognosis is good.

B. MATRIX CELL DAMAGE

Agents that affect the hair matrix lead to patchy or complete alopecia. Agents that cause this damage are most frequently absorbed systemically, and the complaint is of scalp hair coming out "by the roots."

Notable causes are thallium (used in rodenticides), chloroprene dimers (encountered during neoprene manufacture), arsenic, and certain drugs including antimitotic agents (nitrogen mustards, alkylating agents including cyclophosphamide, aminopterin, and methotrexate), atabrine, heparin, colchicine, and oral contraceptives. The hair loss is generally reversible after the medication or environmental exposure is discontinued.

Examination of sufficient shed and plucked hairs may allow one to differentiate between agents that directly poison the hair in the anagen (growth) phase and those which precipitate the telogen (resting) hair phase leading to the loss of "club" hairs. Agents such as antimitotic agents and colchicine cause the former type of damage with hair loss within days to weeks after administration of the agent; oral contraceptives and heparin cause telogen effluvium (hair loss) after a delay of two to four months.

IX. CHANGES IN PIGMENTATION

Numerous phenols and catechols are toxic to pigment cells and produce localized depigmentation. These include hydroquinone, monobenzyl ether of hydroquinone (which is used in rubber as an antioxidant), Paratertiary butylphenyl, Paratertiary amylphenol, and 4 tertiary catechol. Some unrelated agents may also cause depigmentation such as ammoniated mercury. Arsenic may cause both circumscribed areas of pigment loss and a generalized increase in pigmentation. Localized increases in pigmentation result from contact with tars, psoralens, and other materials that cause phototoxic reactions. Such localized hyperpigmentation may also follow cutaneous inflammation. A number of foreign chemicals and drugs cause generalized changes in skin color including busulphan (brown), chlorpromazine and its derivatives (slate gray or purple), and silver (gray black).

X. SKIN CANCER

Skin cancers result from a variety of environmental exposures, generally after a latent period of many years. Causes include contact over a considerable period of time with a variety of tars and pitches, soot, creosote and related materials which contain polycyclic aromatic hydrocarbons. The exposures result in keratoses and squamous cell carcinomata. Inorganic arsenic compounds in medications such as Fowler's solution, industrial and agricultural products, and drinking water may also cause skin tumors including keratoses, squamous cell carcinomas, multiple superficial basal cell epitheliomas, and areas of Bowen's disease (intraepidermal carcinoma). When arsenic is the cause, skin tumors are often multiple and tend to occur on areas of the skin shielded from the sun. Other indices of arsenic toxicity include multiple punctate keratoses on the hands and feet, pigmentary changes and an increased incidence of visceral tumors (lung, esophagus, mouth, urogenital tract, and liver).

Among white populations and especially in sunny areas of the world, skin cancers generally result from the ultraviolet radiation in sunlight. However, the interaction between ultraviolet radiation and certain chemical agents (including some polycyclic aromatic hydrocarbons) can enhance carcinogenesis.

BIBLIOGRAPHY

I. CORROSION AND ULCERATION

Berkhout, P. G., et al.: Treatment of skin burns due to alkyl mercury compounds. Arch. Envir. Health, *3:*592–593, 1961.

Birmingham, D., and Key, M. M.: An outbreak of arsenical dermatosis in a mining community. Arch. Dermatol., *91:*457–464, 1965.

Browne, T. D.: The treatment of hydrofluoric acid burns. J. Soc. Occup. Med., *24:*80–89, 1974.

Curreri, W. P., Asch, M. J., and Pruitt, B. A.: The treatment of chemical burns: specialized diagnostic and prognostic considerations. J. Trauma, *10:* 634–642, 1970.

Fellar, I., Archambeault-Jones, C., and Richards, K. E.: Emergent Care of the Burn Victim. Ann Arbor, National Institute for Burn Medicine, 1977.

Fisher, A. A.: Contact Dermatitis. 2nd ed. Philadelphia, Lea & Febiger, 1973.

Rudowski, W., Nasilowski, W., Zietkiewicz, W., and Zienkiewicz, K.: Burn Therapy and Research. Baltimore, Johns Hopkins University Press, 1976.

Samitz, M. H., and Epstein, E.: Experimental cutaneous chrome ulcers in guinea pigs. Arch. Envir. Health, *5:*463–468, 1962.

Summerlin, W. T., Walder, A. E., and Moncrief, J. A.: White phosphorus burns and massive hemolysis. J. Trauma, *7:*476–484, 1967.

II. ECZEMATOUS DERMATITIS

Adams, R. M.: Occupational Contact Dermatitis, Philadelphia, J. B. Lippincott, 1969.

Emmett, E. A.: Drug Photoallergy. Int. J. Dermatol., *17:*370–379, 1978.

Emmett, E. A., and Suskind, R. R.: Occupational dermatoses. *In* Fitzpatrick, T. B., et al. (eds.):

Dermatology in General Medicine. 2nd ed. New York, McGraw-Hill, 1979.

Fisher, A. A.: Contact Dermatitis. 2nd ed. Philadelphia, Lea & Febiger, 1973.

Fregert, S.: Manual of Contact Dermatitis. Copenhagen, Munksgaard, 1974.

III. FIBERGLASS DERMATITIS

Possick, P. A., Gellin, G. A., and Key, M. M.: Fibrous glass dermatitis. Am. Indust. Hyg. Assoc. J., *31:*12, 1970.

IV. URTICARIA

Odum, R. B., and Maibach, H. I.: Contact urticaria: a different contact dermatitis. *In* Marzulli, F. N., and Maibach, H. I. (eds.): Dermatoxicology and Pharmacology. New York, John Wiley and Sons, 1977.

VI. ACNE OF CHEMICAL ORIGIN

Kimbrough, R. D.: Toxicity of chlorinated hydrocarbons and related compounds. Arch. Envir. Health, *25:*125, 1972.

Kligman, A. M., and Mills, O. H.: Acne cosmetica. Arch. Dermatol., *98:*53, 1972.

Kuratsune, M., Yoshimura, T., Matsuzaka, J., and Yamaguchi, A.: Epidemiologic study on Yusho, a poisoning caused by ingestion of rice oil contaminated with a commercial brand of polychlorinated biphenyls. Envir. Health Persp., *1:*119–128, 1972.

Taylor, J. S., Wuthrich, R. C., Lloyd, K. M., and Poland, A.: Chloracne from manufacture of a new herbicide. Arch. Dermatol., *113:*616, 1977.

X. SKIN CANCER

Emmett, E. A.: Occupational skin cancer. J. Occupat. Med., *17:*44–49, 1975.

21. ANIMAL TOXINS

Irwin B. Hanenson, M.D.

Toxins are produced by animals representing all phyla from unicellular organisms to mammals. The venoms are proteins varying significantly in structure and mechanism of action. This heterogeneity produces a spectrum of medical problems requiring specific as well as supportive therapy.

This chapter will focus on the arthropods, reptiles, and mammals that are responsible for the majority of medically significant poisonings. Emphasis will be placed on clinical identification and management.

I. ARTHROPODA

A. INSECTS

1. Flying Insects

The flying insects include bees, wasps, yellow jackets, and hornets. This group, including ants, is responsible for more deaths from animal toxins than any other group. They account for approximately 40% of the deaths as contrasted to approximately 33% from snakes and 20% from spiders. Death generally occurs more quickly from insect bites than from the other two groups. Insect victims may die within an hour after the sting. The usual period following snake bites is from 6 to 48 hours; following spider bites, approximately 18 hours.

a. Clinical Features

Flying insect stings may present as a small raised erythematous area with a central hemorrhagic zone which represents the site of insertion of the stinger and may contain the stinging element when the patient is seen. Symptoms are pain and itching that is relieved by the application of ice. No other specific treatment is necessary. There is spontaneous resolution of the skin lesion and, ultimately, symptoms.

In the more severe cases, there are marked hypotension, respiratory difficulties, peripheral neuritis, and hemoglobinuria. There may be a sensitivity reaction manifested by collapse of the patient accompanied by bronchoconstriction, pulmonary edema, and edema of the face and lips. Death may occur within an hour.

b. Treatment

Since one is dealing with an anaphylactic reaction which can produce death in over 75% of the victims within one hour and virtually 100% in five hours, it is essential that definitive therapy be instituted immediately.

(1) Administer epinephrine 0.2–0.5 ml. of a 1:1000 solution intravenously. Retain the intravenous line in place for the administration of additional drugs and fluids. If for any reason it is difficult to perform a venipuncture, the drug should be administered subcutaneously.

(2) Establish a patent airway by the insertion of an endotracheal tube. This is to assure adequate oxygenation in the patient with laryngopulmonary edema accompanied by bronchial constriction. The latter would be relieved by the action of epinephrine.

(3) Circulatory collapse should be treated with intravenous fluids, e.g., normal saline, Ringer's lactate.

(4) Antihistamines may be helpful but do not substitute for epinephrine in the more severe cases of intoxication. When indicated, either diphenhydramine (Benadryl), 50 mg., or chlorpheniramine maleate (Chlor-Trimeton), 4 mg., is effective.

(5) Hydrocortisone intravenously may

also be employed in patients with life-threatening cardiovascular collapse. However, this drug, although supportive, does not act quickly enough and should not be considered as a substitute for epinephrine.

In summary, the basic treatment for severe intoxication following insect stings consists of epinephrine accompanied by fluid volume replacement to control the anaphylactic reaction accompanied by circulatory shock.

2. Ants

Ant stings may be painful but are rarely fatal.

a. Clinical Features

Pain and itching occur around the site of the sting, with swelling and possibly blister formation.

b. Treatment

Generally, supportive treatment is adequate. This consists of antihistamines, ice, and pain medication. In anaphylactic-type reactions, epinephrine and steroids may be indicated.

3. Other Insects

Caterpillars, millipedes, and centipedes are those most likely to cause significant clinical problems.

a. Clinical Features

Most commonly noted are redness, swelling, pain, itching, and, occasionally, blister formation. On occasion, tissue necrosis and ulcer formation may occur following caterpillar and centipede bites. Anaphylactic reactions may occur with shock.

b. Treatment

As for other insect bites, basic treatment is supportive and consists of antihistamines, cold application, and analgesics. Epinephrine and steroids should be employed for anaphylactic reactions.

B. ARACHNIDS

1. Spiders

Over 100,000 species of spiders have been identified, making them the most varied, widespread, and numerous animals. They are ubiquitous, extending throughout all life-sustaining areas of the world with the exception of deep water. All spiders produce venom that they inject into their prey to kill and make them available for food.

It has been stated that approximately 50 species of spiders produce human bites. However, severe reactions have been restricted to the genera *Latrodectus* and *Loxosceles*.

a. Latrodectus

This genus is found throughout the United States and Canada. The most common areas of human contact are old wood piles and trash.

Of this genus, the most dangerous to humans is the black widow. Only the female is dangerous. It is black with orange to red markings on the abdomen, shaped in the form of an hourglass. Deaths from this species are rare, occurring primarily in children and elderly people, particularly from multiple bites.

(1) Clinical Features

The bite is characterized by two tiny red marks which identify the entry point of the fangs. Within 30 minutes, there are severe local pains followed by extension of the pain over the entire body including the chest, abdomen, and legs. Nausea, salivation, and sweating also occur. Subsequently, breathing becomes labored, and rigidity of the abdominal, chest, or back muscles can occur. The progression of symptoms occurs rapidly, and coma may occur within 30 minutes. Recovery may begin within several hours and is complete within a week. In summary, the venom causes no tissue necrosis, but it does have a primary neurotoxic effect.

(2) Treatment

(a) For pain give aspirin or a narcotic.

(b) For muscle cramping and spasms, give calcium carbonate, 10 ml. of 10% solution I.V. Administer methocarbomal (Robaxin) 10 ml. I.V. over a 5-minute period followed by 10 ml. in 250 ml. of 5% glucose over 2 hours. If necessary, for the next 24 hours give 80 mg. P.O. every 6 hours.

(c) The antidote is antivenin (Lyovac) 1 unit added to 500 ml. of 5% dextrose in water I.V. over several hours. A skin test of 0.1 mil of a 1:10 dilution in saline intradermally should precede the infusion to test for a serum reaction. Improvement is generally observed within a few hours after the start of the infusion.

b. Loxosceles

This genus, which is also toxic to man, is also found over the entire United States. The species most identified with toxicity is the brown recluse spider. It is relatively small with a light yellow to medium brown body and a darker brown violin-shaped patch on the back. Here too, the female is the more dangerous. The spider lives primarily in undisturbed places such as abandoned houses, cellars, and barns. They are also found in grass and cliffs.

(1) Clinical Features

Initially there is little or no pain. Within a few hours, however, pain develops and is accompanied by blisters, redness, and swelling of the area around the bite. The untreated lesion may continue to increase in size for several days. Necrosis, when it does occur, begins at the center of the bite which becomes indurated and then ischemic. This leads to a necrotic area that detaches, leaving an open ulcer. The ulcer is characterized by its failure to heal, persisting for weeks or even months. Systemic manifestations include fever,

chills, joint pain, vomiting, generalized rash, and delirium. Intravascular hemolysis also occurs. Monitoring of the hemoglobin and hematocrit for 48 hours is recommended.

(2) Treatment

(a) Excision of the bite, including indurated skin and fascia, is helpful because the toxin remains in the fascia for a long time. When the infecting source is removed, the patient's condition will improve and the ulcer heals. Should the ulcer not be excised, it may continue to grow for some time.

(b) Give steroids to control the systemic reaction. They will have no effect on the ulcer.

(c) Give blood transfusion if needed.

(d) Antibiotics will control secondary infection.

(e) Tetanus prophylaxis is necessary.

(f) Dialysis may be necessary if renal shutdown occurs secondary to intravascular hemolysis. Prednisolone, 50 mg. I.V., followed by 25 mg. every six hours, may be beneficial for hemolytic crisis.

C. SCORPIONS

Of the hundreds of species of scorpions, the larger and more poisonous are found in hot, dry climates such as North Africa, the Middle East, and Mexico. They are well adapted to life on the desert. The most poisonous species belong to the family Buthidae and are not found in the United States.

Scorpions have a crablike appearance with eight legs and pincers. They are all venomous. The stinger occurs in the tip of the tail. The sting is painful and the venom may be fatal, but death is rare. For prevention, exercise caution when around scrap lumber and debris in endemic areas.

First aid until arriving at a medical facility after being stung should include hypothermia. Place the extremity in a vessel of ice water until reaching a hospital.

1. Clinical Features

These may be divided into two groups. The first includes all but two species of scorpions. Toxicity is manifested by a severe local reaction, including pain and swelling with ecchymosis. Prickly sensations occur around the mouth and the tongue feels thick. The second group produces a severe systemic reaction with little or no local effect. There may be some pain around the site of the bite, but the major effects are systemic, including respiratory difficulties, sensation of a thick tongue, muscular spasms, drooling, abdominal cramps and distention, convulsions, diplopia, blindness, nystagmus, involuntary passage of urine and feces, hypertension, cardiac arrhythmias, and pulmonary edema.

Duration of symptoms is usually one to two days, but the neurological manifestations may persist up to a week. Fatalities are rare and occur chiefly in children and adults with elevated blood pressure.

2. Treatment

a. Apply a constricting band above the bite to slow absorption of venom.

b. Maintain adequate oxygenation if there is respiratory difficulty.

c. Apply cold packs to the site of the sting to help slow absorption. This may be beneficial if done for the first hour or two after the sting.

d. The antidote is antivenin when available for the particular species.

e. For pain, avoid morphine and morphine derivatives including meperidine (Demerol) because these drugs have a synergistic effect with scorpion venom. Effective relief can be achieved with nerve blocks using Lidocaine.

f. For convulsions, diazepam may be useful. Chlorpromazine has also been reported to be beneficial.

D. TICKS

Ticks are found in damp areas, grass, and weeds. They are attracted by animal odors. Sheep, cattle, and dogs are most often the hosts. Paralysis and death in humans is rare.

The toxicity is the result of a toxin secreted by the pregnant female.

Children are usually the ones affected, but occasional cases have been reported in elderly people.

1. Clinical Features

The symptoms are those of a progressive, ascending motor paralysis. Ataxia, weakness, and paralysis develop 12–24 hours after attachment of the tick. This may be accompanied by respiratory failure. Early clinical manifestations often include irritability, anorexia and leg pain. The patient remains conscious, but speech is impaired and there is difficulty in swallowing.

Differential diagnosis must be made with poliomyelitis, since both occur during the hot months of the year and have similar symptomatology. Tick bites differ from polio in that there is generally absence of fever, normal spinal fluid, and loss of deep tendon reflexes before paralysis. Most definitive in the differential is a careful examination and discovery of a tick.

2. Treatment

a. Locate the tick. Look carefully in hairy areas such as the head, axillae, and perineum. Discovery of one tick does not preclude the presence of others.

b. Remove the tick, making certain the mouth parts are included. This can be done by application of a drop of ether, gasoline, or benzene to the tick or the careful burning of the tick with a lighted cigarette. Wait several minutes after these maneuvers before attempting to pull the tick off. If necessary, excise a small piece of skin with the tick attached.

c. Provide supportive treatment including intravenous fluids and adequate oxygenation by maintaining a patent airway and mechanical ventilation.

II. MARINE ANIMALS

A. FISH

Some fish in tropical climates may become poisonous at certain times of the year by feeding on marine organisms. Others such as puffers, trigger fish, and parrot fish are poisonous throughout the year. Finally, a group including the moray eel, surgeon fish, moon fish, porcupine fish, file fish, and go fish is only toxic a portion of the year in certain localities.

The most common type of fish poisoning is known as "ciguatera" and occurs with fish ordinarily considered to be edible, e.g., grouper, surgeon fish, barracuda, pompono, mackerel, butterfly fish, snapper, sea bass, perch. These fish become poisonous in certain localities.

The puffer group seems to have the most potent toxin, called tetrodotoxin, with a mortality rate as high as 50%. The mortality rate depends on the physical condition of the person, quantity of fish eaten, and the degree of toxicity of the toxin. In general, the mortality is less than 10%.

The toxin present in the flesh or visceral organs of the fish exerts its primary effect on the peripheral nervous system, but the mechanism of action is unknown.

1. Clinical Features

Symptoms of acute poisoning begin 30 minutes to 4 hours after ingestion and include numbness and paresthesias of the face and lips which spreads to the extremities. This is accompanied by nausea, vomiting, diarrhea, dizziness, abdominal pain, and muscular weakness. In severe cases, the symptoms progress to muscular paralysis, dyspnea, and convulsions. Death may occur from convulsions or respiratory arrest within 1–24 hours. If the patient recovers from the acute episode, muscular weakness and the paresthesias may persist for weeks.

2. Treatment

a. Emesis or lavage.
b. Establish an adequate airway and treat respiratory failure to assure optimum oxygenation.
c. For convulsions, give diazepam.
d. For shock, provide volume expanders and pressor agents as indicated.

B. SHELLFISH

Mussels, clams, oysters, and other shellfish may become poisonous during the warm months from feeding on certain dinoflagellates.

1. Clinical Features

The major and most severe toxic effect of shellfish poisoning is respiratory paralysis. There may also be numbness and paresthesias of the lips, tongue, face, and extremities with nausea and vomiting. Convulsions may occur.

Fatality rates are between 1% and 10%. Patient survival for 12 hours is generally followed by complete recovery.

2. Treatment

a. Gastric lavage or emesis.
b. Maintain a patent airway to assure oxygenation with mechanical respirators if necessary.

C. SNAILS, SEA URCHINS, AND CORAL

1. Snails

Marine snails of the genus *Conus* are venomous. Mild intoxication resembles insect stings and requires symptomatic therapy.

More severe intoxications are accompanied by severe pain, numbness, paresthesias, weakness, and paralysis which may involve part or all musculature and may cause difficulty in swallowing, constriction of the chest, visual disturbance, and collapse.

Treatment is entirely symptomatic. No fatalities have been reported in North

America; some deaths have occurred in the South Pacific and Indian Ocean.

2. Sea Urchins

This group causes painful injuries, including dizziness and muscular palsy which lasts for several hours.

Treatment is symptomatic.

3. Coral

The corals produce stinging with hemorrhagic lesions which may lead to necrosis. Intoxication may be more severe with abdominal cramps, chills, and diarrhea.

Treatment is symptomatic.

D. STINGRAY

1. Clinical Features

There is local pain and swelling accompanied by nausea, vomiting, abdominal pain, dizziness, weakness, cramps, sweating, and hypotension. Recovery occurs in 24–48 hours.

2. Treatment

a. Remove foreign materials from wound.

b. Perform surgical debridement if necessary with closure of the wound.

E. SCORPION FISH

1. Clinical Features

There is local pain and swelling with extension to involve the entire extremity.

2. Treatment

a. Treat as for stingray.

b. For pain give analgesics as necessary.

F. JELLYFISH AND PORTUGUESE MAN-OF-WAR

1. Clinical Features

There is urticaria with numbness and pain of the extremity, chest and abdominal pain, abdominal rigidity, and difficulty in swallowing. Death is rare.

2. Treatment

a. For muscular cramps, give 10 ml. of 10% calcium gluconate I.V.

b. Attempt to remove venom locally by application of aromatic spirits of ammonia.

G. STONEFISH

1. Clinical Features

These include intense radiating pain with blanching, then cyanosis of the affected part, nausea, vomiting, fever, delirium, respiratory distress, and convulsions.

2. Treatment

a. Treat as for stingray and scorpion fish.

b. Specific antiserum is available and may be obtained from the Department of Health, Commonwealth Serum Laboratories, Melbourne, Australia.

III. REPTILES

A. SNAKES

Poisonous snakes are more numerous in tropical areas but are also present in most parts of the temperate zone.

Although only a small number of deaths from snakebite occur annually in the United States, there are as many as 30,000–40,000 throughout the world.

Snake venoms are complex protein structures which may be neurotoxic, hemorrhagic, thrombogenic, hemolytic, proteolytic, and bactericidal.

All poisonous snakes have a common characteristic and that is the ability to introduce venom into an animal. This requires fangs. Thus, a poisonous snake must possess fangs. All snakes have small teeth, but these should not be confused with fangs. After an alleged snakebite, it is important to identify fang marks. Although in general there should be two puncture sites, in certain instances, only one fang may have penetrated the skin.

Venomous snakes in the United States are members of the Crotalidae or pit viper family or the Elapidae or coral snake family. The pit vipers have movable fangs, whereas coral snakes have fixed fangs.

1. Pit Vipers

The pit vipers include rattlesnakes, moccasins, and copperheads in the United States and the bushmaster in South America. These snakes are so named because they have a pit below the nostril that is a heat-sensitive device that aids in directing the snake in striking at the victim. Pit vipers are found in almost all of the continental states.

Pit viper venom contains four factors that are present in varying amounts in each species: neurotoxic, spreading, digestive, and hemorrhagic. The systemic reaction is variable even within the same species of snake. Deaths have been reported from hemorrhage or neurotoxin effects.

a. Clinical Features

Symptoms may begin within minutes. The severity of toxicity depends upon the amount of venom injected. Initially, there is discoloration of skin, pain, tenderness, and edema around the site of venom injection. Ecchymosis develops over several hours, and it progresses to hemorrhagic vesiculations. Subsequently, weakness, sweating, nausea, paresthesias, or numbness of the tongue, mouth, or scalp may occur. With severe envenomation, there may be hematemesis, muscle cramping, and possibly paralysis, shock, and convulsions.

b. Laboratory Examination

Measurements should be made for CBC, prothrombin time, partial thromboplastin time, fibrinogen, hematocrit, hemoglobin, platelet count, and serum electrolytes and creatinine. The patient should also be typed and crossmatched for blood.

c. Treatment: First Aid

1. The victim should be moved as little as possible, especially the area of the bite. The recumbent position is preferable. Remove all jewelry and dentures before swelling becomes too severe to do so.

2. The person attending the victim should kill the snake if it can be quickly located and bring the specimen to the hospital for identification. An attempt should be made to at least identify the snake if it cannot be captured or killed. Care should be taken not to touch the snake with the hands.

3. Apply a constricting band (tourniquet) 5–10 cm. proximal to the wound tight enough to impede venous and lymphatic flow but not so tight as to reduce arterial blood flow. A good guide is to apply the ligature loose enough to admit a finger between it and the skin. The ligature should be released for approximately 90 seconds every 10–15 minutes. Do not apply a ligature if more than 30 minutes has elapsed since the bite.

4. Immobilize extremity in position of function.

5. If available, a cold pack may be applied to the wound. Under no circumstances should the wound area be packed in ice or immersed in water.

6. Transport the victim to a medical facility as soon as possible for specific treatment.

7. Do not give the victim anything to drink, especially alcohol.

d. Treatment: Hospital

1. Obtain history including time since bite and whether or not first aid was administered.

2. Identify snake.

3. Search for the fang marks to determine exact location of bite.

4. Provide I.V. infusion in unaffected extremity.

5. Immobilize extremity and, if less than 10 minutes has elapsed since bite occurred, apply constricting ligature, incise fang marks, and remove venom by suction.

6. Skin test for antivenin sensitivity. In those persons who are sensitive to antivenin, desensitization may be carried out by the preparation of a 1:100 solution of antiserum with injections of 0.1, 0.2, and 0.5 ml. of the solution I.V. at 15-minute intervals. This should then be repeated with a 1:10 solution. Keep on hand a 1:1,000 solution of epinephrine in case of an emergency. If you cannot wait for desensitization, epinephrine should be administered prior to and along with the antiserum as needed.

7. There is no evidence to indicate that antihistamines, cortisone, incision and suction 30 minutes after the bite, or cryotherapy is of benefit.

8. Add the appropriate type and amount of antivenin to the intravenous infusion at a rate which would deliver the required amount within three to four hours.

9. Give tetanus prophylaxis.

10. Give analgesics for control of pain. Avoid depressant narcotics.

11. Check vital signs frequently, at least every hour. Also, determine blood count every four hours for hidden bleeding or hemolysis. Maintain blood pressure with intravenous fluids, or if hemoglobin falls below 10 gm., give packed red cells or whole blood to raise the hemoglobin to 12 gm. per 100 ml. Give fibrinogen or platelets if necessary.

12. For respiratory paralysis, maintain a patent airway and support with mechanical ventilation.

13. Check the circulation distal to the bite every hour. An increase in subfascial tension may occlude arterial blood flow with gangrene of the extremity distal to the bite. This increase in tension is due to the development of subfascial edema, and a fasciotomy is indicated. Because of this possible complication, it is advisable following admission to the hospital to obtain a surgical consult for possible fasciotomy and later debridement.

14. Treat renal failure with usual methods including appropriate balance of fluid and electrolytes and hemodialysis.

15. Give antibiotics as indicated.

16. Perhaps the most common error in treating snakebite is the use of insufficient amounts of antivenin.

2. Coral Snakes

This snake is found in essentially the same areas as the pit viper. It is a small, thin snake with a small, round black eye. In contrast to the pit viper, its fangs are fixed, and these snakes therefore do not strike but hold and chew their victim. They usually have alternating red, yellow, and black bands on their bodies and a black head.

a. Clinical Features

The venom of the coral snake has an action which is primarily paralytic. Tissue reaction at the site of the insertion of fangs is generally mild and consists of some pain within a short period of time and a slow onset of swelling. The neurotoxic manifestations appear within one hour but often may be delayed for a longer period of time. General symptoms consist of nausea, salivation, vomiting, weakness, drowsiness, and paralysis of the facial muscles, lips, tongue, and larynx. Blood pressure generally decreases, and respiratory difficulty occurs. In more extreme situations, convulsions may occur with a bulbar-type paralysis and respiratory paralysis. The sensorium generally remains clear until death occurs.

Of significance is the fact that the venom effects, despite complete paralysis, can be reversible.

b. Treatment

All patients should be treated in a medical facility as soon as possible.

a. Check vital signs and provide with supportive therapy. It is important to maintain a patent airway and to assure proper ventilation.

b. Start an intravenous infusion, and after appropriate testing for sensitivity as with the pit viper antivenin, administer it intravenously through the infusion.

c. Wash the area of the bite to remove any unabsorbed venom.

d. Administer tetanus prophylaxis.

Early and adequate specific antiserum treatment will reduce the mortality rate from all snake bites to below 10%.

B. GILA MONSTER

This animal is the only poisonous lizard. It lives in the desert areas of the southwestern United States and northern Mexico. It does not have fangs like snakes, but rather grooves in the front teeth which carry the venom. The venom produces tissue destruction similar to that of a pit viper bite.

1. Clinical Features

Symptoms consist of local swelling and pain which spreads rapidly, nausea, vomiting, shortness of breath, cyanosis, weakness, tachycardia, and scotoma (blinding lights).

2. Treatment

Gila monster bites are rarely fatal. Treatment is, therefore, essentially supportive.

a. If there is copious bleeding at the site of the bite—generally caused by attempting to remove the animal, which tenaciously clings to its victim—simply irrigate the wound with normal saline and apply a pressure dressing. Removal of a tenacious lizard is generally accomplished before arrival at the hospital. It should be done by prying the jaws apart by cutting the muscles of the mouth at the angle of the jaw, or pulling the lizard off, which may be simpler than anticipated because the teeth are easily pulled out. This last maneuver can be best done by grasping the lizard behind the forelegs and pulling it from the victim.

b. Supportive therapy is as for snakebite.

c. There is generally no antivenin readily available.

BIBLIOGRAPHY

Arnold, R. E.: Brown recluse spider bites: five cases with a review of the literature. J. Am. Col. Emerg. Physicians, *5:*262, 1976.

Frazier, C. A.: Insect stings: a medical emergency. J.A.M.A., *235:*2410, 1976.

Russell, F. E.: Pharmacology of toxins of marine organisms. Int. Encyclo. Pharm. Ther., *71*(2):3, 1971.

Southcott, R. V.: Australia venomous and poisonous fishes. Clin. Toxicol., *10:*291, 1977.

Russell, F. E., Carlson, R. W., Wainschell, J., and Osborne, A. H.: Snake venom poisoning in the United States: experiences with 550 cases. J.A.M.A., *233:*341, 1975.

Glass, T. G., Jr.: Early debridement in pit viper bites. J.A.M.A., *235:*2513, 1976.

Poisonous Snakes of the World: a Manual for Use by U.S. Amphibious Forces. Nav. Med. P-5099, Department of the Navy, Bureau of Medicine and Surgery, 1968.

22. PLANT TOXINS

Diana Burton, B.S. Pharm., and Irwin B. Hanenson, M.D.

Drawings by Susan Wilchins, B.F.A.

The National Clearinghouse for Poison Control Centers, in its September 1976 bulletin, reported that plants were among the three substances most frequently ingested by children under five years of age. This is a rise of 20% over the previous year. Plants represent about 4% of accidental poisonings in all age groups in the United States.

The number of deaths from plant ingestions is low. However, the ingestions are of concern not for their lethal qualities but for the morbidity associated with them. The following toxic plants are the most frequently ingested: philodendron, yew, pyracantha*, nightshade, holly, poinsettia, dieffenbachia, black elder, oleander, Jerusalum cherry, jimsonweed, mistletoe (Tables 22-1 and 22-2; Figures 22-1 to 22-11).

Approximately 700 species of North American plants are considered to be poisonous. Toxicity is usually related to the genus, and if one species of a genus is toxic, some or all others in the genus generally display similar toxicity. However, the content of a given poisonous principle, and to some extent its molecular structure, can vary widely in some species depending upon geographic region. Furthermore, within a species there can be variations in absolute quantities and relative proportions of toxic principles deter-

mined by environmental growth factors, maturity of plant, and products of enzymatic action during storage and drying.

Additional factors influencing toxicity are:

1. Individual variation of patient (age, sex, weight).
2. Quantity of plant material ingested.
3. Whether or not the hard coat has been cracked if a seed is ingested. Usually seeds are capable of passing through the alimentary tract without ill effects if not pierced, ground, or chewed.
4. Quantity of poison absorbed by system.

There is only rarely a specific treatment or antidote for plant poisoning. In most cases the approach is supportive. A knowledge of the symptoms and the probable duration and prognosis of the poisoning is helpful. If no symptoms have occurred, and it has been more than 12 hours since ingestion, no treatment is usually necessary. Symptoms from plant ingestions usually appear within 4 hours. If there are no symptoms, and a potentially toxic plant was ingested within 4 hours, syrup of ipecac should be given, the dose adjusted to the weight and age of the patient. If the patient is watched for the next 12 hours, this is sufficient treatment in most cases.

If signs of poisoning are present, or if they develop late, then more definitive treatment is necessary. The symptoms in about three-fourths of plant poisoning cases involve the gastrointestinal tract causing nausea, vomiting, and diarrhea. However, plants that contain alkaloids will cause systemic reactions as well. So if it is not possible to identify the plant in a

---

*Although pyracantha has been reported as both nonpoisonous and poisonous depending upon the source consulted, the National Clearinghouse reports the symptoms of nausea, vomiting, diarrhea, abdominal pains, rash, and edema after ingestion and contact with the plant. No toxic principle has been identified in the plant thus far.

Table 22-1. **The Eleven Most Ingested Toxic Plants**

Plant	Toxic Part	Toxin	Symptoms	Treatment
Philodendron	All parts	Oxalates	See oxalates in text	See oxalates in text
Yew	All parts, especially seeds	Alkaloid taxine	See taxine in text	See taxine in text
Nightshade (includes bittersweet, eggplant, Jerusalem cherry, potato)	Green fruit and spoiled sprouts; ripe fruit harmless	Alkaloid solanine	See solanine in text	See solanine in text
Holly	Berries	Ilicin, ilexanthin, and ilex acid; not identified as to structure and exact action	Nausea, vomiting, diarrhea, and stupor	Gastric lavage and symptomatic care
Poinsettia	White latex exuding from all parts of plant when broken	Not identified	Very similar to oxalates	See oxalates in text
Dieffenbachia	All parts	Oxalates	See oxalates in text	See oxalates in text
Black Elder	All parts except berries	Cyanogenic glycoside sambunigrin	See cyanogenic glycoside in text	See cyanogenic glycoside in text
Oleander	All parts	Cardiac glycosides (neriosdie and oleandroside)	See glycosides in text	See glycosides in text
Jerusalem cherry	Berries	Alkaloid solanine	See solanine in text	See solanine in text
Jimsonweed	Seed	Atropine alkaloids	See atropine alkaloid in text	See atropine alkaloid in text
Mistletoe	All parts, especially berries	Tyramine and beta-phenylethylamine	Increased blood pressure, bradycardia, increased contractions of uterus and intestine	Gastric lavage, supportive care, potassium, procainamide, or quinidine

short period of time by checking with a botanist, poison control center, or library, then treat symptomatically.

The toxic principle has been identified in many of the poisonous plants, and it is now possible to categorize most plants according to their toxic constituent. A number of species of plants contain a toxic substance unique to each; however, there are always exceptions. A large and miscellaneous group of plants contain toxic principles whose nature is not yet fully understood or produce injury in an entirely mechanical manner. A few plants contain two or more toxic principles that are not in the same chemical group; thus, both constituents must be treated. The compounds produced in or absorbed by plants causing the toxic reactions are as follows:

1. Alkaloids
2. Polypeptides and amines
3. Glycosides
   a. Cyanogenetic glycosides
   b. Goitrogenic glycosides
   c. Irritant oils
   d. Coumarin glycosides
   e. Cardiac and saponins
4. Oxalates
5. Resins
6. Phytotoxins
7. Minerals

Table 22-2. Commonly Ingested Plants

Plant	Toxin
Aconitum (Monkshood)	Aconitine alkaloid
Amaryllis	Lycorine alkaloid
Angel's trumpet	Atropine alkaloid
Apple (seed)	Cyanogenic glycoside
Apricot (seed)	Cyanogenic glycoside
Autumn croccus	Colchicine alkaloid
Azalea	Andromedotoxin alkaloid
Beet	Oxalates
Belladonna (deadly nightshade)	Atropine alkaloids
Bitter almond	Cyanogenic glycoside
Black locust	Phytotoxins
Buckeye	Saponins
Buttercup	Irritant oils
Caladium (elephant's ear)	Oxalates
Calla lilly	Oxalates
Castor bean	Phytotoxins
Cherry (seed)	Cyanogenic glycoside
Daffodil	Lycorine alkaloid
Delphinium	Aconitine alkaloid
Devil's ivy (pothos)	Oxalates
English ivy	Saponins
Foxglove	Cardiac glycosides
Glory lilly	Colchicine alkaloid
Hemlock, poison	Coniine alkaloid
Hyacinth	Lycorine alkaloid
Hydrangea	Cyanogenic glycoside
Hyoscyamus (henbane)	Atropine alkaloids
Iris	Resins
Jack-in-the-pulpit	Oxalates
Jonquil	Lycorine alkaloid
Larkspur	Aconitine alkaloid
Lilly-of-the-valley	Cardiac glycosides
Lima bean	Cyanogenic glycoside
Matrimony vine	Atropine alkaloids
Mayapple	Resins
Milkweed	Resins
Monkshood (aconitum)	Aconitine alkaloid
Monstera species	Oxalates
Narcissus	Lycorine alkaloid
Peach (seed)	Cyanogenic glycoside
Plum (seed)	Cyanogenic glycoside
Pokeweed	Saponins and resins
Pothos (devil's ivy)	Oxalates
Privet	Andromedotoxin alkaloid
Rhododendron	Andromedotoxin alkaloid and resins
Rhubarb	Oxalates
Spider lily	Lycorine alkaloid
Syngonium (tri-leaf wonder)	Oxalates
Tuberose	Lycorine alkaloid
Wisteria	Resins

8. Nitrogenous compounds
9. Compounds causing photosensitivity

Because minerals, nitrogenous compounds, and compounds causing photosensitivity occur mostly in grazing food and cause poisonings of a chronic nature in livestock, and thus are not important in human ingestion, they will not be discussed in this chapter.

I. ALKALOIDS

The alkaloids are present in 5–10% of plant species and exert their pharmacological effect in small doses. The alkaloid content of a plant will usually vary little with environmental factors, and the alkaloid is usually distributed throughout all plant parts.

Most alkaloids exert their activity primarily through the nervous system, although the exact mechanism is poorly understood. The rate of onset of symptoms varies according to the mode of ingestion. The systemic effects vary according to the chemical structures of the alkaloid and can be categorized in this manner.

The *atropine*-containing plants produce:

1. Bilaterally, equally dilated pupils
2. Hot, dry flushed skin
3. Increased heart rate
4. Mania, delirium, and visual hallucinations
5. Urinary retention and constipation

Treatment consists of emesis or gastric lavage, and physostigmine given by slow intravenous injection in a dose of 1–4 mg. However, since physostigmine is rapidly destroyed, the dose must be repeated in one to two hours if necessary.

The alkaloid lycorine occurs in the onionlike bulbs of some plants. Severe poisonings have not been reported in humans and symptoms of mild intoxications are severe emesis, shivering, and some diarrhea. Treatment is symptomatic.

The alkaloid cholchicine in some plants

causes acute intoxications and the clinical characteristics are indistinguishable from an overdose of colchicine. The following symptoms of poisoning occur after a latency period of two to six hours and are:

1. Burning of the mouth and throat
2. Dysphagia
3. Intense thirst
4. Nausea followed by violent vomiting
5. Extensive fluid loss, which may lead to shock

The course of intoxication will be prolonged, because colchicine is excreted slowly. Treatment is gastric lavage as soon after ingestion as possible, fluid and electrolyte balance maintenance, and respiratory assistance, if necessary.

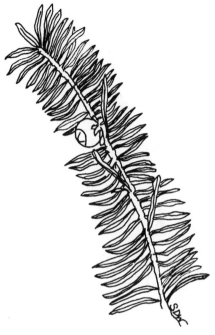

Fig. 22-2. Yew.

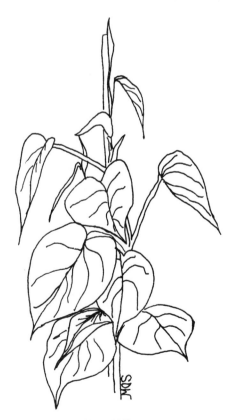

Fig. 22-1. Philodendron.

Aconitine is rapidly absorbed after ingestion or when in contact with mucous membranes. Poisoning by plants containing this alkaloid should be considered a medical emergency and treatment instituted immediately. Symptoms include:

1. Tingling and burning of the lips and mouth with numbness
2. Severe headache with restlessness and confusion
3. Blurring of vision and diplopia
4. Labored respiration
5. Ventricular fibrillation
6. Muscular fasciculations and tonic or clonic convulsions

Gastric lavage should be instituted immediately. The combination of calcium chloride and magnesium sulfate has been the most successful regimen for treatment of the cardiac arrhythmias and conduction disturbances.

The symptoms due to ingestion of

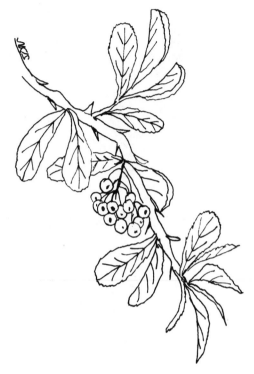

Fig. 22-3. Pyracantha.

1. Increased salivation
2. Nausea, emesis, sometimes diarrhea
3. Sweating
4. Dizziness and sometimes tachypnea

After ingestion, if emesis is not spontaneous, gastric lavage is preferred with a dilute solution of potassium permanganate (1:10,000). Administration of charcoal is an effective adsorbent.

A group of plants commonly known as the solanine group contain the toxic principle solanine. This is actually a glycoalkaloid that yields two components on hydrolysis, a steroidal alkaloid (alkamine) and a sugar. The glycoalkaloid itself is poorly absorbed in the gastrointestinal tract; however, it has a saponinlike character which is responsible for its pronounced irritant action. Therefore, in mild solanine intoxications the predominant

plants containing andromedotoxin resemble those due to aconitine. These include anorexia, excessive salivation, and sometimes emesis and diarrhea. Prickling sensation of the skin is present as is a bradycardia and hypotension. Gastric lavage and symptomatic treatment are recommended. The cardiovascular effects respond to sympathomimetic amines.

A few plants contain the alkaloids cytisine, coniine, nicotine, and lobeline. The concentration varies in different plant parts, with the highest concentration occuring in the mature seeds. The toxicological effect of all four of these alkaloids are very similar and include an action on the central nervous system, the autonomic ganglia, smooth muscle of the intestine, and the striated muscle. Symptoms are as follows:

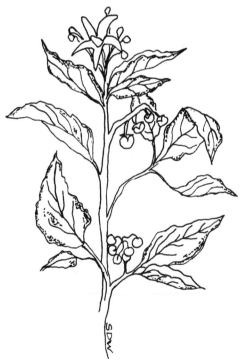

Fig. 22-4. Nightshade.

finding will be gastroenteritis. The free alkamine (the alkaloid) is more readily absorbed and is responsible for most of the systemic reactions.

Many of these plants contain variable amounts of the atropine alkaloids, so signs of mixed intoxications may be seen. The usual signs of solanine intoxication are as follows:

1. Emesis, colic, and diarrhea
2. Rise of body temperature
3. Mild depression and headache

Appropriate management for gastroenteritis is usually all that is required. Treat any systemic involvement symptomatically if it occurs.

The final alkaloid is taxine. Symptoms usually appear within an hour of ingestion and begin with gastrointestinal upset.

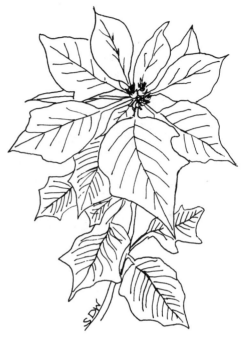

Fig. 22-6. Poinsettia.

There also occurs mydriasis, muscular weakness, and a purple discoloration of the lips. Taxine interferes with cardiac conduction resulting in a slow, irregular pulse. Hypotension and respiratory depression appear secondary to the arrhythmia. Treatment is gastric lavage and symptomatic measures.

II. POLYPEPTIDES AND AMINES

Only a few polypeptides and amines are responsible for toxicity. Those which are of importance in human ingestions include akee plant and mistletoe. The akee plant is native to Africa and rarely seen in the United States. It contains a polypeptide, hypoglycin A, known to cause a hypoglycemic reaction. Mistletoe is one of the eleven most ingested plants and is described in Table 20-1.

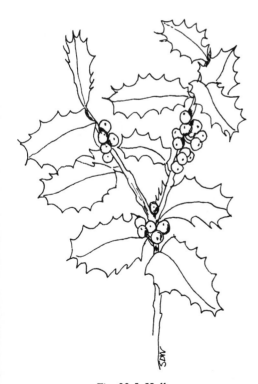

Fig. 22-5. Holly.

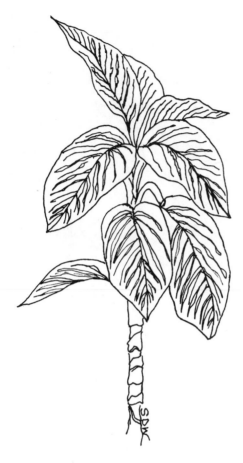

Fig. 22-7. Dieffenbachia.

III. GLYCOSIDES

Glycosides are compounds that yield, on hydrolysis, one or more sugars and one or more other compounds called aglycones. Glycosides are more prevalent in the plant kingdom than are the alkaloids. Toxicity is due to the aglycone component.

The cyanogenetic glycosides yield hydrocyanic acid, a potent respiratory inhibitor, on hydrolysis. This hydrolysis may occur either in the stomach after ingestion or in the plant itself, but only if the plant tissue is disrupted, as may be the case if it is crushed or chewed. There is little free hydrocyanic acid in healthy, actively growing plants.

The cyanogenetic glycosides occur in all plant parts with a high concentration of the glycoside, amygdalin, in the seeds. The hydrolytic enzyme, beta-glucosidase, contained in the plant does not come into contact with the glycoside in healthy plants but is released when the plant cell is disrupted. In many plants which humans consume as food, cooking destroys this enzyme. Because humans have no beta-glucosidase, they are incapable of forming hydrocyanic acid from an intact plant part even though the cyanogenetic glycoside is still present in the plant. Symptoms are as follows:

1. Stimulation of respiration changing to dyspnea

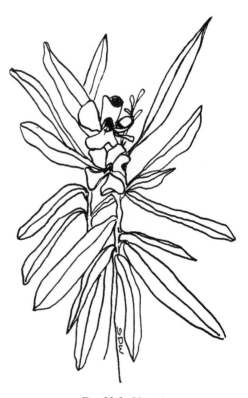

Fig. 22-8. Oleander.

2. Excitement
3. Staggering
4. Paralysis
5. Convulsions, coma, and death

With fatal dose, death occurs within 15 minutes to 3 hours of ingestion and results from anoxia caused by the inhibition of cytochrome oxidase. With nonfatal doses, the inhibition of cellular respiration can be reversed by removal of hydrocyanic acid by respiratory exchange or by a metabolic detoxification process.

Treatment should be started with an inhalation of amyl nitrite and emesis or gastric lavage with a 5% aqueous sodium thiosulfate solution, leaving 200 ml. in the stomach after lavage is completed. Subsequent intravenous injection of sodium nitrite (3% solution, 2.5–5 ml. per minute) plus sodium thiosulfate (50 ml. of a 25% solution I.V.) is indicated. These injections should be repeated if toxic signs persist, using similar or smaller

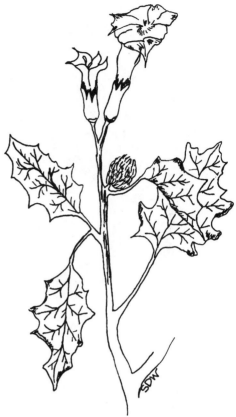

Fig. 22-10. Jimsonweed.

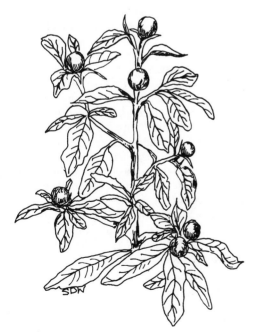

Fig. 22-9. Jerusalem cherry.

doses. Supportive treatment is also indicated.

The goitrogenic glycosides are important only in chronic poisoning of livestock.

A variety of volatile and fixed oils exist in the plant in glycosidic combination, being freed by enzymatic breakdown. Although the glycoside is nonirritant, the oil is a vesicant capable of serious injury to tissue. Treatment is demulcents for gastroenteritis and symptomatic care.

There are several glycosides in the plant kingdom in which the aglycone is a modification of coumarin. These occur mainly in the clovers used as field food

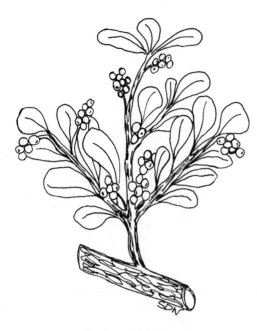

Fig. 22-11. Mistletoe.

for livestock and are rarely responsible for human poisonings.

About 400 cardiac glycosides have been isolated and characterized. The aglycones are responsible for the toxicity; however, the sugar portion is important in increasing the solubility of the molecules. Symptoms after ingestion are as follows:

1. Local irritation to the mucous membranes of mouth and stomach
2. Emesis, abdominal pain, and diarrhea
3. Symptoms of digitalis overdosage

Specific treatment depends upon an electrocardiograph analysis. Saponins are the noncardioactive steroid glycosides. The toxicity of the saponins is the reaction between the saponin and cholesterol in the cell membrane resulting in lysis of erythrocytes. Saponins are not readily absorbed through an intact digestive tract but act as irritants allowing other toxic compounds in the ingested plant to be absorbed. If enough saponin is absorbed through an irritated mucosa, the systemic effect is proportional to the degree of hemolysis.

Demulcents can be given to treat the gastroenteritis, and symptomatic treatment is called for if systemic poisoning occurs.

IV. OXALATES

The organic acid, oxalic acid, occurs in plants in the form of soluble sodium and potassium and insoluble calcium oxalate or acid oxalate crystals. The content of soluble oxalates varies with the location and season, the highest occurring in the late summer and fall. Because oxalates occur in plants as an end product, they tend to accumulate and increase during the life of the plants.

Soluble oxalates may be absorbed rapidly, and absorption of soluble oxalates into the blood correlates directly with a drop in the level of ionic calcium in the serum. This removal of calcium ion by precipitation of the oxalate produces effects due not only to the unavailablility of calcium, but also to an imbalance in monovalent and divalent cations and perhaps pH changes.

The kidney's reaction to soluble oxalates in the circulation is probably of greater importance than the effects of a blood cationic imbalance. Moderate amounts are readily excreted, but larger concentrations result in precipitation of oxalate crystals in the kidney tubules and may occlude the lumen. Microscopic examination of the urine shows proteinuria as well as calcium oxalate crystals and red blood cells. Calculi may also be formed in the urinary tract.

Symptoms are as follows:

1. Burning of the mouth and throat
2. Dullness, depression
3. Colic
4. Dyspnea
5. Tongue swells and speech loss for 2 to 10 days

6. Death if tissues at the back of the throat swell and block air passage

To treat, have the patient rinse the mouth and swallow a solution of aluminum magnesium hydroxide, 30 ml. every two hours. Do not give sodium bicarbonate because the salts formed with the oxalic acid are even more soluble than the acid itself and about as toxic. Give meperidine for pain. Corticosteroids may help edema in throat. This will lessen in about 4 days and be minimal in about 12. Apply wet compresses made with plain water for topical burning.

V. RESINS

Resins and resinoids include an assemblage of polycyclic acids and phenols, alcohols, and complex, neutral substances sharing certain physical characteristics. The exact chemical structure is unknown for many resins. These compounds exert their toxic effect by direct irritation of nervous or muscle tissue. Symptoms include severe gastrointestinal upset with vomiting. Topical contact with the sap of these plants may result in erythematous swelling and blistering of the skin. Treatment is symptomatic.

VI. PHYTOTOXINS OR TOXALBUMINS

Phytotoxins are large complex protein molecules produced by a small number of plants and possess a high degree of toxicity. They are similar to bacterial toxins in structure and cause a somewhat similar physiological reaction—acting as an antigen to elicit an antibody response. It is believed they function as potent proteolytic enzymes breaking down critical proteins and resulting in an accumulation of ammonia. Symptoms are irritation of the gastrointestinal mucosa with hemorrhagic lesions and edematous swelling in several organs after absorption. Treatment is symptomatic.

BIBLIOGRAPHY

Hardin, J. W., and Arena, J. M.: Human Poisoning from Native and Cultivated Plants. Durham, N.C., Duke University Press, 1969.

Kingsbury, J. M.: Poisonous Plants of the U.S. and Canada. Englewood Cliffs, N.J., Prentice-Hall, 1964.

Lampe, K. F., and Fagerstrom, R.: Plant Toxicity and Dermatitis. Baltimore, Williams & Wilkins, 1968.

O'Leary, S. B.: Poisoning in man from eating poisonous plants. Arch. Envir. Health 9:216–242, 1964.

23. ADVERSE DRUG INTERACTIONS

Leonard T. Sigell, Ph.D., and William J. Rietscha, Pharm.D.

An adverse drug interaction can be defined as any undesirable response to a drug that results from the simultaneous or close sequence administration of one or more other substances. Such interactions have been reported for numerous drugs administered along with other drugs or nontherapeutic agents such as foods, tobacco, and alcoholic beverages. They are usually distinguished from in vitro adverse chemical interactions that can alter the effectiveness of administered drugs, for example, incompatible drugs in parenteral fluids.

I. INCIDENCE

It has been surmised that the incidence of such interactions must be great since there is a seemingly endless list of published adverse drug interactions and ample epidemiological evidence of widespread multiple drug usage in our society. In 1977 approximately 2.5 billion prescriptions were written. This amounts to 11 prescriptions per capita. Although the percentage of the population using prescription drugs has not changed significantly in the past 10 years (66%), the number of drugs prescribed per patient has nearly doubled during that period. A plethora of studies have shown that the average hospitalized patient receives 10–12 drugs per stay, elderly patients receive three times as many prescriptions as younger patients, an average of 10 different drug products are used during pregnancy, and about 70% of all "illnesses" are treated with $4–8 billion a year worth of self-prescribed over-the-counter drugs.

Indeed there are nearly 60,000 prescription and 320,000 over-the-counter drug products presently marketed in the United States. Numerous computerized drug interaction alerting systems have been developed to deal with the vast number of reported interactions with these drugs. Many pharmacies maintain computerized or manual "patient drug profiles" which can be scanned for potential interactions. (These would, of course, be of limited value for patients patronizing more than one pharmacy.) There are attempts to encourage the elderly to carry personal drug profile cards and show them to their physician or pharmacist prior to using a new prescription or over-the-counter drug. There is no question that such efforts can help prevent inadvertent prescribing of known interacting drugs.

It is interesting to note that in spite of widespread multiple drug use and implications in the public press of indiscriminate prescribing by physicians, the overall incidence of significant adverse drug interactions appears to be small. There are a handful of well-known, life-threatening interacting combinations, and these appear to be prescribed or used infrequently. One study suggested that less than 7% of all adverse drug reactions can be attributed to a drug interaction; another study reported that the incidence of "significant" adverse drug interactions in hospitalized patients is 0.12%. Although the limited available data are encouraging, they should not be interpreted as a justification for laxity. All reasonable efforts to prevent the inadvertent use of interacting drugs should be encouraged.

II. AWARENESS

Generally, a search for information is warranted when any drug is to be prescribed along with an anticoagulant, anticonvulsant, antihypertensive, diuretic, monoamine oxidase inhibitor, or antimicrobial agent if the effects of the combination are unfamiliar. Table 23-1 is intended as a starting point for such a search. It may also be important to refer to one of the original references cited in the table and/or any of the following sources of additional information. For convenience, the references cited below include information about drug interactions and/or about drug incompatibilities and drug lab test interactions.

Adverse interactions of drugs. Med. Lett. Drugs Ther., *21*:5–12, 1979.

Hansten, P. D.: Drug Interactions: Clinical Significance of Drug-Drug Interactions and Drug Effects on Clinical Laboratory Results. 3rd ed. Philadelphia, Lea & Febiger, 1976.

Evaluations of Drug Interactions. 2nd ed. (and 1978 supplement). Washington, D.C., American Pharmaceutical Association, 1976.

James, J. D., et al.: A Guide to Drug Interactions. New York, McGraw-Hill, 1978.

Powell, M. F., and Lamy, P. P.: Drug-dietary incompatibility. II, Effects on drug therapy. Hosp. Form., *12*:870–874, 1977.

Effects of drugs on clinical laboratory tests. Clin. Chem., *2*(5), 1975.

III. PREVENTION

Many of the following suggestions for avoiding drug interactions and incompatibilities may seem to reflect common sense, but they should not be forgotten or neglected:

A. Obtain and review the patient's drug history including all nonprescription drugs and drugs prescribed by other physicians. (The content of such products should be checked to be certain that they do not contain ingredients that may cause interaction problems.)

B. Avoid multiple drug prescribing whenever possible.

C. Explain to patients why it is important to avoid self-prescribing (check a recent package insert or the *Physicians' Desk Reference* to determine if dietary restrictions are required).

D. When evidence warrants, instruct patients regarding the importance of taking drugs according to directions on the prescription, to take drugs for the prescribed time, not to take other drugs, and to avoid major changes in regular diet.

E. Avoid unfamiliar parenteral drug admixtures unless it is known that they are safe and more effective than single drug therapy.

F. Consider alternate routes or techniques of administration for drugs that may chemically interact.

G. Do not use solutions in which a visual change has occurred upon mixing unless it is known that the change is expected and is not harmful.

H. When prescribing drugs known to have a potential for producing adverse interactions, carefully and frequently monitor the response to treatment (e.g., perform more frequent coagulation tests in patients receiving anticoagulants and other drugs).

I. Do not consider published reports of adverse drug interactions as absolute contraindications to the use of a particular drug combination. Many publications or reports of drug interactions are questionable in quality and validity. Furthermore, some of the reported interactions are the result of the formulation rather than the active drug. Since formulations change, the same trade name drug may no longer cause the alleged interaction.

J. When possible, consider using equally effective and safe, noninteracting drugs.

K. When ordering or interpreting laboratory tests, consider the possibility of drug interactions affecting the test result.

IV. MECHANISMS

In Table 23-1, information is offered about the proposed or known mechanisms for producing certain interactions. The letters and numbers used refer to the following mechanisms:

A. Interference with drug absorption
B. Displacement from binding sites
   1. Drug A displaces drug B

Table 23-1. Drug Interactions

Drug Combination	Reported Effects	Possible Mechanism	Comments	Reference
Antimicrobial Cephalosporins	↑Nephrotoxicity with aminoglycosides, ethacrynic acid, furosemide	F	Avoid cephaloridine. Monitor renal function.	39 40
Aminoglycosides	↑Nephrotoxicity with cephalosporins, ↑ototoxicity with ethacrynic acid	F	Avoid cephaloridine. Monitor renal function.	39 41 42
	↑Muscular blockade with surgical muscle relaxants	D	Use with extreme caution. Toxicity with anticholinesterase and calcium has been tried.	43 44
Amphotericin B	+Curariforms = ↑curariform effects +digoxin = ↑digoxin toxicity	hypokalemia induced	Monitor potassium.	45
Chloramphenicol	+Oral anticoagulant = ↑anticoagulant effect +Phenytoin = ↑phenytoin toxicity	C-2 C-2	Monitor patient closely. Monitor for toxicity; ↓ dose of phenytoin.	6 17
Isoniazid	+Disulfiram = psychoses and ataxia +Phenytoin = phenytoin toxicity	F C-2	Use with caution. Monitor for toxicity of ↓ dose of phenytoin. Important in slow acetylators.	46 20
Rifampin	+Oral contraceptives = menstrual irregularities and ↑ incidence of pregnancy +Oral anticoagulant ↓ anticoagulant effect	C-1 C-2	Avoid concomitant use. Do not start or stop rifampin unless patient is monitored.	47 48 14
Tetracycline	↓TCN absorption	A	Do not administer within an hour or two of antacids in aluminum, magnesium, or calcium or products with iron or dairy products.	49
Antihypertensives, (ESP. Guanethidine) Amphetamines	↓	D	Avoid concurrent use of amphetamines.	21
Ephedrine		D	Monitor for ↓ control of hypertension.	21
Levarterenol	↓ cardiac arrythmias possible	D = 3	Use cautiously and in small doses.	22
Methylphenidate	↓	D = 2	Avoid concurrent use of methylphenidate.	27, 24
Tricyclic antidepressants	↓	D	Doxepin, <100 mg./day, produces less hypotension. Avoid concurrent use.	24, 25, 26
Sympathomimetic amines (OTC cold preps)	↓	D	Avoid concurrent use.	21

Diuretics

Drug	Effect		Code	Management	Ref
Potassium-depleting					
Digoxin	Arrhythmias			Potentially serious if severe. Replace K+.	27
Lithium	Lithium toxicity			Avoid long-term concurrent therapy.	28
Potassium-sparing					
Potassium chloride	Hyperkalemia			Potentially life threatening. Avoid K+ supplement.	29
Anticoagulants	Hypokalemia				
Allopurinol		↑	C-4	Use caution. May need ↓ dose of anticoagulant.	1
Anabolic Steroids		↑	F	Monitor patient. Avoid oxymetholone; ↓anticoagulant dose.	2, 3, 4
Barbiturates		↓	C-2, A	Dose related. Use caution when stop or start barbiturate therapy. Use benzodiazepines.	5, 11
Chloramphenicol		↑	C-4	Closely monitor patient. Use chloramphenical discriminantly.	6
Clofibrate		↑	B-2	Monitor patient; ↓dose of anti-coagulant.	7
Dextrothyroxine		↑	F	↓dose of anticoagulant.	8
Disulfiram		↑	C-4	Monitor patient.	9
Glutethimide		↓	C-2	Use benzodiazepines.	10
Neomycin		↑	F	Assure adequate vitamin K intake.	11
Phenylbutazone		↑	B-2	Avoid. Consider ibuprofen.	11, 12
Phenytoin	Phenytoin intoxication		F	Avoid and monitor closely.	13
Rifampin		↓	C-2	Do not start or stop rifampin unless patient is monitored.	14
Salicylates		↑	B-2	Use acetaminophen. Avoid large doses of salicylates.	11, 15
Thyroid hormones		↑	F	Hypothyroid → warfarin resistant; erythyroid → NML response. Monitor patient on thyroid therapy closely.	16
MAO Inhibitors					
Amphetamines	Hypertensive, arrhythmias, cerebral hemorrhage		C-3	Avoid concurrent use	3
Tricyclic antidepressants	Convulsions		F	Avoid large doses. Give drugs orally. Monitor patient. Use only if experienced. Avoid tranylcypromine, imipramine	31, 32

(Continued on overleaf)

Table 23-1. Drug Interactions (Continued)

Drug Combination	Reported Effects	Possible Mechanism	Comments	Reference
Hypoglycemics	Hypoglycemia	F	Monitor for hypoglycemia; ↓dose of hypoglycemic	33
Insulin	Hypoglycemia	F	Monitor for hypoglycemia; ↓dose of hypoglycemic	33
L-dopa	Hypertension, flushing	D	Avoid. Use phentolamine to tx.	34
Meperidine	Hypertension, sweating, rigidity	C-3 F	Avoid meperdine. Use other morphine cautiously.	35
Sympathomimetic amines	Hypertension	C-3	Generally avoid. Patient should consult with M.D. or pharmacist before use of OTC prep.	36, 37
Tyramine in food, beer, and wine	Hypertension	C-3	Low tyramine diet	38
Anticonvulsants				
Alcohol (chronic misuse)	↓Phenytoin levels	C-2	Monitor phenytoin levels in alcoholic.	19
Anticoagulants	Phenytoin intoxication	C-4	Avoid. Monitor closely.	13
Chloramphenicol	Phenytoin intoxication	C-4	Monitor for toxicity; ↓dose of phenytoin.	17
Disulfiram	Phenytoin intoxication	C-4	Monitor for toxicity; ↓dose of phenytoin.	18
Isoniazid	Phenytoin intoxication	C-4	Monitor for toxicity; ↓dose. Important in slow acetylators.	20
Dopamine	+Phenytoin = hypotension	F	Avoid or use with extreme caution.	50

2. Drug B displaces drug A
C. Altering drug metabolism
1. Drug A induces metabolism of drug B
2. Drug B induces metabolism of drug A
3. Drug A inhibits metabolism of drug B
4. Drug B inhibits metabolism of drug A
D. Competition at site of action
E. Altering drug excretion
F. Other

It is important to realize that the likelihood of occurrence of an interaction in a particular patient will depend upon a number of patient and drug factors. The presence of certain diseases (e.g., hyperthyroidism or hypothyroidism, diabetes, alcoholism) can affect the clinical consequences of an interacting combination as can the patient's renal and hepatic function, serum protein levels, genetic makeup, and age. Drug dosage and intervals between doses, the duration of therapy (some combinations produce one effect early in therapy and the opposite effect with continuing use), the route of administration (e.g., antacids plus oral versus parenteral tetracycline), and even the dosage form in certain instances can be important factors.

Table 23-1 is not intended to be a complete reference to all drug interactions. Only the drug interactions with potential major clinical significance are included with a reference to one or more of the original reports. The comments section is intended to enable the prescriber to interpret the potential significance of the interacting combination and to suggest some alternatives to certain interacting drugs.

As with all such charts, it is merely a quick reference and will not necessarily contain all the information needed for arriving at a therapeutic decision. Furthermore, significant new interactions are continually being reported, and known in-

teractions may have inadvertently been omitted from the table. When the prescribing of unfamiliar drug combinations not listed in Table 23-1 is being considered, the prescriber is encouraged to check the references cited earlier and to obtain information (and evidence to support that information) from a pharmacist, drug information center, or the manufacturer of one or more of the drugs.

TABLE REFERENCES

1. Vesell, E. S., et al.: Impairment of drug metabolism in man by allopurinol and nortriptyline. N. Engl. J. Med., 283:1484, 1970.
2. Murakamn, M., et al.: Effects of anabolic steroids on anticoagulant requirements. Jap. Circ. J., 29:243, 1965.
3. Robinson, B. H. B., et al.: Decreased anticoagulant tolerance with oxymetholone (letter). Lancet, 1:1352, 1971.
4. Longridge, R. G. M., et al.: Decreased anticoagulant tolerance with oxymetholone (letter). Lancet, 2:90, 1971.
5. Cucinell, S. A., et al.: Drug interactions in man: lowering effect of phenobarbital on plasma levels of bishydroxycoumarin (Dicumarol) and diphenylhydantoin (Dilantin). Clin. Pharmacol. Ther., 6:420, 1965.
6. Christensen, L. K., and Skousted, L.: Inhibition of drug metabolism by chloramphenicol. Lancet, 2:1397, 1969.
7. Solomon, R. B., and Rosner, F.: Massive hemorrhage and death during treatment with clofibrate and warfarin. N.Y. State J. Med., 73:2002, 1973.
8. Owens, J. C., et al.: Effect of sodium dextrothyroxine in patients receiving anticoagulants. N. Engl. J. Med., 266:76, 1962.
9. O'Reilly, R. A.: Interaction of sodium warfarin and disulfiram (Antabuse®) in man. Ann. Intern. Med., 78:73, 1973.
10. MacDonald, M. G., et al.: The effects of phenobarbital, chloral betaine, and glutethimide administration on plasma levels and hypothrombinemic responses in man. Clin. Pharmacol. Ther., 10:80, 1969.
11. Udall, J. A.: Drug Interference with warfarin therapy. Clin. Med. 77:20, 1970.
12. Aggeler, P. M., et al.: Potentiation of anticoagulant effect of warfarin by phenylbutazone. N. Engl. J. Med., 276:496, 1967.
13. Hansen, J. M., et al.: Dicumarol-induced diphenylhydantoin intoxication. Lancet, 2:265, 1966.
14. O'Reilly, R. A.: Interaction of sodium warfarin

and rifampin: studies in man. Ann. Intern. Med., *81:*337, 1974.

15. O'Reilly, R. A., et al.: Impact of aspirin and chlorthalidone on the pharmacodynamics of oral anticoagulant drugs in man. Ann. N.Y. Acad. Sci. *179:*173, 1971.

16. Walters, M. D.: The relationship between thyroid function and anticoagulant therapy. Am. J. Cardiol., *11:*112, 1963.

17. Christensen, L. K., and Skousted, L.: Inhibition of drug metabolism by chloramphenicol. Lancet, *2:*1397, 1969.

18. Olesen, O. V.: Disulfiram (Antabuse) as inhibitor of phenytoin metabolism. Acta Pharmacol. Toxicol., *24:*317, 1966.

19. Kater, R. M. H., et al.: Increased rate of clearance of drugs from the circulation of alcoholics. Am. J. Med. Sci., *258:*35, 1969.

20. Brennan, R. W., et al.: Diphenylhydantoin intoxication attendant to slow inactivation of isoniazid. Neurology, *20:*687, 1970.

21. Gulati, O. D., et al.: Antagonism of adrenergic neuron blockage in hypertensive subjects. Clin. Pharmacol. Ther., *7:*510, 1966.

22. Muelheims, G. H., et al.: Increased sensitivity of the heart to catecholamine-induced arrhythmias following guanethidine. Clin. Pharmacol. Ther., *6:*757, 1965.

23. Deshmankar, B. S., and Lewis, J. A.: Ventricular tachycardia associated with the administration of methylphenidate during guanethidine therapy. Can. Med. Assoc. J., *97:*1166, 1967.

24. Mitchell, J. R., et al.: Antagonism of the antihypertensive action of guanethidine sulfate by desipramine hydrochloride. J.A.M.A. *202:*973, 1967.

25. Fawn, W. E., et al: Doxepin: effects on transport of biogenic amines in man. Psychopharmacologia, *22:*111, 1971.

26. Stone, C. A., et al.: Antagonism of certain effects of catecholamine-depleting agents by antidepressant and related drugs. J. Pharmacol. Exp. Ther., *114:*196, 1964.

27. Binnion, P. F.: Hypokalemia and digoxin-induced arrhythmias. Lancet, *1:*343, 1975.

28. Petersen. V., et al.: Effect of prolonged thiazide treatment on renal lithium clearance. Br. Med. J., *3:*143, 1974.

29. Greenblatt, D. J., et al.: Adverse reactions to spironolactone: a report from the Boston Collaborative Drug Surveillance Program (Abstr.). Clin. Pharmacol. Ther., *14:*136, 1973.

30. Brownlee, G., et al.: Potentiation of amphetamine and pethidine by monoamine oxidase inhibitors. Lancet, *1:*669, 1963.

31. Brachfeld, J., et al.: Imipramine-tranylcypromine incompatability, near fatal toxic reaction. J.A.M.A., *186:*1172, 1963.

32. Schuckit, U., et al.: Tricyclic antidepressants and monoamine oxidase inhibitors: combination therapy in the treatment of depression. Arch. Gen. Psychiat., *24:*509, 1971.

33. Cooper, A. J., et al.: Potentiation of insulin hypoglycemia by M.A.O.I. antidepressant drugs. Lancet, *1:*407, 1966.

34. Hunter, K. R., et al.: Monoamine oxidase inhibitors and L-dopa. Br. Med. J., *3:*338, 1970.

35. Vigran, I. M.: Dangerous potentiation of meperidine hydrochloride by pargyline hydrochloride. J.A.M.A., *187:*953, 1964.

36. Elis, J., et al.: Modification by monoamine oxidase inhibitors of the effect of some sympathomimetics on blood pressure. Br. Med. J., *2:* 75, 1967.

37. Cuthbert, M. P., et al.: Cough and cold remedies: potential danger to patients on monoamine oxidase inhibitors. Br. Med. J., *1:*404, 1969.

38. Pettenger, W. A., et al.: Supersensitivity to tyramine during monoamine oxidase inhibition in man: mechanism at the level of the adrenergic neuron. Clin. Pharmacol. Ther., *9:*341, 1968.

39. Borrow, S. N.: Anuria and acute tubular necrosis associated with gentamicin and cephalothin. J.A.M.A., *222:*1546, 1972.

40. Dodds, M. G., et al.: Enhancement by potent diuretics of renal tubular necrosis induced by cephaloridine. Br. J. Pharmacol., *40:*227, 1970.

41. Mathog, R. H., et al.: Ototoxicity of ethacrynic acid and aminoglycoside antibiotic in uremia. N. Engl. J. Med., *280:*1223, 1969.

42. Prazma, J., et al.: Ethacrynic acid ototoxicity potentiation by kanamycin. Ann. Otol. Rhinol. Laryngol., *83:*111, 1974.

43. Pittinger, C. B., et al.: Antibiotic induced paralysis. Anesth. Analg. *49:*487, 1970.

44. Warner, W. A., et al.: Neuromuscular blockage associated with gentamicin therapy. J.A.M.A., *215:*1153, 1971.

45. Miller, R. P., et al.: Amphotericin B toxicity: a follow-up report of 53 patients. Ann. Intern. Med., *71:*1089, 1969.

46. Whittington, H. G., et al.: Possible interaction between disulfiram and isoniazid. Am. J. Psychiatry, *125:*1725, 1969.

47. Nocke-Findr, L., et al.: Effect of rifampin on menstrual cycle and on estrogen excretion in patients taking oral contraceptives. Dtsch. Med. Wochenschr., *98:*1521, 1973.

48. Anon.: Rifampin, "pill" do not go well together (Medical News). J.A.M.A., *227:*608, 1974.

49. Neuvonen, P., et al.: Interference of ions with the absorption of tetracycline in man. Br. Med. J., *4:*532, 1970.

50. Bivins, B. A., Rapp, R. P., Griffen, W. O., et al.: Dopamine-phenytoin interaction: a cause of hypotension in the critically ill. Arch. Surg., *113:*245–249, 1978.

24. LOCATING TOXICOLOGIC INFORMATION

E. Don Nelson, Pharm.D.

There are several references, textbooks, and information systems that may be used in specific toxicologic emergencies. Unfortunately, at present there is no one source that adequately fulfills all of the information needs of the physician dealing with the wide variety of toxicologic emergencies. Although there are a vast number of possible toxicology reference sources, most poison control centers and emergency departments operate within a restricted budget, and must rely on a limited number of references. The major references in current use are: (1) textbooks, (2) card systems, (3) computer-generated microfilm systems, (4) individually designed file systems, (5) consultants, (6) drug or chemical manufacturers, and (7) other poison control centers or drug and poison information centers.

I. CARD SYSTEMS

Card systems are more easily updated than textbooks but can be frustrating and time-consuming when the cards are misfiled. The most common card file system presently in use is that of the National Clearinghouse for Poison Control Centers. The cards are mailed free of charge to centers which are listed with the agency. The reliability of the information contained on the cards is variable since the data is supplied by the drug manufacturers in most cases. Although manufacturers give an accurate list of ingredients in a product, the treatment recommendations may not be as reliable because they are not subjected to a uniform review process.

The Federal Food and Drug Administration (FDA) Clinical Experience Abstract cards may be useful in drug overdoses or adverse drug reactions but seldom in chemical poisonings. Any person or institution can request to be placed on the mailing list. These cards are perforated and mailed in packages. They need to be separated and filed alphabetically by the generic name of the substance to be easily located when needed. The primary intent of these cards is to report adverse clinical experiences with drugs. The system is by no means comprehensive.

II. TEXTS AND REFERENCE BOOKS

Textbooks suffer from obsolescence and several years often elapse between editions. They are useful to persons who wish to review various aspects of clinical toxicology. The text and reference books of primary interest to poison control centers are listed in the Bibliography.

III. COMPUTER-GENERATED MICROFILM SYSTEMS

These systems use microfilmed computer printouts to provide a resource which is quite useful to poison control centers. "Poisindex" and "ToxiFile" are the microfilm systems in greatest use today. They can be easily updated as product, ingredient, or treatment information changes. The more expensive Poisindex system has about 88,000 product listings with more informative treatment protocols than the ToxiFile system. The ToxiFile system lists ingredients on about 33,000 different products. Much of the information contained in the ToxiFile

Table 24-1. Evaluation of Four Resources by Eight Raters Searching for Answers to 24 Poison Information Questions

	Search Time (Mean, in sec)		No. of Pages Searched (mean)		FREQUENCY (%) OF FINDING CONTENT AND/OR MANAGEMENT INFORMATION	CONTENT INFORMATION (AS MEAN)*	MANAGEMENT INFORMATION (AS MEAN)†
	ALL SEARCHES	SEARCHES WHERE INFORMATION FOUND	ALL SEARCHES	SEARCHES WHERE INFORMATION FOUND			
Poisindex	149	155	2.5	2.5	92.2	1.48	1.46
Clinical Toxicology of Commercial Products	128‡	148	3.6§	4.2§	74.0	1.18§	1.12§
ToxiFile	127‡	150	2.4	2.7‖	69.3	1.03§	1.19§
National Clearinghouse Cards	74§‖#	87§‖#	1.4§‖	1.6§‖#	57.8	0.89§	1.04§

*On a scale of 0=no information, 1=contents only, 2=contents and amounts.
† On a scale of 0=no information, 1=management for general class of compounds, 2=management for specific compound.
‡ Differs from Poisindex $P < .02$.
§ Differs from Poisindex $P < .001$.
‖ Differs from Clinical Toxicology of Commercial Products, $P < .001$.
Differs from ToxiFile, $P < .001$.

system is the same as that found on the National Clearinghouse cards. Both Poisindex and ToxiFile systems have periodically reviewed management protocols, poisonous plants and animals, and lists of drug and chemical manufacturers.

In a study conducted to compare the usefulness of currently available toxicologic information resources, Yokel et al. compared Poisindex, ToxiFile, Clinical Toxicology of Commercial Products, and the National Clearinghouse cards. The results of that study are summarized in Table 24-1.

The Poisindex system was most often useful in providing ingredient information in a series of twenty-four cases randomly selected from the records of the University of Cincinnati Drug and Poison Information Center. Although the poison control information required varies somewhat from one location to another, the results of the study are probably applicable to most poison control centers and emergency departments in the United States.

IV. INDIVIDUALLY DESIGNED FILE SYSTEMS

Such systems are restricted to centers large enough to have a staff to file data and periodically review the selection and evaluation of papers and documents to be incorporated into the system for updating information.

V. CONSULTANTS

The consultant is an important source of toxicologic information. In each area of the country there are physicians with expertise in clinical toxicology who serve as valuable resources in the management of toxicologic emergencies. Each poison control center should be prepared with a list

of local and national consultants who can be called on whenever specific problems occur.

VI. DRUG AND CHEMICAL MANUFACTURERS

When a manufacturer is used as a source of toxicologic information, one should clearly ascertain the qualifications of the person who is serving as the consultant for a particular problem. It should be noted that manufacturers are in a delicate legal position when dealing with intoxications caused by their products. This could result in a biased response which may be unintentional. A list of drug manufacturers appears in the front of the Physician's Desk Reference. Partial lists of drug and chemical manufacturers are located in *Clinical Toxicology of Commercial Products,* Poisindex, ToxiFile, and in other references.

VII. OTHER POISON CONTROL CENTERS OR DRUG AND POISON INFORMATION CENTERS

Poison control centers are listed in the current *American Druggist Blue Book* or *Red Book* which can be found in any pharmacy. In addition, listed below are drug and poison information centers which provide 24-hour service.

Although a computer information system which will meet most poison control and emergency toxicology needs is not yet available, there is progress in that direction. However, at the present time the physician who is treating drug and poison emergency problems must be familiar with a number of different systems to obtain information. An alternative is to have 24-hour access to a comprehensive regional information center.

24-HOUR DRUG AND POISON INFORMATION CENTERS

ARKANSAS

Poison Control-Drug Information Center
University of Arkansas for Medical Sciences
4301 West Markham
Little Rock, Arkansas 72201

Phone: (501) 666–5352

CALIFORNIA

Drug Information Analysis Center
Valley Medical Center
445 South Cedar Avenue
Fresno, California 93702

Phone: (209) 252–2888
or
(209) 251–4833,
ext. 2468

CONNECTICUT

Drug Information Service
University of Connecticut Health Center
Farmington, Connecticut 06032

Phone: (203) 674–2782
or
(203) 674–2783

IDAHO

Idaho Drug Information Service
St. Anthony Community Hospital
650 North 7th Street
Pocatello, Idaho 83201

Phone: (800) 632–9490
or
(208) 232–2733,
ext. 244 or 245

ILLINOIS

Drug Information and Poison Control Center
Brokaw Hospital
Virginia and Franklin Streets
Normal, Illinois 61761

Phone: (309) 829–7685,
ext. 223

Rockford Drug Information Center
Swedish American Hospital
1400 Charles Street
Rockford, Illinois 61101

Phone: (815) 968–6898,
ext. 635

IOWA

Drug Information and Poison Control Center
University of Iowa Hospitals and Clinics
Iowa City, Iowa 52242

Phone: (319) 356–2600

LOUISIANA

Drug Information and Poison Control Center
St. Francis Hospital
309 Jackson Street
Monroe, Louisiana 71201

Phone: (318) 325–6454,
7 AM to midnight,
(318) 325–2611,
ext. 146 or 147,
other times

MICHIGAN

Poison Information Center
Pharmacy Clinic Riverside Center
777 W. Riverside Drive
Ionia, Michigan 48846

Phone: (616) 527–0110,
ext. 255

Poison Information
Bronson Methodist Hospital
252 E. Lovell Street
Kalamazoo, Michigan 49006

Phone: (616) 383–6409

Drug and Poison Information Center
St. Lawrence Hospital
1210 West Saginaw
Lansing, Michigan 48914

Phone: (517) 372–3610,
ext. 305

Drug Information Center
William Beaumont Hospital
3601 West 13 Mile Road
Royal Oak, Michigan 48072

Phone: (313) 549–7000,
ext. 565

Drug Information Service
Providence Hospital
16001 West Nine Mile Road
Southfield, Michigan 48075

Phone: (313) 424–3125

NEW MEXICO

Poison Information Center
New Mexico Poison, Drug Information and
    Medical Crisis Center
2211 Lomas Blvd., N.E.
Albuquerque, New Mexico 87106

Phone: (505) 843–2551

OHIO

Drug and Poison Information Center
234 Goodman Street
Room E 7-8
Cincinnati, Ohio 45267

Phone: (513) 872–5111

Drug Information-Poison Control Center
Bethesda Hospital
2951 Maple Avenue
Zanesville, Ohio 43701

Phone: (614) 454–4221

OREGON

Drug Information Service
Oregon State University
Corvallis, Oregon 97331

Phone: (503) 754–3535
or
(800) 452–2201

PENNSYLVANIA

Drug and Poison Service
Hamot Medical Center
201 State Street
Erie, Pennsylvania 16512

Phone: (814) 455–6711,
ext. 529

SOUTH CAROLINA

Drug and Poison Information Service
Medical University of South Carolina
80 Barre Street
Charleston, South Carolina 29401

Phone: (803) 792–3896
and
(803) 792–4201
for poison infor-
mation

Drug and Poison Information
University of South Carolina
Columbia, South Carolina 29208

Phone: (803) 765–7539

UTAH

Poison Information Center
Intermountain Regional Poison Control
    and Drug Information Service
50 North Medical Drive
Building 428
Salt Lake City, Utah 84132

Phone: (801) 581–2151

WISCONSIN

Drug Information and Poison Control Center
University of Wisconsin
University Hospital
1300 University Avenue
Madison, Wisconsin 53706

Phone: (608) 262–1315,
drug information,
(608) 262–3702,
poison control

BIBLIOGRAPHY

Arena, J. M.: Poisoning: Toxicology-Symptoms-Treatments. 3rd ed. (American Lectures in Living Chemistry Ser.) Springfield, Ill., Charles C Thomas, 1976.

Cooper, P.: Poisoning by Drugs and Chemicals. 3rd ed. Chicago, Year Book Medical Publishers, 1974.

Gosselin, R., et al.: Clinical Toxicology of Commercial Products. 4th ed. Baltimore, Williams & Wilkins, 1976.

Grant, W. M.: Toxicology of the Eye: Drugs, Chemicals, Plants, Venoms. 2nd ed. Springfield, Ill., Charles C Thomas, 1974.

Kingsbury, J. M.: Poisonous Plants of the United States and Canada. 3rd. ed. Englewood Cliffs, N. J., Prentice-Hall, 1964.

Patty, F. A.: Industrial Hygiene and Toxicology. 2 vols., 2nd ed. New York, Interscience Publishers, 1967.

Yokel, R. A., Sigell, L. T., and Nelson, E. D.: A comparison of four toxicology resources for information retrieval rates and times. Pediatrics, 92:145, 1978.

25. ANALYTICAL TOXICOLOGY

Michael Hassan, B.S., and Amadeo J. Pesce, Ph.D.

Recent interest in clinical toxicology has led to the demand for qualitative and quantitative analyses of exogenous chemicals in the body. The analytical procedures are still not considered routine because of the sophisticated equipment and techniques. This has led to the development of regional facilities that provide such service without costly duplication of instruments and technical staff.

The laboratory services are dictated by the needs of the community and area physicians. Drugs account for more accidental and suicidal poisonings than nontherapeutic agents, and therefore make up the majority of tests.

This chapter gives generalized information regarding the operation of the clinical toxicology laboratory, emphasizing the proper samples for analysis and their storage, methods and techniques used by the laboratory, and the interpretation of data.

I. TEST ORDERING: PROPER INFORMATION AND SPECIMENS OF CHOICE FOR ANALYSIS

As in all areas of laboratory testing, obtaining the proper samples for analysis is of utmost importance. The selection of specimens is based on several factors, including the ease of collecting the sample, the amount of sample which can be obtained, the concentration of chemical found in the sample, and whether the sample contains the parent compound and its metabolic products. The body fluids most readily available and useful are urine, blood, and stomach contents. Advantages and disadvantages of each of these fluids are outlined in Table 25-1.

In addition to the factors mentioned above, the time after ingestion or exposure to the toxic compound and the rate at which the compound is absorbed also determine the fluid of choice. Gastric fluid is usually a good source of unmetabolized parent compound, provided the sample is collected relatively soon after ingestion of the compound. Approximately 50–100 ml. of the emesis or initial lavage fluid should be collected.

Blood and urine specimens are used most often in toxicological analyses. Urine (50–100 ml.) is the specimen of choice for most screening procedures. If urine is to be used, the laboratory not only must have knowledge of the properties of the toxic chemical and metabolites but must also be familiar with normal urinary constituents and metabolic products that may interfere with the analytical procedure.

The most useful laboratory information on the effect of toxic agents is offered by quantitative analyses on blood. The decision to use whole blood, plasma, or serum is dependent on the material to be analyzed. There are no significant differences in the concentration of compounds, between plasma and serum. However, there are notable differences between these fluids and whole blood. If a compound is not present to a large extent in red blood cells, then using the cells (whole blood) for analysis results in a dilution of the specimen. Serum or plasma concentrations may thus be as much as 15% greater than a whole blood specimen value. On the other hand, some poisons are found in high concentration in the red blood cell. For these toxins, whole blood is the sample of choice. An example is lead, which is bound primarily to red blood cells, and analysis of plasma or serum therefore, would be worthless. Other compounds for which whole blood

Table 25-1. **Specimens of Choice for Toxicological Analysis**

Sample	Advantages	Disadvantages
Urine	Easy to obtain in high volume. Most compounds found in sufficient concentration to enable identification. Quantitation helpful in monitoring the excretion of certain metals.	Contains many metabolic products which may interfere with identification. Parent compound may not be present. Quantitation offers little correlation with dosage.
Serum Plasma Blood	Usually contains parent compound. Quantitative level may assist with patient management (therapeutic and toxic levels often known).	Limitation of sample volume. Analytical procedures not available for all compounds (concentration of some compounds too low for measurement).
Gastric lavage, fluid or emesis	Parent compound present. Quantitative level will enable estimation of amount of compound recovered from the stomach.	Substances which are quickly absorbed will be missed by a "gastric" screen. Substances which are not orally ingested will not be detected. Quantitation offers no correlation with dosage.

analysis is required include carboxyhemoglobin, methemoglobin, and cyanide. A common practice of many laboratories is to request a heparinized whole blood sample for most of their test procedures, thus providing the option of either using whole blood or plasma.

Each laboratory will have its guidelines for obtaining specimens for toxicological testing. Table 25-2 is an example of a laboratory specimen guideline.

Once the samples have been collected, it is good practice to consider all compounds for analysis to be sensitive to

Table 25-2. **Example of Specific Specimens Required for Toxicological Analysis**

Test	Sample	Preservative or Anticoagulant	Volume Required	Comments
Comprehensive drug screen	Urine	None	50 ml. minimum	Send initial specimen if available if quantitation desired.
	Gastric	None	50 ml. minimum	
	Serum	None	3 ml.	
Qualitative analysis of one drug or drug group	Urine	None	50 ml.	Specify drug or group.
Quantitative analysis of one drug	Serum	None	2 ml.	Specify drug.
Quantitative lead	Blood	Heparin	5 ml.	Collect blood in lead-free tube.*
	Urine	None	100 ml. minimum	Collect 24-hour sample in lead-free container.* Record total volume.
Quantitative analysis for other metals (Hg, As, etc.)	Urine	None	100 ml. minimum	Collect 24-hour sample* and record total volume.
Quantitative analysis of carbon monoxide, methemoglobin	Blood	EDTA	3 ml.	Send to laboratory immediately.
Quantitative alcohol	Blood	NaF	3 ml.	Send to laboratory immediately.

* Acid-washed containers.

Table 25-3. **Laboratory Methods and Instruments**

Method	Instrument Required	Comments
Thin-layer chromatography	None	Primarily a qualitative method; subjective interpretation involved; ideal for drug screening
Gas chromatography	Gas chromatograph	Qualitative and quantitative analysis of volatile compounds of molecular weight less than 800
Liquid chromatography	High-pressure liquid chromatograph	Quantitation of a variety of compounds including those with molecular weights greater than 800
Mass spectrometry	Gas chromatograph, mass spectrometer	Objective analytical tool for qualitative identification and quantitation; requires high degree of operator training
Ultraviolet spectroscopy	Ultraviolet spectrophotometer	Specific quantitation and for screening or confirmation of pure compounds which absorb ultraviolet light
Visible spectroscopy	Colorimeter, visible spectrophotometer	Quantitation of compounds which absorb light in the visible wavelength region
Infrared spectroscopy	Infrared spectrometer	Confirmation analyses; requires pure sample at relatively high concentration; for compounds which absorb light in the infrared region
Atomic absorption spectroscopy	Atomic absorption spectrophotometer	Quantitation of a variety of metals
Fluorometry	Fluorometer, spectrofluorometer	Quantitation of compounds which are naturally fluorescent or which can be made to fluoresce
Enzyme immunoassay	Spectrophotometer (heated cuvette)	Qualitative and quantitative testing for drugs; available in kit form
Radioimmunoassay	Gamma counter	Qualitative and quantitative testing for drugs; available in kit form
Hemaglutination inhibition	None	Qualitative identification of selected drug groups; available in kit form
Minimum inhibitory concentration technique	None	Quantitative antimicrobic susceptibility; determination of antibiotic concentrations

heat, light, and pH changes. Specimens should be delivered to the laboratory as promptly as possible. On receipt, they must be properly stored if there is to be a delay in testing. Plasma or serum, once separated from red blood cells by centrifugation, should be frozen (−18°C.). Whole blood is refrigerated (4–6°C) or frozen. Urine and gastric samples should be filtered and refrigerated or frozen with no preservatives added. In general, most drugs and metals will be stable for months if properly stored. Volatile compounds (i.e., glycols, hydrocarbons) will remain stable for several weeks.

Laboratory service is greatly improved if historical and clinical information is obtained from the referring physician. An example, would be a salicylate overdose. Informing the analyst of the suspected drug will enable identification and quantitation of this compound to be completed

Table 25-4. **Classification of Potential Poisons**

1. Nonvolatile organic drugs
   a. Acidic (salicylates, barbiturates hydantoins)
   b. Neutral (carbamates)
   c. Basic (major tranquilizers, amphetamines, narcotics)
2. Volatile compounds (alcohols, glycols, hydrocarbons)
3. Gases (carbon monoxide)
4. Metals (lead, mercury, arsenic, iron, cadmium)
5. Miscellaneous compounds (insecticides, pesticides)

within minutes. If this information is not available, it may require a complete toxic screen and several hours to obtain the same data.

II. LABORATORY TECHNIQUES AND METHODS

The toxicology laboratory utilizes a wide variety of instruments and techniques to identify and quantitate poisons in biological samples. As in other areas of

laboratory medicine, no one instrument or technique can be used to satisfy every analytical need. Table 25-3 lists laboratory methods and instruments.

Most analytical procedures require isolation of the suspected compound from the biological fluid. The isolation procedure used is dependent on the chemical nature or classification of the compound. Table 25-4 classifies into groups potential poisons based on chemical properties.

Once the compounds have been isolated and concentrated, the analysis can be performed.

The laboratory will usually attempt to identify the unknown poison or poisons before employing techniques to quantitate specific compounds in the biological fluid (except for therapeutic monitoring). A request for analysis of a particular drug or poison, as suggested by the patient history, often allows the laboratory to employ a method which is relatively quick, sensitive, and specific for that compound. In contrast, when no history is available, a

Table 25-5. **Examples of Specific Screening Tests**

Compound	Sample Required	Test	Test Time (min.)	Comments
Alcohol	1 ml. serum or 1 ml. urine	Microdiffusion	15–30	Nonspecific for ethanol
Carbon monoxide	1 ml. whole blood	Microdiffusion	60–120	Test is sensitive to 10% carboxyhemoglobin.
Cholinesterase (organophosphate insecticide exposures)	1 ml. serum	Acholest	30	Semiquantitative
Heavy Metals (antimony, arsenic, bismuth, mercury)	20 ml. urine	Reinsch	60–120	Will not react with normal urinary concentrations
Imipramine	1 ml. urine	Forrest	5	Phenothiazines may interfere.
Iron	0.5 ml. serum	Bathophenanthroline	15	Will not react with normal serum concentration
Phenothiazine (mellaril, thorazine, trilafon)	1 ml. urine	FPN	5	Nonspecific
Salicylate (sodium salicylate, salicylic acid)	0.5 ml. serum	Ferric nitrate	5	High specificity and sensitivity

Table 25-6. **Therapeutic and Normal Levels of the More Common Agents in Plasma or Blood**

Compound	Level*	Compound	Level
Acetaminophen	Up to 20; (< 50, 10 hr. postingestion)	Isoniazid	0.5–12
		Isopropanol	None
Amikacin	15–30	Lead	Up to 0.4 (blood); up
Amitriptyline	0.09–0.3		to 80 µg./24 hrs.,
Amobarbital	Up to 10		(urine)
Aminolevulinic acid	Up to 0.1	Lidocaine	2–6
Arsenic	<0.1 (blood) <100 µg./24 hr. (urine)	Lithium	0.5–1.3 µg./L.
		Mephobarbital	15–40
Benzene	None	Mephenytoin	5–16
Beryllium	None	Meprobamate	Up to 20
Bromide	Up to 1,000	Mercury	0.05 (blood); 5 µg./L.
Butabarbital	Up to 10		(urine)
Butalbital	Up to 10	Methaqualone	Up to 5
Cadmium	0.5–11 µg./L. (urine)	Methanol	None
Carbamazepine	4–8	Methsuximide	10–40
Carbon monoxide		(as *N*-demethylsuximide)	
Smokers	Up to 8%	Methyprylon	Up to 10
Nonsmokers	Up to 2%	Nortriptyline	0.05–0.14
Carbon tetrachloride	None	Pentobarbital	Up to 6
Chloral hydrate	Up to 10	Phenobarbital	15–40
(as trichloroethanol)		Phensuximide	40–60
Chloramphenicol	Up to 40	Phenylbutazone	Up to 100
Chlordiazepoxide	Up to 3	Phenytoin	10–20
Chlorpromazine	Up to 0.5	Primidone	5–15
Clonazepam	Up to 0.12	Procainamide	4–8
Clorazepate	0.1–0.7	Propoxyphene	Up to 0.5
(as demethyldiazepam)		Propanolol	0.025–0.050
Cyanide	<0.1 (blood)	Pseudocholinesterase	1800–4800 mIu./ml.
Desipramine	0.15–0.3	Quinidine	3–6
Diazepam	Up to 2	Salicylate	100–200
Digitoxin	0.014–0.03	Secobarbital	Up to 6
Digoxin	0.001–.002	Sulfadiazine	80–150
Disopyramide	2–4	Sulfamethoxazole	80–150
Doxepin	Up to 0.2	Sufanilamide	100–150
Ethanol	None	Sufathiazole	80–150
Ethchlorvynol	Up to 10	Sulfisoxazole	90–100
Ethosuximide	40–80	Theophylline	10–20
Ethylene glycol	None	Thiocyanate	Up to 10
Flurazepam	Up to 0.020	(metabolite of nitroprusside)	
Fluoride	Up to 0.5	Thiopental	Up to 4
Gentamycin	Up to 10	Thioridazine	0.3–1.0
Gluthethimide	Up to 6	Tobramycin	Up to 10
Gold	2–10	Toluene	None
Imipramine	0.04–0.4	Valproic acid	50–120
Iron	0.5–1.6		

*Reported in micrograms per milliliter unless stated otherwise.

complete screen may be requested. The major disadvantage of such a screen is the prolonged time required for obtaining data. Table 25-5 gives examples of some of the common rapidly performed tests.

Currently it is impossibile for laboratories to quantitate all drugs or toxic agents that may be present in serum body fluids. Laboratories may offer quantitative tests for therapeutic drug monitoring (phenytoin, phenobarbital). In addition, if therapeutic and toxic levels are known for a given compound, the laboratory results may have interpretative value. It follows, therefore, that the priority for which quantitative tests are developed by the laboratory is influenced by those compounds which show a correlation between blood levels and clinical effect.

III. INTERPRETATION OF DATA

Information from toxicological analysis should have clinical value, just as is the case for other laboratory tests.

In considering qualitative test results, the agents identified influence how the data can be utilized. If the compounds are nontherapeutic, such as benzene or ethylene glycol, then their presence can be interpreted as the cause of clinical toxicity. On the other hand, if drugs are involved, their identification does not establish that they are etiological unless the clinical symptoms are known to be associated with the particular compounds.

Qualitative analysis may not specifically identify the toxic agent. If the compound has been entirely converted to its metabolites, the laboratory may be unable to determine the original substance. This is especially true when urine specimens are being analyzed for drugs with similar metabolic pathways, such as oxazepam and diazepam, which may only be identified by class (i.e., benzodiazepine derivatives). Blood analysis also does not necessarily assure identification of the actual parent compound. This can be seen in the conversion of chloral hydrate to trichloroethanol, or of clorazepate to demethyldiazepam.

A more comprehensive discussion of quantitative data, and the interpretation of blood levels in particular, can be found in the literature. Of importance is a basic understanding of the specific laboratory methods being employed. Therapeutic tables should not be used without a firsthand knowledge of the values considered "normal" by the laboratory whose services are being utilized.

Table 25-6 lists therapeutic or normal concentrations of the more common agents in plasma or blood. Toxic and lethal concentrations are not specifically indicated because of individual variations in these levels. However, values above those listed should be considered abnormal.

BIBLIOGRAPHY

Clarke, E. G. C.: Isolation and Identification of Drugs, London, Pharmaceutical Press, 1969.

Davies, D. S. (ed.): Biological Effects of Drugs in Relation to Their Plasma Concentrations, Baltimore, University Park Press, 1973.

Kaye, S. (ed.): Handbook of Emergency Toxicology. 3rd ed. Springfield, Ill., Charles C Thomas, 1970.

Sunshine, I. (ed.): Methodology for Analytical Toxicology, Cleveland, CRC Press, 1975.

Winek, C. L.: Tabulation of therapeutic toxic and lethal concentrations of drugs and chemicals in blood. Clin. Chem., *22:*6, 832, 1976.

INDEX

Numerals in *italics* indicate a figure; "t" following a page number indicates a table.